RiA2 1989 Dec

Geriatric Psychiatry
and
Psychopharmacology
A Clinical Approach

Michael A. Jenike

YEAR BOOK MEDICAL PUBLISHERS, INC.
CHICAGO • LONDON • BOCA RATON

OCLC: 19456243

This book is dedicated to:

my courageous parents who have not only survived my father's near-fatal automobile accident but also made a remarkable recovery and are enjoying life again,
and
my 98-year-old great aunt, Mrs Min Cleverly, who still lives alone in a small town in southern England and serves as an inspiration for my work with elderly persons,
and
Thomas P. Hackett, chairman of Psychiatry at MGH, who passed away recently at the much too young age of 59. He was an inspiration to me and a driving force for our department. He is sorely missed.

ABOUT THE AUTHOR

Michael A. Jenike, MD, is presently research psychiatrist at Massachusetts General Hospital and Associate Professor of Psychiatry at Harvard Medical School. He was the Director of the Inpatient Psychiatric Service at Massachusetts General Hospital for five years from 1982 to 1987 and was Co-Director of the Geriatric Psychiatry Memory Disorders Clinic for seven years. He has directed the Obsessive-Compulsive Disorders Clinic for the past five years.

A psychiatrist with extensive experience in clinical geriatric psychopharmacology, Dr Jenike has conducted a number of research studies in clinical psychopharmacology and has published over 130 scientific and clinical papers. He edited the monthly newsletter *Massachusetts General Hospital Topics in Geriatrics* for six years and is presently Co-Editor of the psychiatry section of *Scientific American Medicine* and Editor-in-Chief of the *Journal of Geriatric Psychiatry and Neurology*. He is a member of a number of professional societies including the American Geriatrics Society, the Gerontological Society of America, the American Psychiatric Association, the American Medical Association, and the Academy of Psychosomatic Medicine.

Dr Jenike has lectured nationally and internationally to physicians and mental health professionals on the topics of obsessive-compulsive disorders, affective illness, geriatric psychopharmacology, and Alzheimer's disease and has conducted a number of symposia on the pharmacologic and nonpharmacologic treatment of psychiatric illness.

CONTENTS

Since the *Handbook of Geriatric Psychopharmacology* was written in 1985, the field of geriatrics has continued to grow at a rapid rate. Although many of the general principles remain the same, numerous specifics have changed. Novel drugs and new reports of side effects allow for better treatment of our elderly patients who suffer from psychiatric illnesses. As the absolute number of elderly people grows in the United States, the need for clinicians to acquire a specialized body of knowledge becomes more pronounced.

Because pharmacologic and nonpharmacologic therapy intertwine in the treatment of psychiatric disorders in the elderly, we have decided not to simply do a second edition of the *Handbook* which focused mainly on drug treatments, but to elaborate on a number of relevant issues. This book is an attempt to organize the large body of relevant data into usable information for clinicians and to address directly some of the difficult treatment decisions that face the clinician. Physicians and health care workers of all disciplines come into contact with elderly patients who may be depressed, demented, anxious, or psychotic. Insomnia and the sequelae of toxic drug interactions are frequently encountered. Sadness, depression, and in some cases even psychosis may be helped by certain psychotherapeutic interventions or environmental manipulation.

The earlier book, *Handbook of Geriatric Psychopharmacology,* was an attempt to recommend specific medications for particular situations in order to maximize therapeutic benefits and minimize unwanted side effects. Reviews for that book were overall very positive and a number of helpful suggestions were generated. Rather than write a second edition that solely focused on psychopharmacology, we felt that it would be more helpful to update the information in that book and expand it to include a number of other issues relevant to the psychiatric and medical care of elderly patients. Chapters from *Handbook of Geriatric Psychopharmacology* have been integrated into this book and modified to include new and updated data. More information has been added in reference to classification of the relevant disorders and DSM-III-R categories are used when relevant. In addition, this new book contains sections on alcoholism and drug abuse, delirium, use of neuroimaging techniques, and psychotherapy.

We have not attempted to cover every relevant topic and welcome suggestions of other major areas that readers might find of use in future editions of this book.

I wish to express my thanks to my secretary, Jane Borstel, who has been magnificent and an inspiration to us all in the face of extreme personal tragedy. Thank you to my chief research technician, Amy Holland, whose dedicated efforts are greatly appreciated. I am most appreciative of the efforts of my colleagues, Dr Marilyn Albert, whose intellect and enthusiasm viii

have contributed greatly to my understanding of and interest in dementing patients and their families, and to Dr Lee Baer who generously shares his extensive knowledge of science, computers, and study design.

A special thanks to my wife, Nancy, and my three children, Lisa, Eric, and Sara, who generously gave me the time to work on this book.

I sincerely hope you enjoy reading this book and that it serves you well as a source of helpful information which benefits your elderly patients.

Michael A. Jenike, MD

1

Introduction

EMPATHY

The following poem was found among the personal possessions of an elderly woman who had died in a nursing home in Scotland. Her words remind us of our obligations to understand, comfort, and maximize quality of life in our elderly patients.

A Crabbit Old Woman Wrote This
What do you see, nurses, what do you see?
Are you thinking when you look at me—
A crabbit old woman, not very wise,
Uncertain of health, with far-away eyes,
Who dribbles her food and makes no reply
When you say in a loud voice,
"I do wish you'd try."
Who seems not to notice the things that you do,
And forever is losing a stocking or shoe.
Who unresisting or not, lets you do as you will,
With bathing and feeding, the long day to fill.
Is that what you're thinking,
   is that what you see?
Then open your eyes, nurse,
   you're not looking at me.
I'll tell you who I am as I sit here so still,
As I rise at your bidding, as I eat at your will.
I'm a small child of ten with a father and mother,
Brothers and sisters, who love one another;
A young girl of sixteen with wings on her feet,
Dreaming that soon now a lover I'll meet;
A bride soon at twenty—my heart gives a leap,
Remembering the vows that I promised to keep;
At twenty-five now I have young of my own,
Who need me to build a secure happy home:

A woman of thirty, my young now grow fast,
Bound to each other with ties that should last;
At forty, my young sons have grown and are gone,
But my man's beside me to see I don't mourn;
At fifty once more babies play round my knee,
Again we know children, my loved one and me.
Dark days are upon me, my husband is dead,
I look at the future, I shudder with dread.
For my young are all rearing young of their own.
And I think of the years and
   the love that I've known.
I'm an old woman now and nature is cruel—
'Tis her jest to make old age look like a fool.
The body is crumbled, grace and vigor depart,
There now is a stone where I once had a heart.
But inside this old carcass a young girl still dwells,
And now and again my battered heart swells.
I remember the years, I remember the pain,
And I'm loving and living life over again.
I think of the years all too few—gone too fast,
And accept the stark fact that nothing can last.
So open your eyes, nurses, open and see
Not a crabbit old woman, look close—see ME.

DEMOGRAPHY AND GOALS

Until the twentieth century, diseases of the elderly were not a significant concern. Before the turn of the century, average life expectancy was quite low, and many of the problems associated with an aging population did not exist. By 1900, with the introduction of significant public health measures, the average life span had increased to approximately 65 years (Thal, 1988). With the introduction of antibiotics and other modern medical technologies, longevity increased even more. As a result of such advances the average life span for persons born in the 1980s will be more than 80 years.

More than 25 million Americans are presently over the age of 65 years, roughly 11% of the United States population, and they spend about one-fourth of the national total for medication (Vestal, 1984). It is estimated that by the year 2030, nearly 52 million people—17% of the population—will exceed the age of 65. As we all know far too well, the elderly suffer from many concurrent acute and chronic diseases. In one study of 200 consecutively admitted patients, 78% had at least four major diseases, 38% had six or more, and 13% had eight or more (Wilson et al, 1962). The elderly are clearly more susceptible to disease and are also more vulnerable to side effects from the medications used to treat these illnesses. Fewer than 5% of those over the age of 65 abstain from all drug use (Guttmann, 1978).

Superimposed on these physical ailments, mental illness in the elderly is common. A National Institute of Mental Health (NIMH) study of approximately 10,000 people aged 18 years and older found that about 19% of the

United States population—approximately 29 million people—are suffering from a mental illness (Anonymous, Psychiatric News, 1984). Depression is common, with depressive symptoms reported in as many as 20% of healthy adults (Busse, 1978). Alzheimer's disease is now believed to be present in 5% to 7% of those over the age of 65, and in 20% of those over the age of 80. Over 10 billion of the 21 billion dollars spent on nursing care in the United States in 1982 was expended on patients with dementing illnesses and about half of all nursing home beds are occupied by dementing patients. Many dementing patients suffer from superimposed treatable symptoms such as depression, agitation, confusion, insomnia, and/or psychosis.

Anxiety disorders are extremely common in the elderly and in the NIMH study they were found to be the most common psychiatric disorders in the United States. Sleep disorders occur as a primary disorder or may accompany anxiety, depression, or dementia. In one large survey, 40% of subjects over the age of 50 complained of insomnia (Bixler et al, 1979).

Because of the prevalence of psychiatric disorders and symptoms in the elderly, every practicing clinician is confronted with these complicated situations. Psychotropic drugs are now among the most frequently prescribed medications in the aged (Greenblatt et al, 1975; Parry et al, 1973; Vestal, 1984). Unfortunately, many of these drugs have side effects, and considerable clinical skill and knowledge are required in order to maximize effectiveness and minimize unwanted effects (Salzman, 1984; Jenike, 1988). Side effects can also be used therapeutically. For instance, a depressed patient with pronounced secondary sleeplessness will benefit much from a sedating antidepressant given near bedtime.

The elderly not only are more sensitive to the adverse effects of psychotropic agents, but also exhibit an increased variability of response to these drugs. Interindividual differences are much more pronounced in the elderly than they are in the young. Many elderly patients will need doses of medication similar to what younger patients need; on the other hand, others may need one-tenth the dosage.

This book presents an approach to the elderly patient with psychiatric symptoms which will allow the clinician to optimally manage the elderly patient in order to maximize benefit and minimize unwanted effects.

GUIDELINES FOR PRESCRIBING PSYCHOTROPIC DRUGS IN THE ELDERLY

A few general principles should be kept in mind when prescribing psychotropic drugs to the elderly:

1. *Take a careful history.* It is necessary to know what concomitant illnesses the patient has and it is crucial that the clinician know what medications have been taken. For instance, giving meperidine hydrochloride (Demerol) for pain relief to a patient experiencing a myocardial infarction who

has been taking a monoamine oxidase inhibitor (MAOI) may be fatal. Many psychotropic agents produce anticholinergic effects that may add to an anticholinergic load from other agents, such as antihistamines or cardiac antiarrhythmic agents.

2. *Diagnose prior to treatment.* This is imperative to avoid the inappropriate use of psychotropic medication. For example, if severe insomnia is secondary to depression, benzodiazepines may worsen the overall clinical situation, while a sedating antidepressant will treat the underlying disorder. Treating uncomplicated anxiety with neuroleptics is inappropriate and may result in irreversible neurologic sequelae. A recent report of 42 patients with tardive dyskinesia who were seen in movement disorder clinics in various centers found that 19 had been inappropriately treated with neuroleptics (Burke et al, 1982). Of these, 6 patients had been treated for anxiety; 6, for depression; 4, for behavioral disturbances associated with mental retardation; and 3, for an acute psychotic episode precipitated by emotional stress.

3. *Evaluate potential for noncompliance.* Make the therapeutic regimen as simple as possible. Explain which medications are to be taken, the dosage, and the timing to both the patient and the family. Write down the dosing schedule. Choose the most appropriate dosage form; liquids may be more suitable for a patient who has trouble swallowing. Encourage patients to destroy or return discontinued medication. In patients who are confused or demented, be sure that adequate supervision is present.

4. *Do not avoid the use of psychotropic agents just because of age.* These drugs can be used safely in the elderly, and older patients deserve relief of symptoms of depression, psychosis, and severe anxiety. Avoiding the use of these agents, when they are required, contributes to suffering and may lead to death by suicide, malnutrition, and stress-related disorders.

5. *Use a low dose initially.* Because interindividual differences are so great in the elderly, the clinician should start with very low doses and titrate up gradually. Try to identify signs and symptoms that can be followed such as sleep disturbance, anorexia, hallucinations, or aggressive behavior. With some drugs, measuring blood levels may be useful. Once a drug has reached steady-state levels, which takes about five half-lives, the plasma level may help the clinician to determine whether enough drug is being given to achieve a therapeutic effect (Vestal, 1984). If the patient is not responding and not having significant side effects, increase the dose, keeping in mind that some elderly patients will require the same dosage as young adults.

6. *Know the pharmacology of the drug prescribed.* It is best to be familiar with the use of a few drugs in each class. The clinician needs to be aware of altered dosing schedules in the elderly and changes in half-life, elimination, and protein binding. Potential interactions with other drugs as well as toxicity and side effects must be kept in mind.

7. *Monitor drugs on a regular basis.* This is extremely important, especially when more than one physician may be prescribing medication or when

neuroleptics are being used. It is not uncommon for medications to be continued for many months after the indication has resolved.

8. *Avoid polypharmacy*. Not infrequently, patients receive two or more drugs that are the same type, or that have similar and additive side effects, perhaps prescribed by the same or different clinicians.

9. *Optimize the patient's environment*. Environmental manipulation (eg, increasing the level of care for a dementing patient) may alleviate anxiety, loneliness, depression, and even psychosis. Optimize the patient's physical condition and encourage social activities and exercise whenever possible. Provide supportive individual and family psychotherapy when needed.

10. *Watch for drug side effects*. Most psychotropic agents have side effects that can be of major significance. Many of these may not be present when the drug is started and frequent monitoring is necessary.

COMPLIANCE

General nonadherence to treatment ranges from 25% to 50% among outpatients. Reviewing the literature on compliance, Blackwell (1976) found several factors that contribute to treatment adherence including age, sex, race, and socioeconomic status of the patient; drug regimen; clinic management; patient attitudes; and physician behavior. Patients who continued in treatment had physicians who had a positive attitude and who were optimistic about the treatment outcome. Providing reassurance about medication side effects and inquiring about progress also improved compliance. Adherence was adversely affected when multiple medications were given, when drugs were given in divided doses, or when instructions to patients were complex.

The data from a number of studies affirm a commonsense approach to improving compliance: keep treatment methods and explanations simple, provide positive reinforcement for compliance, and inquire about progress (Walker et al, 1984).

Providing the patient with an explanation of the illness, the course of treatment, and a rationale for drug dosage and choice enhances compliance. In reference to medication prescribing Walker and associates (1984) recommended explanations, when applicable, to the patient: "You have an illness that is related to an imbalance in certain biochemical substances in your nervous system. The medication will return the biochemicals to a proper range so that you will begin feeling normal again." The physician can then explain about the initial side effects of any medication and reassure the patient that the side effects will subside within a few weeks as the patient begins to feel better. The advantages of a particular medication should be reviewed. It is very helpful to the elderly patient if pertinent aspects of the medication and plan of attack on the disease are written down. For some medications, such as the MAOIs, the patient should carry a card or note in his or her wallet and wear a bracelet that

6

warns against the administration of contraindicated drugs, such as meperidine (Demerol) or pressor amines.

Neil and associates (1979) noted that complex treatment regimens decrease patient compliance and that the longer the duration of treatment, the more it is likely that tedious instructions will be circumvented.

With delusional elderly patients, it is not necessary to confront the delusions initially; both physician and patient can agree that the goal of treatment may be to get rid of the animal that is living on the patient's shoulder without having to argue the reality of the situation. It is real to the patient. This approach will enhance compliance.

REFERENCES

Anonymous: 19% of Americans have mental illness NIMH finds. *Psychiatric News* Nov 2, 1984, p. 1.

Bixler EO, Kales A, Soldatos CR, et al: Prevalence of sleep disorders in the Los Angeles metropolitan area. *Am J Psychiatry* 136:1257, 1979.

Blackwell B: Treatment adherence. *Br J Psychiatry* 129:513–531, 1976.

Burke RE, Fahn J, Janovic J, et al: Tardive dyskinesia and inappropriate use of neuroleptic drugs. *Lancet* 1:1299, 1982.

Busse EW: The Duke Longitudinal Study. I: Senescence and senility, in Katzman R, et al (eds): *Alzheimer's Disease: Senile Dementia and Related Disorders*. New York, Raven Press, 1978.

Greenblatt DJ, Shader RI, Koch-Weser J: Psychotropic drug use in the Boston area: A report from the Boston Collaborative Drug Surveillance Program. *Arch Gen Psychiatry* 32:518–523, 1975.

Guttmann D: A study of drug-taking behavior of older Americans, in Beber CR, Lamy PP (eds): *Medication Management and Education in the Elderly*. Amsterdam, Excerpta Medica, 1978.

Jenike MA: Assessment and treatment of affective illness in the elderly. *J Geriatr Psychiatry Neurol* 1:89–107, 1988.

Neil JF, Licata SM, May SJ, et al: Dietary noncompliance during treatment with tranylcypromine. *J Clin Psychiatry* 40:33–37, 1979.

Parry HJ, Baiter MB, Mellinger GD, et al: National patterns of psychotherapeutic drug use. *Arch Gen Psychiatry* 28:769–776, 1973.

Salzman C: *Clinical Geriatric Psychopharmacology*. New York, McGraw-Hill Book Co, 1984.

Thal LJ: Dementia update: Diagnosis and neuropsychiatric aspects. *J Clin Psychiatry* 49:5 (Suppl):5–7, 1988.

Vestal RE (ed): *Drug Treatment in the Elderly*. Boston, ADIS Health Science Press, 1984.

Walker JI, Davidson J, Zung WWK: Patient compliance with MAO inhibitor therapy. *J Clin Psychiatry* 45(7, Sec 2):78–80, 1984.

Wilson LA, Lawson IR, Braws W: Multiple disorders in the elderly. A clinical and statistical study. *Lancet* 2:841-847, 1962.

2

Mental Status and Neuropsychiatric Examination of the Geriatric Patient

MENTAL STATUS EXAMINATION

It is essential that the patient's illness be correctly diagnosed as successful treatment depends to a major extent on the adequacy of the initial evaluation of social and psychological functioning. Pfeiffer (1980) noted that while the diagnosis may be based largely on the presence of specific psychological symptoms, the prognosis will depend heavily on the social context in which those psychological symptoms exist. This chapter largely focuses on the identification of particular neuropsychiatric problems. Management issues are covered in later chapters.

The elderly patient's psychiatric history is of utmost importance; it is often necessary to question family members or others who know the patient well (such as the primary caregivers in the nursing home). The patient's previous level of functioning, as well as coping styles, requires careful assessment. For instance, if one is called to evaluate a hospitalized patient for dementia and it turns out that one week ago he was working and functioning well, it is likely that the patient is delirious and not demented; identifying potentially treatable disorders rather than chronic management becomes the main focus of attention.

A number of questions can be helpful in assessing baseline social functioning. Does the patient live alone? Does she have friends? Does he belong to any social organizations? Is he married?

Before psychotropic medication is begun, it is necessary to decide who will be following and who, if anyone, will be supervising the administration of medication.

Each elderly patient and, if any cognitive disturbance is present, at least one primary caregiver should be questioned in reference to symptoms of cognitive dysfunction, affective illness, and psychosis (CAP is a useful mnemonic).

Cognitive Assessment

General Clinical Assessment
Several tests of cognition are available but are time-consuming and require some expertise to interpret (Jenike, 1988a). Some simple screening tests of cognitive dysfunction include the Mini-Mental State Exam (MMSE) (Folstein et al, 1975), the Short Portable Mental Status Questionnaire (Pfeiffer, 1975), Mental Status Questionnaire (Kahn et al, 1960), Blessed Dementia Scale (Blessed et al, 1968), East Boston Memory Test (Scheer et al, in press), and the Set Test (Isaacs and Kennie, 1973).

Two tests that are easily performed and are valid detectors of organic brain disease in the elderly are the Set Test and the MMSE. Deficiencies on either examination correlate with dementia and necessitate a thorough medical workup (see chapter 5). The MMSE is more commonly used.

Set Test: The Set Test was developed in 1972 as a specific screening test for dementia in the elderly (Isaacs and Kennie, 1973). The test is performed by asking the patient to name ten items in each of four categories: (1) fruits, (2) animals, (3) colors, and (4) towns (FACT is a helpful acronym). One point is given for each correct item and scoring is from 0 to 40.

In the original study, Isaacs and Kennie tested 189 individuals over the age of 65 who were also evaluated for dementia, intelligence, physical illness, affective disorder, and social class. They found that a score of less than 15 corresponded closely to a clinical diagnosis of dementia. No one scoring more than 25 was found to be demented. Scores from 15 to 24 showed some association with dementia. Thus, a patient scoring less than 15, and possibly less than 25, should be thoroughly evaluated.

Mini-Mental State Exam: The Mini-Mental State Exam (MMSE), like the Set Test, is a valid detector of organic disease in elderly patients (Folstein et al, 1975). The test requires five to ten minutes to administer and consists of 11 categories of questions with 30 responses. It is specifically a test of cognitive aspects of mental function and does not evaluate mood, logic, or abnormal mental experiences.

Folstein et al (1975) showed that this test is both reliable and valid. In their initial study, patients with dementia had a mean score of 9.7, those with depression and secondary cognitive impairment (pseudodementia) had a mean score of 19, those with uncomplicated depression had a mean score of 25, and normals a mean score of 27.6. They also showed that patients with pseudodementia raised their scores after treatment with antidepressants and/or electroconvulsive therapy.

Clinically, it is best not to use a particular score on this exam as a cutoff point, above which you do not have to worry about the presence of dementia.

Some very bright individuals will receive a full score of 30 but it will be clear from their history that they are having a loss of cognitive functioning and a decision not to perform further workup would be ill advised; conversely, some patients with little education or awareness might perform poorly despite the absence of dementia. Recent data suggest that elderly persons with a poor educational background (ie, 0–8 years) perform differentially more poorly on a broad range of cognitive tasks than elderly persons with a good educational background (ie, 10–16 years) (Anthony et al, 1982). The MMSE should be used as a clinical screening tool and evaluated in the context of the rest of the mental status examination and the history of present illness.

The MMSE is performed as shown in Figure 2-1 (Keller and Manschreck, 1979; Murray, 1987): Mini-Mental State Exam (Folstein et al, 1975).

Neuropsychiatric Assessment

The tests just mentioned are useful screening examinations that aid in detecting specific areas of cognitive dysfunction. When deficits are found or if the patient's history suggests that cognitive deficits may be present (even if MMSE is normal), neuropsychiatric evaluation will help to further evaluate possible areas of deficit. Detailed discussion of cognitive testing is available elsewhere (see Albert and Moss, 1988, or Lezak, 1983, for excellent discussions). In this section, we will give a broad overview of neuropsychological areas that the clinician might expect the neuropsychologist to cover.

Neuropsychologists are trained not only to identify areas of poor functioning but also to suggest ways that patients can work around such deficits. For example, one elderly dementing woman, with only mild memory deficits, was told that she could still continue to drive and to knit because her memory difficulties were quite minor. Her family members had difficulty understanding why she had trouble dressing herself but still was able to remember with great vividness events that occurred ten years ago. This led them to think that the patient could do many tasks but "wasn't really trying." On further testing, it was determined that she had quite pronounced visuospatial difficulties despite very mild memory deficits and that it was impossible for her to knit and probably unsafe for her to drive. Explaining how apparently discrepant abilities were consistent with what was known of her brain functioning helped the family to readjust their expectations and begin to think of how to capitalize on areas of preserved ability. She was advised to spend more time on her hobby of listening to classical music and to stay involved in her social clubs. The earlier recommendations were inappropriate and only led to increased frustration with her disabilities, because the clinician was telling her that she should still be able to knit and perform other tasks that required visuospatial skills.

Albert (1988) recommended evaluating the elderly patient in six broad areas of function: attention, language, memory, visuospatial ability, conceptualization, and general intelligence. These will be briefly reviewed.

Patient _____
Examiner _____
Date _____

"MINI-MENTAL STATE"*

Maxi-mum score	Score	
		Orientation
5	( )	What is the (year) (season) (date) (day) (month)?
5	( )	Where are we? (state) (country) (town) (hospital) (floor).

Registration

| 3 | ( ) | Name 3 objects: 1 second to say each. Then ask the patient all 3 after you have said them. Give 1 point for each correct answer. Then repeat them until he learns all 3. Count trials and record. |

Trials _____

Attention and Calculation

| 5 | ( ) | Serial 7's. 1 point for each correct. Stop after 5 answers. Alternatively spell "world" backwards. |

Recall

| 3 | ( ) | Ask for the 3 objects repeated above. Give 1 point for each correct. |

Language

| 9 | ( ) | Name a pencil, and watch (2 points) |

Repeat the following "No ifs, ands or buts." (1 point)
Follow a 3-stage command:
"Take a paper in your right hand, fold it in half, and put it on the floor" (3 points)
Read and obey the following:

Close your eyes (1 point)

Write a sentence (1 point)
Copy design (1 point)
Total score
ASSESS level of consciousness
along a continuum _____

Alert Drowsy Stupor Coma

Figure 2–1   Mini-Mental State Examination (reproduced with permission from Folstein et al, 1975).

INSTRUCTIONS FOR ADMINISTRATION OF
MINI-MENTAL STATE EXAMINATION

Orientation

(1) Ask for the date. Then ask specifically for parts omitted, e.g., "Can you also tell me what season it is?" One point for each correct.

(2) Ask in turn "Can you tell me the name of this hospital?" (town, country, etc.). One point for each correct.

Registration

Ask the patient if you may test his memory. Then say the names of 3 unrelated objects, clearly and slowly, about one second for each. After you have said all 3, ask him to repeat them. This first repetition determines his score (0–3) but keep saying them until he can repeat all 3, up to 6 trials. If he does not eventually learn all 3, recall cannot be meaningfully tested.

Attention and calculation

Ask the patient to begin with 100 and count backwards by 7. Stop after 5 subtractions (93, 86, 79, 72, 65). Score the total number of correct answers.

If the patient cannot or will not perform this task, ask him to spell the word "world" backwards. The score is the number of letters in correct order. E.g., dlrow = 5, dlorw = 3.

Recall

Ask the patient if he can recall the 3 words you previously asked him to remember. Score 0–3.

Language

Naming: Show the patient a wrist watch and ask him what it is. Repeat for pencil. Score 0–2.

Repetition: Ask the patient to repeat the sentence after you. Allow only one trial. Score 0 or 1.

3-Stage command: Give the patient a piece of plain blank paper and repeat the command. Score 1 point for each part correctly executed.

Reading: On a blank piece of paper print the sentence "Close your eyes", in letters large enough for the patient to see clearly. Ask him to read it and do what it says. Score 1 point only if he actually closes his eyes.

Writing: Give the patient a blank piece of paper and ask him to write a sentence for you. Do not dictate a sentence, it is to be written spontaneously. It must contain a subject and verb and be sensible. Correct grammar and punctuation are not necessary.

Copying: On a clean piece of paper, draw intersecting pentagons, each side about 1 in., and ask him to copy it exactly as it is. All 10 angles must be present and 2 must intersect to score 1 point. Tremor and rotation are ignored.

Estimate the patient's level of sensorium along a continuum, from alert on the left to coma on the right.

Attention: Attention, often evaluated first, must be preserved for any other tasks to be performed adequately and if the subject has problems keeping his or her mind on the task for a few minutes at a time, it will not be possible to assess other areas of function. Auditory and visual attention can be assessed easily by tests of digit span and letter cancellation (a patient is asked to draw a line through a certain letter that is scattered throughout a page of numerous letters).

Language: Language testing for aphasia should include an evaluation of comprehension, repetition, reading, writing, and naming. Several standardized batteries are available for this purpose (Goodglass and Kaplan, 1972; Kertesz, 1980). Albert (1988) recommended that, if aphasia has been ruled out or is not suspected, then confrontation naming (Kaplan et al, 1983) should almost always be part of the assessment of an older individual, as decreases in naming ability occur with age and are also a prominent symptom of a number of disorders common among the elderly, such as Alzheimer's disease. (See Albert and Helm-Estabrooks, 1988, for a comprehensive and up-to-date review of aphasia.)

Memory: Testing of memory is probably the most essential of all the tests in the elderly since memory dysfunction occurs in almost all of the cognitive disorders associated with aging (Albert, 1988). The assessment of memory is complicated by the fact that changes in memory capacity occur as people age and thus careful testing by a knowledgeable neuropsychologist is required to differentiate normal from pathological memory performance. Albert (1988) noted that there are a number of good memory tests which can be used, including the Wechsler Memory Scale (Wechsler, 1945), Rey Auditory Verbal Learning Test (Rey, 1964), Selective Reminding Test (Buschke and Fuld, 1974), and the Delayed Recognition Span Test (Moss et al, 1986).

Visuospatial abilities: Assessment of visuospatial ability may be more difficult in the elderly than in the young because of the prevalence of visual deficits in some patients (Albert, 1988). In the previously discussed cognitive tests, function can be evaluated either orally or visually.

Figure copying is the method of assessment that is most likely to yield useful information about level of functioning.

Conceptualization: This is evaluated by assessing concept formation, abstraction, set shifting, and set maintenance (Albert, 1988). Some of the commonly used tests include the Similarities subtest of the Wechsler Adult Intelligence Scale-Revised (WAIS-R) (Wechsler, 1981), Proverbs Test (Gorham, 1956), Trail Making Test (Reitan, 1958), Modified Card Sorting Test (Nelson, 1976), and the Visual-Verbal Test (Feldman and Drasgow, 1951).

General intelligence: Albert (1988) also recommended that, in addition to the areas of assessment just mentioned, general intelligence should be estimated so that one can determine whether the individual has access to previously acquired knowledge. She recommended the Vocabulary subtest of the WAIS-R as a well-known tool to make a quick estimate of intelligence quotient (IQ).

Assessing Symptoms of Affective Illness

As discussed in more detail in chapter 4, depression in the elderly may present with various clinical symptoms such as chronic pain, multiple somatic complaints, or even dementia (pseudodementia). Although some elderly depressed individuals present atypically, most can be diagnosed according to the Washington University research criteria, which form the basis for the *Diagnostic and Statistical Manual of Mental Disorders,* revised, ed 3 (DSM-III-R) criteria (Spar and LaRue, 1983).

A helpful mnemonic, developed by Dr Carey Gross at Massachusetts General Hospital, that outlines the clinical picture of major depression is SIG E CAPS (prescription for energy capsules): Sleep, Interest, Guilt, Energy, Concentration, Appetite, Psychomotor, and Suicide. Each of these corresponds to one of the DSM-III-R criteria for major depression (Jenike, 1988).

To elaborate, depressed patients generally complain of insomnia, typically with early awakening in the morning; occasionally, however, hypersomnia is the problem. They lose interest in usually stimulating activities—job, hobbies, social activities, and sex. Guilty ruminations and feelings of self-reproach are the rule. Depressed patients have no energy and feel fatigued all day. They frequently report an inability to concentrate, with slowed or mixed-up thinking (cognitive changes associated with severe depression are reviewed below and in chapter 5). They usually have a poor appetite with associated loss of weight, although occasionally they overeat. Psychomotor retardation is usually observed, but agitated depressions in the elderly are not uncommon. They may have recurrent thoughts of suicide or death and may feel that life is not worth living or wish that they were dead. A patient with at least five of these eight criteria is depressed and if his dysphoric emotional state has persisted for two to four weeks, he needs treatment.

Assessing Psychotic Symptoms

Each elderly patient should be evaluated for the presence of psychotic symptoms including hallucinations which may be auditory, visual, olfactory, or tactile; ideas of reference (eg, TV, radio, or other people talking about the patient), thought insertion (eg, hearing others' thoughts), thought withdrawal (eg, others can hear patient's thoughts), or paranoia. It is not uncommon for the patient to deny such symptoms and it is of utmost importance that a primary caregiver or someone who is familiar with the patient's recent behavior be questioned about these symptoms. The evaluation of psychotic symptoms is covered in more detail in chapter 6.

Example of Using CAP To Formulate
Differential Diagnostic Possibilities

Whenever elderly patients are evaluated by any physician, questions concerning cognition, affective state, and psychotic symptoms (CAP) should be part of the examination. To illustrate how a brief but thorough mental status exam can help pin down the diagnosis with a complicated patient, consider the case of an 86-year-old gentleman who is brought into the emergency room by his daughter. He is pacing around the room with vigor and cannot sit still. A pained look on his face suggests at least confusion, but perhaps even great fear.

The physician on duty speaks to his daughter and finds that the patient is not taking medication, has no history of serious medical or psychiatric illness, and the physician proceeds to interview the patient. Slowly the patient completes the MMSE and is found to be completely oriented and able to remember all three memory items after three minutes. He received a score of 28, having missed the county (which his daughter also did not know) and one item on serial 7's. This five-minute exam ruled out the presence of severe cognitive deficit.

Questions concerning affective symptoms are directed at the daughter and the patient. It turns out that the patient's wife died last year and that he is now having difficulty eating and sleeping and has lost over 20 pounds in the last five weeks. Energy level is low, he is psychomotorically agitated, but he can concentrate if he has to. He is very uninterested in his usual hobbies and feels quite guilty about some of his earlier activities. He denies thoughts of suicide. The patient clearly meets DSM-III-R criteria for a major depressive episode.

The patient denies psychotic symptoms and says "I'm not crazy doc!" when asked about hallucinations, ideas of reference, thought withdrawal or insertion, or paranoia. His daughter asks the physician if she can speak to him alone and they step out of the room despite mild protests by the patient. The daughter becomes tearful and relates that her father has been yelling and swearing into the kitchen sink because he feels that "little people" are living in the sink. He has thrown glass cups into the sink and often boils water and pours it into the sink in an effort to kill these people. In addition, her father feels that the Internal Revenue Service has hired detectives to follow him because he fabricated a business trip on his tax return about 35 years ago.

The physician makes the correct diagnosis of an agitated major depressive episode with psychotic features (eg, psychotic or delusional depression). The patient is hospitalized immediately and started on 25 mg of nortriptyline, an antidepressant, and 0.5 mg of haloperidol, an antipsychotic medication. A medical workup is done to rule out an organic or neurologic explanation for the psychiatric symptoms.

By systematically evaluating this patient, the most likely diagnosis was determined. If the patient had been seen alone, the physician would have missed the presence of psychotic symptoms and would have had little idea of the course of the depressive symptoms; this points out the importance of getting a history from someone other than the patient. The absence of deficits on the MMSE indicated that this patient was not agitated and pacing secondary to a dementing illness such as Alzheimer's disease. The fact that the patient was not taking any medication ruled out akathisia (see chapter 6) secondary to antipsychotic medication.

MEDICAL, PSYCHIATRIC, AND COGNITIVE HISTORY

Evaluation of geriatric patients must include a good history, and especially if the patient has any evidence of cognitive dysfunction, it is necessary, as noted already, for the history to be corroborated by someone other than the patient, preferably by both medical records and a person familiar with the patient (Albert, 1988). While some family members may have difficulty attending an evaluation session, it is imperative that every effort be made to obtain necessary information. If possible, several family members should be present because each person tends to have a slightly different perspective to the symptoms and the course of the problems. Often family members will be more open when the patient is not in the room. For example, they may be reluctant to discuss psychotic or cognitive symptoms in the presence of the patient if the patient gets angry or upset when confronted by such problems.

History of previous and present diseases and medication use is important as a wide variety of systemic illnesses and drugs can cause neuropsychiatric changes. The patient's past drinking and smoking habits should be noted and if the patient was a heavy drinker, quantification of the amount ingested should be attempted; keep in mind that such patients generally tend to underestimate intake (see chapter 10).

Information concerning the medical, neurologic, and psychiatric history, as well as cause of death of immediate family members, is often relevant. A standardized form for recording family history, developed by Breitner and Folstein (1984), is in the appendix.

Obtaining a history of any cognitive deficits often presents a clinical challenge, as patients by definition will have difficulty remembering and some family members may be very poor historians; in addition, subtle cognitive changes are often overlooked or attributed to the aging process. Albert (1988), noting that a comprehensive cognitive history should include information concerning the progression of behavioral change, stated that family members may not know how to isolate important aspects of the medical history or how to focus on individual cognitive functions in isolation from one another. For example, the family may state that the first symptom of disease was the patient's anxiety and depression about work, and only when specifically asked they remember several episodes that preceded the onset of work-related anxiety in which the patient could not remember how to deal with a complex situation or how to use new equipment. Family members may use words imprecisely and the clinician must ask for specific examples when terms like "memory difficulties," "nervous breakdown," or "senility" are used.

When cognitive deficits are present, questions about when the deficits began and how they have progressed are of utmost importance for diagnostic purposes. For example, in Alzheimer's disease, insidious onset with a gradually progressive course is the rule while in multi-infarct dementia, stepwise progression is more likely. However, an acute urinary infection in an Alzheimer's patient may produce a sudden loss of function; generally, however, once the infection is cleared the patient's behavioral state will return to baseline. In addition, superimposed psychiatric symptoms (eg, depression or hallucinations) may also produce stepwise deterioration, so special care is required to determine the underlying cause of stepwise deterioration of cognitive function (Albert, 1988). Some dementing illnesses (for example, Creutzfeldt-Jakob disease), are notable by their rapid rate of progression. Acute confusional states (see chapter 9) generally have an acute onset as well.

Also the nature of the behavioral changes that are present at the time of interview and earlier in the course of the disease may yield diagnostic clues. For example, a symptom of Pick's disease is generally thought to be a change in personality with poor judgement and inappropriate behavior early in the illness, while in Alzheimer's disease gradually progressive decline in the ability to learn new information may be the earliest sign of illness.

Information about how the patient is functioning in his or her own environment is useful. A substantial discrepancy between functional performance of the patient and level of cognitive disability suggests the presence of a psychiatric illness. For example, an apparently mildly demented patient with a MMSE score of 26 who cannot cook and wants to stay in bed all day may well be depressed rather than have an early dementing illness.

SUMMARY

The general assessment of the elderly patient sets the stage for a diagnosis and ultimately sound treatment. Three main areas of functioning need to be assessed in every elderly patient regardless of presenting symptom or complaint. CAP (ie, cognition, affect, psychosis) is a mnemonic which helps the clinician to remember the major categories that need to be assessed.

Cognitive status is best evaluated by using one of the brief screening tests which are in wide usage; the MMSE, which takes less than ten minutes to perform in most patients, is commonly used and is discussed in detail.

Affective state is best evaluated by inquiring into the elements of DSM-III-R which can be remembered at the bedside by use of the mnemonic SIG E CAPS (ie, sleep, interest, guilt, energy, concentration, appetite, psychomotor, suicide). The presence of psychotic symptoms should be evaluated by asking about hallucinations, ideas of reference, thought insertion and withdrawal, and paranoia.

Because elderly patients may be unaware of particular symptoms (eg, in dementia) or be evasive about some symptoms (eg, psychosis), it is important to speak to at least one other family member or someone else who knows the patient well and can describe the history of the present illness.

History of previous and present diseases and medication use must be obtained as a wide variety of systemic illnesses and drugs can cause neuropsychiatric changes. The patient's past drinking and smoking habits should be noted and if the patient was a heavy drinker, quantification of the amount ingested should be attempted. Information concerning any medical, neurologic, and psychiatric history, as well as cause of death, of immediate family members is often relevant. Information about how the patient is functioning in his or her own environment is useful.

Further medical and psychiatric workup as well as treatment are based on this initial assessment. Reasonable treatment is unlikely to follow incomplete or inaccurate diagnosis.

REFERENCES

Albert ML, Helm-Estabrooks N: Diagnosis and treatment of aphasia: Part I and Part II. *JAMA* 259:1043–1047, 1205–1210, 1988.

Albert MS, Moss MB: *Geriatric Neuropsychology*. New York, Guilford Press, 1988.

Albert MS: Assessment of cognitive dysfunction, in Albert MS, Moss MB (eds): *Geriatric Neuropsychology*. New York, Guilford Press, 1988.

Anthony JC, LeResche L, Niaz U, et al: Limits of the Mini-Mental State as a screening test for dementia and delirium among hospital patients. *Psychol Med* 12:397–408, 1982.

Blessed G, Tomlinson BE, Roth M: The association between quantitative measures of dementia and of senile changes in the cerebral gray matter of elderly subjects. *Br J Psychiatry* 114:797–811, 1968.

Breitner JC, Folstein M: Familial Alzheimer dementia: A prevalent disorder with specific clinical features. *Psychol Med* 14:63–80, 1984.

Buschke H, Fuld PA: Evaluating storage, retention, and retrieval in disordered memory and learning. *Neurology* 11:1019–1025, 1974.

Feldman MJ, Drasgow JA: A visual-verbal test for schizophrenia. *Psychiatric Q* 25 (Suppl):55–64, 1951.

Folstein MF, Folstein SE, McHugh PR: Mini-Mental State Exam: A practical method for grading the cognitive state of patients for the clinician. *J Psychiatry Res* 12:189–198, 1975.

Goodglass H, Kaplan E: *The Assessment of Aphasia and Related Disorders*. Philadelphia, Lea and Febiger, 1972.

Gorham DR: A proverbs test for clinical and experimental use. *Psychol Rep* 1:1–12, 1956.

Isaacs B, Kennie AT: The Set Test as an aid to the detection of dementia in old people. *Br J Psychiatry* 123:467–470, 1973.

Jenike MA: Alzheimer's disease. *Sci Am Med* 9:1–4, 1986.

Jenike MA: Assessment and treatment of affective illness in the elderly. *J Geriatr Psychiatry Neurol* 1:89-107, 1988.

Jenike MA: Alzheimer's disease—What the practicing clinician needs to know. *J Geriatr Psychiatry Neurol* 1:37–46, 1988a.

Kahn RL, Goldfarb AL, Pollack M, et al: Brief objective measures for the determination of mental status in the aged. *Am J Psychiatry* 111:326–328, 1960.

Kaplan E, Goodglass H, Weintraub S: *Boston Naming Test*. Philadelphia, Lea and Febiger, 1983.

Keller MB, Manschreck TC: The biologic mental status examination, in Lazare A (ed): *Outpatient Psychiatry*. Baltimore, Williams and Wilkins, 1979, pp 203–214.

Kertesz A: *Western Aphasia Battery*. London, Ontario, University of Western Ontario, 1980.

Lezak M: *Neuropsychological Assessment*. New York, Oxford, 1983.

Moss M, Albert M, Butters N, et al: Differential patterns of memory loss among patients with Alzheimer's disease, Huntington's disease and alcoholic Korsakoff's syndrome. *Arch Neurol* 43:239–246, 1986.

Murray GB: Confusion, delirium, and dementia, in: *Massachusetts General Hospital Handbook of General Hospital Psychiatry*, ed 2. Littleton, Mass, PSG Publishing, 1987.

Nelson HE: A modified card sorting test sensitive to frontal lobe defects. *Cortex* 12:313–324, 1976.

Pfeiffer E: SPMSQ: Short Portable Mental Status Questionnaire. *J Am Geriatr Soc* 23:433–441, 1975.

Pfeiffer E: The psychosocial evaluation of the elderly patient, in Busse EW, Blazer DG (eds): *Handbook of Geriatric Psychiatry*. New York, Van Nostrand Reinhold Co, 1980, pp 275–284.

Reitan RM: Validity of the Trail Making Test as an indication or organic brain damage. *Percept Mot Skills* 8:271–276, 1958.

Rey A: *L'examen clinique en psychologie*. Paris, Presses Universitaires de France, 1964.

Sheer PA, Albert MS, Funkenstein H, et al: Correlates of cognitive function in an elderly community population. *J Epidemiol* (in press).

Spar JE, LaRue A: Major depression in the elderly: DSM III criteria and the dexamethasone suppression test as predictors of treatment response. *Am J Psychiatry* 140:844–847, 1983.

Wechsler D: A standardized memory scale for clinical use. *J Psychol* 19:87–95, 1945.

Wechsler D: *WAIS-R Manual*. New York, Psychological Corporation, 1981.

APPENDIX
Alzheimer Dementia Risk Questionnaire[1]

Let me begin asking you a couple of questions about *subject*.

1. To the best of your knowledge, has *subject* ever had:

	Yes	No
a. High blood pressure?	1	2
b. A stroke?	1	2
c. Diabetes or "sugar"?	1	2
d. A drinking problem?	1	2
e. A head injury that resulted in loss of consciousness for more than a second or two?	1	2
f. A psychiatric illness that required hospitalization (other than the present problem)?	1	2
g. Any other neurological diseases or disorders of the brain such as a brain tumor, multiple sclerosis, or Parkinson's disease?	1	2

2. What was the last year of school that *subject* completed?
   - 1–12. Last grade completed
   - 14.   Some college
   - 16.   College graduate
   - 17.   Graduate degree

3. Before he or she became ill, was *subject* able to read and write?   Yes No
       1   2

4. Could you tell me the last address where *subject* lived before he or she first entered a nursing home?

5. What type of work did *subject* do before this illness began or before he or she retired? (IF MORE THAN ONE JOB, ASK FOR THE JOB SUBJECT HELD LONGEST)
   Homemaker   Student
   Disabled   Other

        Yes No

5a. Was *subject* ever married?   1   2

5b. IF YES: What type of work did *subject's* spouse do?
   (IF MORE THAN ONE JOB, ASK FOR THE JOB SPOUSE HELD LONGEST. IF MORE THAN ONE SPOUSE, CODE FOR SPOUSE WITH HIGHEST PRESTIGE JOB.)
   Homemaker   Student
   Disabled   Other

5c. IF NO: What type of work did *subject's* father do?
   (IF MORE THAN ONE JOB, ASK FOR JOB FATHER HELD LONGEST.)
   Disabled
   Other

---

[1]From J.C. Breitner and M. Folstein, Familial Alzheimer dementia: A prevalent disorder with specific clinical features. *Psychol Med* 1984;14:63–80. Copyright 1984 by Cambridge University Press. Reprinted with permission.

6. Now I'd like to ask you some questions about *subject's* recent illness and in particular about the time when you or your family first noticed some specific changes. Have you noticed:

	Yes	No	If yes: mo/yr change began
a. A change in *subject's* personality (eg, a change in tidiness, restlessness, irritability, loss of concern for others)?	1	2	____/____
b. Loss of memory?	1	2	____/____
c. Difficulty in speech or finding words?	1	2	____/____
d. Loss of ability to read (eg, stopped reading books or newspapers)?	1	2	____/____
e. Loss of ability to write (eg, stopped writing notes or letters)?	1	2	____/____
f. Loss of ability to cook or dress self?	1	2	____/____
g. Loss of control of bladder or bowels?	1	2	____/____

7. To the best of your recollection, when was the last time *subject* was really well or his or her old self?

____/____
mo/yr

8. When would you say you first noticed a change?

____/____
mo/yr

9. What was the first change (SYMPTOM) that you noticed?

Now I'd like to ask you a few questions about *subject's* children.

10a. How many children did *subject* have, including those who died in infancy or childhood, but not including stillbirths and abortions?

_____
no. children

IF NO CHILDREN, SKIP TO Q 11.

10b. Could you tell me the names of all these children, living or deceased, in order of their birth, starting with the oldest?

10c. What is the birthdate of *child?*

10d. What is the sex of *child?*

10e. Is *child* still alive?

10f. What is the current age of each child? (IF CHILD IS DECEASED, RECORD AGE AT DEATH.)

10g. IF DECEASED: What was the cause of *child's* death?

10h. Have any of these children suffered from any of the following?
   1. Mental retardation (Down's syndrome, mongolism as a cause, if known)
   2. Birth defects (eg, congenital heart disease, spina bifida, etc)
   3. Malignancy of blood forming organs or lymphatics (eg, leukemia or lymphoma, by type if possible, Hodgkin's disease, multiple myeloma, Waldenstorm's macroglobulinemia, etc)
   4. Central nervous system or brain disease (eg, epilepsy, amyotrophic lateral sclerosis, Parkinson's disease, multiple sclerosis, etc. DO NOT INCLUDE "BAD NERVES," ETC)

5. Symptoms of mental deterioration such as:
   a. Memory loss (ML)
   b. Loss of ability to read (RL) or write (WL)
   c. Difficulty finding words, speaking nonsense words, etc (SL)
   d. Difficulty with cooking or dressing (due to apraxia) (CD)
   e. Loss of control of bowels or bladder (IN) (LIST ONLY IN PRESENCE OF
      OTHER ASSOCIATED SYMPTOMS OF DEMENTIA.)

IF NO SYMPTOMS OR CONDITIONS, SKIP TO Q 11.

10b Name of child (last name, first name; if female, maiden name)	10c Birth-date (mo/day/yr)	10d Sex (M = 1; F = 2)	10e Living? (Yes = 1; No = 2)	10f Age	10g Cause of death
1					
2					
3					
4					
5					
6					

10h

ALL APPLICABLE CONDITIONS OR SYMPTOMS WITH DATE OF ONSET (mo/yr). Be as specific as possible. (If positive response in 1–5, administer SUPPLEMENTAL FORM for relative with condition.)

1
2
3
4
5
6

Now I'd like to ask you the same questions about *subject's* brothers and sisters.

11a. How many brothers and sisters did *subject* have, including those who may have died at any time after birth? (DO NOT INCLUDE HALF-SIBLINGS OR STEP-SIBLINGS.)

_____
no. siblings

IF NO SIBLINGS, SKIP TO Q 12.

11b. Could you tell me the names of all brothers and sisters, living and deceased, from the oldest to the youngest? Please include subject but do not include any step-brothers or sisters or half-brothers or sisters.

11c. What is the birthdate of *sibling?*

11d. What is the sex of *sibling?*

11e. Is *sibling* still alive?

11f. What is the current age of each sibling? (IF SIBLING IS DECEASED, RECORD AGE AT DEATH.)

11g. IF DECEASED: What was the cause of *sibling's* death?

11h. Have any of these brothers or sisters suffered from any of the following?
  1. Mental retardation (Down's syndrome, mongolism as a cause, if known)
  2. Birth defects (eg, congenital heart disease, spina bifida, etc)
  3. Malignancy of blood forming organs or lymphatics (eg, leukemia or lymphoma, by type if possible, Hodgkin's disease, multiple myeloma, Waldenstorm's macroglobulinemia, etc)
  4. Central nervous system or brain disease (eg, epilepsy, amyotrophic lateral sclerosis, Parkinson's disease, multiple sclerosis, etc. DO NOT INCLUDE "BAD NERVES," ETC)
  5. Symptoms of mental deterioration such as:
    a. Memory loss (ML)
    b. Loss of ability to read (RL) or write (WL)
    c. Difficulty finding words, speaking nonsense words, etc (SL)
    d. Difficulty with cooking or dressing (due to apraxia) (CD)
    e. Loss of control of bowels or bladder (IN) (LIST ONLY IN PRESENCE OF OTHER ASSOCIATED SYMPTOMS OF DEMENTIA.)

IF NO SYMPTOMS OR CONDITIONS, SKIP TO Q 12.

11b Name of sibling (last name, first name; if female, maiden name)	11c Birth- date (mo/day/yr)	11d Sex (M = 1; F = 2)	11e Living? (Yes = 1; No = 2)	11f Age	11g Cause of death
1					
2					
3					
4					
5					
6					

11h

ALL APPLICABLE CONDITIONS OR SYMPTOMS WITH DATE OF ONSET (mo/yr). Be as specific as possible. (If positive response in 1–5, administer SUPPLEMENTAL FORM for relative with condition.)

1
2
3
4
5
6

12a. What are the names of *subject's* biological parents, living or deceased?

12b. What was the birthdate of *parent?*

12c. FILL IN SEX.

12d. Is *parent* still alive?

12e. What is the current age of each parent? (IF DECEASED, RECORD AGE AT DEATH.)

12f. IF DECEASED. What was the cause of *parent's* death?

12g. Has either parent suffered from any of the following?
 1. Mental retardation (Down's syndrome, mongolism as a cause, if known)
 2. Birth defects (eg, congenital heart disease, spina bifida, etc)
 3. Malignancy of blood forming organs or lymphatics (eg, leukemia or lymphoma, by type if possible, Hodgkin's disease, multiple myeloma, Waldenstorm's macroglobulinemia, etc)
 4. Central nervous system or brain disease (eg, epilepsy, amyotrophic lateral sclerosis, Parkinson's disease, multiple sclerosis, etc. DO NOT INCLUDE "BAD NERVES," ETC)
 5. Symptoms of mental deterioration such as:
   a. Memory loss (ML)
   b. Loss of ability to read (RL) or write (WL)
   c. Difficulty finding words, speaking nonsense words, etc (SL)
   d. Difficulty with cooking or dressing (due to apraxia) (CD)
   e. Loss of control of bowels or bladder (IN) (LIST ONLY IN PRESENCE OF OTHER ASSOCIATED SYMPTOMS OF DEMENTIA.)

IF NO SYMPTOMS OR CONDITIONS. SKIP TO Q 13.

12a Name of parent (last name, first name; if female, maiden name)	12b Birth- date (mo/day/yr)	12c Sex (M = 1; F = 2)	12d Living? (Yes = 1; No = 2)	12e Age	12f Cause of death
1					
2					

12g
ALL APPLICABLE CONDITIONS OR SYMPTOMS WITH DATE OF ONSET (mo/yr). Be as specific as possible. (If positive response in 1–5, administer SUPPLEMENTAL FORM for relative with condition.)

1

2

13a. Was *subject* ever married? _____ (no. of times)

IF NO SKIP TO Q 14.

13b. What are the names of all of *subject's* marriage partners (INCLUDING COMMON LAW), whether living or deceased?

13c. What was the birthdate of *partner?*

13d. Is *partner* still living?

13e. What is the current age of each partner? (IF DECEASED, RECORD AGE AT DEATH.)

13f. When did this marriage (cohabitation) begin?

13g. IF APPLICABLE. When did *subject* separate from this partner? (Separation includes divorce, *de facto* or legal separation, death, institutional placement of partner or subject, etc)

13h. IF DECEASED: What was the cause of *partner's* death?

13i. Have any of *subject's* partners suffered from the following?
  1. Mental retardation (Down's syndrome, mongolism)
  2. Birth defects (eg, congenital heart disease, spina bifida, etc)
  3. Malignancy of blood forming organs or lymphatics (eg, leukemia or lymphoma, by type if possible, Hodgkin's disease, multiple myeloma, Waldenstorm's macroglobulinemia, etc)
  4. Central nervous system or brain disease (eg, epilepsy, amyotrophic lateral sclerosis, Parkinson's disease, multiple sclerosis, etc. DO NOT INCLUDE "BAD NERVES," ETC)
  5. Symptoms of mental deterioration such as:
     a. Memory loss (ML)
     b. Loss of ability to read (RL) or write (WL)
     c. Difficulty finding words, speaking nonsense words, etc (SL)
     d. Difficulty with cooking or dressing (due to apraxia) (CD)
     e. Loss of control of bowels or bladder (IN) (LIST ONLY IN PRESENCE OF OTHER ASSOCIATED SYMPTOMS OF DEMENTIA.)

13b Name of partner (last name, first name; if female, maiden name)	13c Birth-date (mo/day/yr)	13d Living? (Yes = 1; No = 2)	13e Age	13f Marriage began?	13g Marriage end?	13h Cause of death
1						
2						
3						
4						

13i

ALL APPLICABLE CONDITIONS OR SYMPTOMS WITH DATE OF ONSET (mo/yr). Be as specific as possible. (If positive response in 1–5, administer SUPPLEMENTAL FORM for relative with condition.)

1
2
3
4

14. Could you tell me the name of another family member who is knowledgeable about *subject's* family's medical history?

3

Metabolic Changes with Aging

OVERVIEW

Certain drugs are more likely to be toxic in the elderly because of physiologic concomitants of aging. To use psychopharmacologic agents wisely in the elderly patient, changes in drug absorption, distribution, protein binding, hepatic metabolism, and renal excretion (Table 3-1) must be taken into account when the physician is planning type and dosage of any psychotropic drug. Changes in receptor sensitivity and brain neurotransmitters have also been reported (Jenike, 1982a; Vestal, 1984; Greenblatt et al, 1982; Salzman, 1984).

AGE-RELATED CHANGES IN DRUG PHARMACOKINETICS

A number of age-related changes affect how psychopharmacologic agents are handled in the elderly. They are briefly reviewed in this chapter.

Absorption

Overall, changes in absorption are the least important physiologic alterations accompanying aging. In general, gastric pH is higher and intestinal blood flow is reduced. Also, gastric emptying is delayed, gastrointestinal (GI) motility is decreased, and the number of absorbing cells is lower in the elderly. Decreased active transport with increased age is well documented, but because most psychotropic agents are passively diffused, this is of little or no consequence. Clearly, more research is needed in this area, but the available data suggest that age alone produces few changes in the gut that are of clinical significance in terms of drug metabolism (Plein and Plein, 1981; Schumacher, 1980).

Table 3-1
Altered Metabolism with Aging

Absorption
Distribution
Protein binding
Hepatic metabolism
Renal excretion
Receptor sensitivity
Brain enzyme systems
Decreased acetylcholine and dopamine
Increased monoamine oxidase

Distribution

Distribution changes are, on the other hand, clinically very important in the elderly. On the average, elderly patients tend to be smaller than younger patients and standard drug doses might be expected to result in higher blood and tissue levels (Greenblatt et al, 1982).

As humans age, total levels of body water decrease, lean body mass is reduced, and body fat increases (Bruce et al, 1980; Novak, 1972; Forbes and Reina, 1970). From the ages of 20 to 60 years, the percentage of total body water may decrease from 25% to 18%. Drugs such as ethanol which are distributed in body water will have higher levels per unit dose in an elderly person because of an apparent decrease in the size of their reservoir (Vestal et al, 1977).

In the same period, the proportion of total body fat may increase from 10% to 50% (Greenblatt et al, 1982). This increases the volume of distribution of lipid-soluble drugs, such as desmethyldiazepam, a metabolite of diazepam (Valium), and contributes to greatly prolonged drug half-life (Greenblatt et al, 1980 and 1981; Allen et al, 1980). From Figure 3-1, it can be seen that drug half-life is raised by an increase in the volume of distribution or by a decrease in creatinine clearance (Greenblatt et al, 1982). For example, as a consequence of changes in volume of distribution and clearance, the half-life of diazepam metabolites is prolonged from an average of 20 hours at the age of 20 years to 90 hours at the age of 80 years (Rosenbaum, 1979). Because it takes about four to five half-lives to reach a steady state, diazepam's metabolites will not

$$T_{\frac{1}{2}} = \frac{Vd \times k}{Ccl}$$

where $T_{\frac{1}{2}}$ = half-life

Vd = volume of distribution

k = constant

Ccl = creatinine clearance

Figure 3-1 Relation of drug half-life to volume of distribution and renal clearance.

reach a steady blood level with daily dosing in an average elderly person until between two and three weeks. With drugs such as flurazepam (Dalmane), which have metabolites with mean half-lives of more than 200 hours, a steady-state level may not be reached until after six weeks when the patient takes the drug each night to avoid insomnia (see chapter 8). It is not surprising then, that patients may not be symptomatic of benzodiazepine toxicity until long after the drug is started and clinicians and patients may not associate the drug with symptoms such as lethargy, drowsiness, depression, ataxia, and confusion. Elderly patients who have been hospitalized are frequently sent home with instructions to take nightly doses of long-acting benzodiazepines and, as a consequence of these age-associated metabolic changes, they may have signs of toxicity as the weeks progress.

Serum albumin levels are reduced by 15% to 25% in the elderly (Schumacher, 1980; Bender et al, 1975; Hayes et al, 1975), and because many psychotropic drugs bind to albumin, this may be clinically important. Free drug concentration is an important determinant of drug distribution, elimination, and action. The less albumin available for drug binding, the more free drug is available to body tissues where sites of action may be located.

Increased availability of free drug may make the elderly patient more susceptible to adverse effects or more vulnerable to the effects of multiple drug therapy on drug binding. Some experts believe, however, that these age-associated changes do not change clinical drug effects, as the free drug concentration at steady state is a function of dose and clearance, not the unbound fraction (Greenblatt et al, 1982).

Hepatic Metabolism

Psychotropic drugs are primarily removed from the circulation by the liver, which produces active and inactive metabolites, and by the kidney, which excretes some unchanged drugs as well as hepatic metabolites.

In persons who are older than 65, compared to a person who is aged 25 years old, hepatic blood flow is decreased by 40% (Bender, 1965; Geokas and Haverback, 1969). This is at least partially the result of an age-associated decline in cardiac output. Also, liver size in relation to body mass decreases with age (Vestal, 1984).

Antipyrine is useful for studying hepatic metabolism as it is minimally protein bound and is mostly metabolized by the liver (Vestal, 1984). One large study of antipyrine metabolism revealed an interindividual variation of sixfold in similarly aged subjects (Vestal et al, 1975). However, only 3% of the variance in liver metabolic clearance could be explained by age alone. These data confirm the frequent clinical impression that no consistent generalizations hold true in reference to hepatic metabolism in the elderly (Jenike, 1982a and 1983).

Because of this great clinical variation among similarly appearing elderly patients, physicians frequently see 80-year-old patients who require doses comparable to those given to 25-year-old patients while others require one-tenth the dosage. For example, some elderly patients reach therapeutic blood levels of desipramine (Norpramin) when they take a daily dose of 10 mg while others may require 200 mg.

The metabolism of most psychotropic drugs is primarily by the hepatic microsomal enzymes (Veith, 1984) and tobacco smoking may cause less induction of these enzymes in the elderly than in younger patients (Vestal and Wood, 1980). Long-term alcohol use can induce liver microsomal activity and increase the rate of psychotropic drug metabolism after alcohol is out of the system. While alcohol is still in the blood, microsomal enzymes are inhibited (Vestal et al, 1977; Sellers and Holloway, 1978; Sellers et al, 1980; Sandor et al, 1981).

Renal Excretion

In contrast to the variable and unpredictable changes in hepatic metabolism, renal concomitants of aging are well studied and easily measured, and are consistent. The glomerular filtration rate (GFR) decreases by approximately 50% by the age of 70 (Papper, 1978; Rowe and Besdine, 1982). From the age of 20 to 80 years, there is a 20% decrease in kidney size and a 30% loss in the number of functional glomeruli (Davies and Shock, 1950; Rowe, 1978).

The creatinine clearance of healthy kidneys declines by 0.5 to 1.0 mL/min/1.73 m^2/year. Renal plasma flow also declines during these years by 1.5% to 2.0%/year (Bender, 1965; Schumacher, 1980). If kidney damage or disease is superimposed on these normal changes, it will further lower the age-related reduced clearance. For drugs whose clearance is partly or entirely by renal excretion of the intact drug, clearance will predictably decline approximately in proportion to the reduced GFR.

Serum creatinine concentration alone is often a poor guide to the evaluation of renal status in the elderly as it may be normal in the face of greatly reduced renal function. Lean body mass decreases with age and produces a concomitant lowering of the daily creatinine production. Because the serum creatinine concentration depends on creatinine production as well as renal clearance, a decline in renal function in an elderly patient may not yield an elevated creatinine concentration. Creatinine clearance based on 24-hour urinary excretion, as well as on serum creatinine concentration, is a far more accurate indicator of kidney function (Greenblatt et al, 1982). Figure 3-2 gives an often used formula that estimates true creatinine clearance in relation to age

$$Ccl = \frac{(140 - age) \times body\ weight\ (kg)}{72 \times serum\ creatinine}$$

Figure 3-2　Computing creatinine clearance (Ccl).

in men. For women, multiply the computed creatinine clearance by 0.85 (Jenike, 1982b).

Changes in renal excretion are known to be important for digoxin, procainamide, penicillins, and aminoglycosides (Jenike, 1982a; Greenblatt et al, 1982). It is less well known, however, that metabolism of long-acting benzodiazepines is profoundly altered by age-related changes in renal clearance. For example, as mentioned earlier, the half-lives of diazepam metabolites are increased from an average of 20 hours at the age of 20 to 90 hours at the age of 80, largely because of changes in renal excretion.

Lithium carbonate (Eskalith and others), a drug with a very limited range of tolerable plasma levels, undergoes over a 30% to 50% reduction in renal clearance when comparing patients aged 25 years to those aged 75 years (Lehman and Merten, 1974). Roughly a one-third to one-half reduction in dosage is needed to maintain comparable blood levels in the elderly (Hewick and Newbury, 1976).

RECEPTOR SENSITIVITY AND NEUROTRANSMITTERS

Much research is being directed to understanding age-related changes in receptors and brain neurotransmitters (Salzman, 1984). In theory, a reduced sensitivity to pharmacologic agents could be postulated as a result of a decreased number of receptors, decreased availability of enzymes to mediate the effect of the drug, and increased resistance to drug diffusion through tissues. Results of studies with isoproterenol hydrochloride (Isuprel) and propranolol hydrochloride (Inderal) indicated that the elderly are indeed more resistant to the effects of these two compounds (London et al, 1976; Vestal et al, 1979). The dose of isoproterenol needed to increase heart rate by 25 beats per minute is four to six times higher in old persons as compared to young ones (Vestal et al, 1979). On the other hand, many drugs demonstrate a heightened response with age. Common examples include sedatives (Reidenberg et al, 1978; Giles et al, 1978), narcotics (Bellville et al, 1971; Kaiko, 1980), and anticoagulants (Husted and Andreasen, 1977; Shepherd et al, 1977; Hotraphinyo et al, 1978).

The number of muscarinic (the primary acetylcholine receptors in the central nervous system) cholinergic receptor binding sites in the normal human brain decreases with age (Bender, 1974); thus the reduction in acetylcholine neurotransmission during normal aging may therefore result partially from reduced binding at muscarinic receptor sites. The activity of the enzyme responsible for the manufacture of acetylcholine, choline acetyltransferase, decreases during the natural aging process (Bartus et al, 1982; Coyle, 1983; Davies, 1979) and dramatically decreases in patients with Alzheimer's disease (see chapter 5). When psychotropic drugs are taken, these changes may predispose the normal elderly patient to adverse anticholinergic effects in the central nervous system (CNS) such as confusion, delirium, and psychosis (eg, hallucinations). Patients with Alzheimer's disease also have striking loss of cholinergic cells in the basal forebrain as well as further decrements in the activity of choline acetyltransferase (Davies, 1979); thus, any drug with anticholinergic effects will further impair an already damaged system (Jenike, 1986) (see chapter 5).

There are other reports of decreased levels of dopamine and acetylcholine in the CNS which may make the elderly more sensitive to drug side effects (Robinson et al, 1972; Horita, 1978).

As humans age, most neurotransmitters and enzyme levels appear to decrease (Goodnick and Gershon, 1984). Recently, however, it has been demonstrated that with age there is a marked increase in monoamine oxidase (MAO) levels in human plasma, platelets, and brain (Gottfries et al, 1983). Norepinephrine concentrations correlate negatively and 5-hydroxyindoleacetic acid concentrations correlate positively with brainstem MAO activity. This suggests that MAO plays a major role in regulating intracellular biogenic amines. There is a linear decrease of norepinephrine levels with age and this is consistent with the hypothesis that these age-related decrements in norepinephrine levels are a consequence of the also age-related increase in MAO activity (Jenike, 1985). If biogenic amines are indeed lowered by increased activity of MAO in elderly patients, this could lead to low concentrations of CNS norepinephrine and/or serotonin which could make the elderly particularly vulnerable to depression. This age-related increase in MAO activity has been shown to be even more pronounced in demented patients and it has been suggested that MAO inhibitors (MAOI) may be particularly useful in treating depressed patients who have Alzheimer's disease (Jenike, 1984 and 1985) (see chapter 4).

Other neurotransmitter alterations occur with age, but the significance of these at present is not clear. For a further review of age-related neurotransmitter changes see Salzman (1984).

SUMMARY

With aging, there are major changes in the body that affect the manner in which psychopharmacologic agents are metabolized. Alterations in absorption are of little importance. Changes in hepatic metabolism are variable with aging, and interindividual differences far outweigh age-related alterations. On the other hand, alterations in drug distribution, renal function, and brain enzyme systems and neurotransmitters are consistent and of major consequence. In contrast to most brain enzyme systems, MAO is increased and this may have important consequences, such as an increased tendency for the elderly, particularly those who are demented, to suffer from clinical depression.

REFERENCES

Allen MD, Greenblatt DJ, Harmatz JS, et al: Desmethyldiazepam kinetics in the elderly after oral prazepam. *Clin Pharmacol Ther* 28:196–202, 1980.

Bartus RT, Dean RL, Beer R, et al: The cholinergic hypothesis of geriatric memory dysfunction. *Science* 217:408–416, 1982.

Bellville JW, Forrest WH, Miller E, et al: Influence of age on pain relief from analgesics: A study of postoperative patients. *JAMA* 217:1835–1841, 1971.

Bender AD: The effect of increasing age on the distribution of peripheral blood flow in man. *J Am Geriatr Soc* 13:192–198, 1965.

Bender AD: Pharmacodynamic principles of drug therapy in the aged. *J Am Geriatr Soc* 22:296–303, 1974.

Bender AD, Post A, Meier JP, et al: Plasma protein binding of drugs as a function of age in adult human subjects. *J Pharm Sci* 64:1711–1713, 1975.

Bruce A, Anderson M, Arvidsson B, et al: Body composition. Prediction of normal body potassium, body water and body fat in adults on the basis of body height, body weight and age. *Scand J Clin Lab Invest* 40:461–473, 1980.

Coyle JT: Alzheimer's disease: A disorder of cortical cholinergic innervation. *Science* 219:1184–1190, 1983.

Davies DF, Shock N: Age changes in glomerular filtration rate, effective renal plasma flow, and the tubular excretory capacity in adult males. *J Clin Invest* 29:496, 1950.

Davies P: Neurotransmitter-related symptoms in SDAT. *Brain Res* 171:319–327, 1979.

Forbes GB, Reina JC: Adult lean body mass declines with age: Some longitudinal observations. *Metabolism* 19:653–663, 1970.

Geokas MC, Haverback BJ: The aging gastrointestinal tract. *Am J Surg* 117:881–892, 1969.

Giles HG, MacLeod SM, Wright JR, et al: Influence of age and previous use on diazepam dosage required for endoscopy. *Can Med Assoc J* 118:513–514, 1978.

Goodnick P, Gershon S: Chemotherapy of cognitive disorders in geriatric subjects. *J Clin Psychiatry* 45:196–209, 1984.

Gottfries CG, Adolfsson R, Aquilonius SM, et al: Biochemical changes in dementia disorders of Alzheimer's type (AD/SDAT). *Neurobiol Aging* 4:261–271, 1983.

Greenblatt DJ, Allen MD, Harmatz JS, et al: Diazepam disposition determinants. *Clin Pharmacol Ther* 27:301–312, 1980.

Greenblatt DJ, Divoll M, Puri SK, et al: Clobazam kinetics in the elderly. *Br J Clin Pharmacol* 12:631–636, 1981.

Greenblatt DJ, Sellers EM, Shader RI: Drug disposition in old age. *N Engl J Med* 306:1081–1088, 1982.

Hayes MJ, Langman MJS, Short AH: Changes in drug metabolism with increasing age: phenytoin clearance and protein binding. *Br J Clin Pharmacol* 2:73–79, 1975.

Hewick DS, Newbury PA: Age: Its influence on lithium dosage and plasma levels. *Br J Clin Pharmacol* 3:354, 1976.

Horita A: Neuropharmacology and aging, in Roberts J, Adelman RC, Cristalato VJ (eds): *Pharmacological Intervention in the Aging Process.* New York, Plenum Press, 1978.

Hotraphinyo K, Triggs EJ, Maybloom B, et al: Warfarin sodium: Steady-state plasma levels and patient age. *Clin Exp Pharmacol Physiol* 5:143–149, 1978.

Husted S, Andreasen F: The influence of age on the response to anticoagulants. *Br J Clin Pharmacol* 4:559–565, 1977.

Jenike MA: Using sedative drugs in the elderly. *Drug Ther* 12:186–190, 1982a.

Jenike MA: Using digoxin in the elderly. *Massachusetts General Hosp Topics Geriatr* 1:21–23, 1982b.

Jenike MA: Treatment of anxiety in elderly patients. *Geriatrics* 38:115–120, 1983.

Jenike MA: Monoamine oxidase inhibitors in elderly depressed patients. *J Am Geriatr Soc* 32:571–575, 1984.

Jenike MA: MAO inhibitors as treatment for depressed patients with primary degenerative dementia (Alzheimer's disease). *Am J Psychiatry* 142:763–764, 1985.

32

Jenike MA: Alzheimer's disease. *Sci Am Med* 9:1–4, 1986.

Kaiko RF: Age and morphine analgesia in cancer patients with postoperative pain. *Clin Pharmacol Ther* 28:823–827, 1980.

Lehman K, Merten X: Die Elimination von Lithium in Abhdngigkeit vom Lebensalter bei Gesunden und Niereninsuffizienten. *Int J Clin Pharmacol Ther Toxicol* 10:292–298, 1974.

London GM, Safar ME, Weiss YA, et al: Isoproterenol sensitivity and total body clearance of propranolol in hypertensive patients. *J Clin Pharmacol* 16:174–179, 1976.

Novak LP: Aging, total body potassium, fat-free mass, and cell mass in males and females between ages 18 and 35 years. *J Gerontol* 27:438–443, 1972.

Papper S: *Clinical Nephrology*. Boston, Little, Brown, 1978.

Plein JB, Plein EM: Aging and drug therapy, in Eisdorfer C (ed): *Annual Review of Gerontology and Geriatrics*. New York, Springer-Verlag, 1981, vol 2, p 211.

Reidenberg MM, Levy M, Warner H, et al: Relationship between diazepam dose, plasma level, age, and central nervous system depression. *Clin Pharmacol Ther* 23:371–374, 1978.

Robinson DS, Davis JM, Nies A, et al: Aging, monoamines and MAO levels. *Lancet* 1:290–291, 1972.

Rosenbaum JF: Anxiety, in Lazare A (ed): *Outpatient Psychiatry*. Baltimore, Williams and Wilkins Co, 1979, pp 252–256.

Rowe JW: The influence of age on renal function. *Res Staff Phys* 24:49–55, 1978.

Rowe JW, Besdine EW: *Health and Disease in Old Age*. Boston, Little, Brown. 1982.

Salzman C: Neurotransmission in the aging central nervous system, in Salzman C (ed): *Clinical Geriatric Psychopharmacology*. New York, McGraw-Hill Book Co, 1984, pp 18–31.

Sandor P, Sellers EM, Dumbrell M, et al: Effect of short- and long-term alcohol use on phenytoin kinetics in chronic alcoholics. *Clin Pharmacol Ther* 30:390–397, 1981.

Schumacher GE: Using pharmacokinetics in drug therapy: VII: Pharmacokinetic factors influencing drug therapy in the aged. *Am J Hosp Pharm* 37:559–562, 1980.

Sellers EM, Giles HG, Greenblatt DJ, et al: Differential effects on benzodiazepine disposition by disulfiram and ethanol. *Arzneimittelforsch* 30:882–886, 1980.

Sellers EM, Holloway MR: Drug kinetics and alcohol ingestion. *Clin Pharmacokinet* 3:440–452, 1978.

Shepherd AMM, Hewick DS, Moreland TA, et al: Age as a determinant of sensitivity to warfarin. *Br J Clin Pharmacol* 4:315–320, 1977.

Veith RC: Treatment of psychiatric disorders, in Vestal RE (ed): *Drug Treatment in the Elderly*. Boston, ADTS Health Science Press, 1984, pp 317–337.

Vestal RE: Geriatric clinical pharmacology: An overview, in Vestal RE (ed): *Drug Treatment in the Elderly*. Boston, ADTS Health Science Press, 1984, pp 12–28.

Vestal RE, McGuire EA, Tobin JD, et al: Aging and ethanol metabolism. *Clin Pharmacol Ther* 21:343–354, 1977.

Vestal RE, Norris AH, Tobin JD, et al: Antipyrine metabolism in man: Influence of age, alcohol, caffeine, and smoking. *Clin Pharmacol Ther* 18:425–434, 1975.

Vestal RE, Wood AJJ, Shand DG: Reduced beta-adrenoreceptor sensitivity in the elderly. *Clin Pharmacol Ther* 26:181–186, 1979.

Vestal RE, Wood AJJ: Influence of age and smoking on drug kinetics in man: Studies using model compounds. *Clin Pharmacokinet* 5:309–318, 1980.

4

Affective Disorders in the Elderly

OVERVIEW

Among the elderly, affective disorders constitute the most commonly encountered psychiatric illness; studies of incidence, unfortunately, are scarce and complete data concerning the prevalence rate are unavailable (Georgotas, 1983). Estimates for the presence of affective disorders in elderly hospitalized and community-dwelling residents range from 10% to 65% (Butler, 1975 and 1975a). Gurland (1976) more conservatively estimated the prevalence of severe depression to be about 2% to 3% after the age of 65 years and the rate for definite, but mild, depression, is 3% to 4%. European studies have reported prevalence rates of 2% to 10%; in one Swedish study, lifetime risks of depression were estimated to be 8.5% for men, and 17.7% for women up to the age of 80 (Essen-Moller et al, 1956). Studies looking specifically at depressive symptoms, rather than diagnoses, may tend to overestimate prevalence because of the high incidence in the elderly of transient depressive episodes, lasting a few hours to a few days, which are not incapacitating enough to be diagnosed as depressive disorders by most clinicians (Georgotas, 1983).

According to most studies, women tend to have higher rates of depression than men in almost all age groups below the age of 65, but after this age, the frequency of depression in men increases so that the rates tend to approach each other or even reverse (Gurland, 1976).

As many as 20% to 35% of elderly patients with concurrent medical illness are depressed (Anonymous, 1979; Moffie and Paykel, 1975). Those who are older than 65 account for about 11% of the US population, but account for about 25% of all suicides (Busse and Pfeiffer, 1977; Sendbuehler and Goldstein, 1977). White men older than age 65 have a suicide rate four times that of the national average, twice as high as that of women of the same age (Resnick and Cantor, 1967 and 1967a).

Depressed elderly patients are often malnourished and agitated for months or even years (Jefferson and Marshall, 1981) and untreated major depression lowers life expectancy and is associated with a greater risk for cardiac disease (Kay and Bergman, 1966; Avery and Winokur, 1976; Tsuang et al, 1980). Depression in a person with a dementing illness can present special challenges. In view of the effective therapies available for depression, it is especially crucial to make the diagnosis and proceed with treatment (Jenike, 1988 and 1988a).

RECOGNIZING DEPRESSION

DSM-III-R Criteria

Sadness is common in the elderly and it is not clear how normal sadness and clinical depression are related (Klerman, 1976); clinicians do not agree on the full range of affective phenomena to be diagnosed as pathological. With this controversy in mind, I will discuss diagnostic criteria that have been agreed upon and clinical clues that are a function of experience. Clinicians may have to perform therapeutic drug trials on elderly patients even if they do not meet full criteria for major depression.

In older age groups, the depressed patient may not admit to the symptoms of depression itself but rather to the accompanying anxiety, somatic or hypochondriacal symptoms, or to loss of concentration and difficulty with memory (Georgotas, 1983). Often somatic complaints predominate in elderly depressed patients (Fogel and Kroessler, 1987). Thus, depression in the elderly may present with various clinical pictures such as chronic pain, multiple somatic complaints, or even dementia (pseudodementia). Depression is, in fact, the main cause of a treatable dementia in the elderly (Wells, 1963 and 1979; Feinberg and Goodman, 1984; Cole et al, 1983).

Although some elderly depressed individuals present atypically, many can be diagnosed according to the Washington University research criteria, which form the basis for the DSM-III-R criteria (Table 4–1; Spar and LaRue, 1983). A helpful mnemonic, developed by Dr Carey Gross at Massachusetts General Hospital, that outlines the clinical picture of major depression is SIG E CAPS (eg, a prescription for energy capsules): Sleep, Interest, Guilt, Energy, Concentration, Appetite, Psychomotor, and Suicide (Figure 4–1). Each of these letters corresponds to one of the DSM-III-R criteria for major depression (Jenike, 1988). To elaborate, depressed patients generally complain of insomnia, typically with early awakening in the morning; occasionally, however, hypersomnia and daily lethargy are the problems. They lose interest in usually stimulating activities—job, hobbies, social activities, and sex. Guilty ruminations and feelings of self-reproach are the rule. Depressed patients have no energy and feel fatigued all day. They frequently report an inability to concentrate, with slowed or mixed-up thinking (cognitive changes associated with

Table 4–1
Diagnostic Criteria for Major Depressive Episode

Note: A "major depressive syndrome" is defined as criterion A below.

A. At least five of the following symptoms have been present during the same two-week period and represent a change from previous functioning; at least one of the symptoms is either (1) depressed mood, or (2) loss of interest or pleasure. (Do not include symptoms that are clearly due to a physical condition, mood-incongruent delusions or hallucinations, incoherence, or marked loosening of associations.)

  (1) depressed mood (or can be irritable mood in children and adolescents) most of the day, nearly every day, as indicated either by subjective account or observation by others

  (2) markedly diminished interest or pleasure in all, or almost all, activities most of the day, nearly every day (as indicated either by subjective account or observations by others of apathy most of the time)

  (3) significant weight loss or weight gain when not dieting (eg, more than 5% of body weight in a month), or decrease or increase in appetite nearly every day (in children, consider failure to make expected weight gains)

  (4) insomnia or hypersomnia nearly every day

  (5) psychomotor agitation or retardation nearly every day (observable by others, not merely subjective feelings of restlessness or being slowed down)

  (6) fatigue or loss of energy nearly every day

  (7) feelings of worthlessness or excessive or inappropriate guilt (which may be delusional) nearly every day (not merely self-reproach or guilt about being sick)

  (8) diminished ability to think or concentrate, or indecisiveness, nearly every day (either by subjective account or as observed by others)

  (9) recurrent thoughts of death (not just fear of dying), recurrent suicidal ideation without a specific plan, or a suicide attempt or a specific plan for committing suicide

B. (1) It cannot be established that an organic factor initiated and maintained the disturbance

  (2) The disturbance is not a normal reaction to the death of a loved one (uncomplicated bereavement)

  Note: Morbid preoccupation with worthlessness, suicidal ideation, marked functional impairment or psychomotor retardation, or prolonged duration suggest bereavement complicated by major depression.

C. At no time during the disturbance have there been delusions or hallucinations for as long as two weeks in the absence of prominent mood symptoms (i.e., before the mood symptoms developed or after they have remitted).

D. Not superimposed on schizophrenia, schizophreniform disorder, delusional disorder, or psychotic disorder NOS.

severe depression are reviewed later in this chapter). They usually have a poor appetite with associated weight loss, although occasionally they overeat. Psychomotor retardation is usually observed, but agitated depressions in the elderly are not uncommon. They may have recurrent thoughts of suicide or death and may feel that life is not worth living or wish that they were dead. A patient with at least five of these eight criteria meets DSM-III-R criteria for

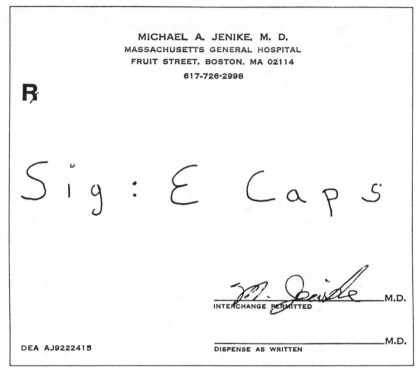

MICHAEL A. JENIKE, M. D.
MASSACHUSETTS GENERAL HOSPITAL
FRUIT STREET, BOSTON, MA 02114
617-726-2998

R̸

Sig : E Caps

_____ M.D.
INTERCHANGE PERMITTED

_____ M.D.
DISPENSE AS WRITTEN

DEA AJ9222415

Figure 4–1 A helpful mnemonic.

a major depressive episode, and if the dysphoric emotional state has persisted for two to four weeks, he or she needs treatment.

Of interest, crying is not necessarily a manifestation of depression as will be discussed.

Diagnostic Clues

Another clue to recognizing depression is the presence of multiple somatic complaints in several body systems. When a patient's complaints do not fit a recognizable pattern or when chronic pain is a component, depression should be suspected and the SIG E CAPS criteria should be investigated.

Crying in Medically Ill Patients: Not Necessarily Depression

Crying in medically ill patients is not uncommon and, because it is not always a manifestation of depression, may present a diagnostic dilemma for the clinician. In an effort to clarify the relationship of crying to depression in medically ill patients, Green and associates (1987) evaluated prospectively all hospitalized patients who were referred to the psychiatric consultation service with a primary symptom of crying. Forty-six patients were referred for a presumed diagnosis of depression because crying was a prominent symptom. They found, however, that crying was often due to the presence of neurologic disease, which was vastly underestimated by the referring physicians.

Suspecting that many of the consultation requests to evaluate "depressed," crying patients would actually turn out to be cases of neurologically induced emotionality, Green and associates conducted their 18-month prospective study on all patients referred to the psychiatric consultation service. From this population, patients who were referred because of crying became the principal subjects of the study. They divided all the crying patients into two groups: (1) "prominent criers" —if they were referred because of crying, because crying dominated the recent history, or because crying occurred during repeated psychiatric evaluations; and (2) "nonprominent criers"—if crying occupied a minor part of the recent history and minimally occurred during the course of bedside psychiatric evaluation. Patients in this second group had not been referred for crying. Over the 18-month study period, 296 consultations were done for 276 consecutively referred patients. Forty-six (17%) of these were prominent criers and 17 (6%) were nonprominent criers. The mean age of the prominent criers was 57 years; the median age of the overall group was 60 years.

Green and associates found that only a minority of the prominent criers had psychiatric disorders alone. Of these nine patients, three had major depression, one had atypical depression, two had an anxiety disorder, and three had adjustment disorders. The majority of prominent criers had a psychiatric disorder plus a medical or neurologic condition that did or could in theory contribute to a tendency to cry easily (for example, patients withdrawing from alcohol or taking steroids). Fifteen prominent criers (33%) had neurologic disorders and no discernible psychiatric disorder.

Of interest, the authors identified two male patients for whom easy crying was a long-standing personality trait. They referred to this as "essential crying" and noted that this was a previously undescribed entity. These men reported lifelong abrupt outbursts of crying, with tears, that occurred several times a day, usually in response to internal and environmental cues such as thoughts of home or family. They described their mood during the crying bouts as sad, and the bouts were embarrassing to them. One patient reported that his father, brother, paternal uncle, and three daughters had the same trait.

It is not uncommon to see crying patients in the hospital, and it is clear from this report that effective therapy for patients who cry depends on proper identification of the cause of crying. Many patients have structural or metabolic brain dysfunction and not a primary psychiatric disorder. In fact, neurologic disorders were more likely than psychiatric disorders to produce crying. They also found that bilateral cerebral disease was the most common neurologic cause of crying. It is generally believed that bilateral corticobulbar tract lesions are necessary determinants of pathological crying. These tracts apparently subserve a voluntary cortical pathway to inhibit limbic and hypothalamic input to the brain stem motor nuclei controlling the various motor aspects of crying. In patients with bilateral corticobulbar tract lesions, Green and associates (1987) noted that crying could be provoked by minor emotional stimuli or even by emotionally neutral auditory stimuli (a slammed door, for example). Pseudobulbar palsy resulting from bilateral corticobulbar lesions from strokes, motor neuron disease, multiple sclerosis, and other disorders is the classic syndrome in which pathological crying is seen.

Pseudobulbar palsy, which leads to such inappropriate affect and fluctuation (lability) of emotions, is said to originate from damage to the frontal lobe, or, less often, injury to the upper part of the brain stem. Patients may cry, or less often, laugh in response to minimal provocation. In addition, as a manifestation of their emotional lability, they appear to switch readily between euphoria and depression. The term pseudobulbar palsy has become the commonly accepted explanation for unwarranted emotional states in patients with brain damage.

Green and colleagues noted observable characteristics that distinguished crying due to psychiatric disorders from that due to neurologic disorders. Crying that was inappropriate to the stimulus occurred more commonly in the neurologic-disorder group, and appropriate crying occurred more commonly in the psychiatric-disorder group. In addition, there was a high rate of abrupt onset and stereotyped crying (episodes identical in appearance from one episode to the next) in patients who exhibited crying that was inappropriate to a stimulus.

Green and associates (1987) concluded with recommendations for evaluation of the patient in whom crying is a major symptom. It is important to avoid any a priori assumptions about the crying, such as thinking that sadness is understandable and natural, given the patient's circumstances. The history should include inquiries into the context of the crying episodes, the mood at the time of crying, the patient's premorbid crying behavior, and the presence of symptoms of affective or neurologic disorder. They also recommend a complete neurologic and mental status examination, with special emphasis on the cognitive examination. Several crying episodes should be observed to see whether the crying is appropriate to the context, how abrupt it is in onset, and how stereotyped the episodes are.

Since people typically associate crying with sadness, sometimes family members misinterpret crying in a patient with a neurologic or dementing disorder as a manifestation of depression, but they are usually easily convinced that the patient is not depressed when it is pointed out, by questioning the patient in front of family members, that the patient is not sad while crying.

What if the Terminally Ill Patient Wants To Die?

One might think it quite natural for a terminally ill patient to want to die; results of a recent study, however, dispute this inclination. Brown and associates (1986) noted that the prevalence of depression and suicidal thinking among terminally ill people has become an important topic and that a voluntary euthanasia movement is growing. Organizations such as the Voluntary Euthanasia Society in the United Kingdom and the Hemlock Society in the United States offer the basic assumption that people facing serious life problems, especially those with a painful, disfiguring, or disabling terminal illness, should be given encouragement and assistance in thinking of suicide as a rational solution. They found a paucity of data, however, on the mental state of those who are terminally ill.

In Finland, Achte and Vauhkonen (1971) studied 100 persons affected by cancer and found none who expressed suicidal thoughts, although one man later killed himself. Another group, also in Finland, found that the suicide rate was 1.3 times higher among male cancer patients and 1.9 times higher among female cancer patients than the rate in the general population (Luohivuori and Hakama, 1979).

Clinicians frequently encounter patients who wish to die. As noted already, suicidal thinking is one of the DSM-III-R criteria for depression, but it does not by itself justify a diagnosis of depression. In trying to evaluate the presence of depression in terminally ill patients who wish to die, Brown and colleagues (1986) noted special difficulties in evaluating the DSM-III-R criteria as anorexia, weight loss, insomnia, reduced energy, and concentration difficulties are also common features of chronic debilitating disease. They gave a self-assessment instrument (Beck Depression Inventory) to terminally ill patients and performed a short interview to evaluate whether patients wished to die and whether they suffered from depression. After they eliminated patients with an impaired sensorium during initial screening, the final sample consisted of 22 men and 22 women with a mean age of 63 years. All patients had terminal cancer, except one who had severe hypertensive heart disease.

Brown and associates found that of the 44 patients, 34 had never thought of suicide or wished for death to come early. No patient asked for mercy killing and only one was actively suicidal at the time of interview. Two had formerly been suicidal but were no longer so at the time of interview. Seven patients desired or had desired death but not by suicide. All of the patients who had desired death were found to have severe depressive illness. Of the 44 terminally ill patients, 11 were severely depressed. None of the patients who did not have clinical depression had thoughts of suicide or wished death would come early.

Suicidal thoughts and desire for death appear to be linked exclusively to depression. Patients with terminal illness who were not mentally ill were no more likely than the general population to wish for premature death. When the clinician is faced with the terminally ill patient who wants to die, clinical depression should be strongly suspected and the SIG E CAPS criteria should be carefully investigated. Aggressive treatment of the mental disorder should be attempted in order to maximize the patient's quality of remaining life.

EVALUATION AND DIFFERENTIAL DIAGNOSIS

Overview

Fogel and Kroessler (1987), in reviewing some of the complicated issues that arise when depression and medical illness occur together in the elderly, made a number of helpful suggestions. Evaluating their experience on a combined medical-psychiatric unit, they recommended that the clinician not presume that the patient's medical problems are stable or even that they are fully known, and that the clinician perform a thorough physical examination, neurologic examination, and laboratory workup. Systematic, structured, cognitive assessment is invaluable in diagnosis and management, provided that the results are properly interpreted. Beyond the identification of gross delirium and dementia, cognitive assessment permits the identification of patients with mild-to-moderate dementia or focal neurologic lesions that may interfere with psychotherapy or adherence to medical treatment regimens. Cognitive deficits found during neuropsychologic screening of patients who are actively depressed should serve only as a baseline and should not be used for the definitive diagnosis of dementia. Depressed patients with cognitive impairment should be retested after maximum remission of their mood disorder.

A meticulous neurologic exam, for example, may uncover parkinsonism, tardive dyskinesia, or previously unsuspected deficits in higher cortical function (Fogel and Kroessler, 1987). Gait disturbances may be the primary physical sign of organic illnesses ranging from hypothyroidism to normal pressure hydrocephalus. Results of prior laboratory tests should be reviewed, and claims that results are "essentially normal" should not be taken at face value. For example, hypothyroidism cannot be ruled out without determining the level of thyroid-stimulating hormone (TSH), and a normal level of serum B_{12} does not conclusively rule out neuropsychiatric B_{12} deficiency.

Fogel and Kroessler (1987) also recommended a high level of suspicion for drug toxicity and drug interaction. When possible, drug levels should be obtained. One cannot assume that the physician prescribing any medication will be familiar with the range of neuropsychiatric side effects. When the contribution of a drug to the psychiatric syndrome is in doubt, it should be discontinued if possible and a less psychotoxic substitute found.

When it has been determined that a patient is depressed, it is necessary to rule out both medical and psychiatric causes.

Psychiatric Differential Diagnosis

Some psychiatric conditions that can include depression are manic-depressive disease, schizophrenia, psychotic depression, borderline personality disorder, alcoholism, and unresolved grief (Jenike and Anderson, 1984).

In manic-depressive disorders, the depressive state is indistinguishable from other types of depression, and a history of a manic episode in the patient or in his family is the key to diagnosis.

A schizophrenic may appear depressed but at some time will have delusions, hallucinations, or a thought disorder. Hallucinations are characteristically auditory (visual hallucinations suggest a medical cause) and the patient may believe that others can hear what he is thinking (thought broadcasting) or that they are putting thoughts or ideas into his head (thought insertion). Ideas of reference (eg, television or radio communicating about him or talking to him directly) and paranoia are common.

Some alcoholics have a primary affective disorder that they are attempting to treat by drinking. A careful history of alcohol intake is mandatory in depressed patients (see chapter 10).

Grieving patients may appear depressed and they frequently experience shortness of breath, frequent sighing, an empty feeling in the abdomen, lack of muscular strength, and extreme tension (Lazare, 1979). Often they feel that every task is a major effort and that life has no meaning. Sometimes the bereaved takes on traits of the deceased or the symptoms of his last illness. Uncomplicated grief may last six months or more. In one follow-up study, 17% of bereaved persons were clinically depressed one year after the death of a spouse or close family member (Clayton, 1974).

When taking the history, the physician should inquire about recent illnesses and operations, mental status changes, and current drug and medication use. The patient's support systems—the availability and reliability of family or friends—should be evaluated. Psychiatric syndromes causing depression can be largely eliminated from the differential diagnosis by asking about prior manic or psychotic episodes, present disturbing thoughts, recent deaths of people close to the patient, and alcohol use.

Medical Differential Diagnosis

Many physical illnesses may be associated with depression and should be considered in the workup of all depressed patients (Table 4–2) (Anderson, 1979; Jenike and Anderson, 1984). Although it is clearly impractical to rule out all potential causes of depression, the physician must look for certain life-threatening conditions. These include diuretic-induced hypokalemia or hyponatremia, Addison's disease, hypoparathyroidism, severe anemia, pneumonia, myocardial infarction, congestive heart failure, uremia, hepatic encephalopathy, Wernicke's encephalopathy, meningitis, and encephalitis.

Table 4–2
Medical Causes of Depression

Deficiency States
Pellagra
Pernicious anemia
Wernicke's encephalopathy

Drugs and Medication
Alcohol
Amphetamines
Antihypertensive agents
  Clonidine
  Diuretics—hypokalemia*
  or hyponatremia*
  Guanethidine
  Methyldopa
  Propranolol
  Reserpine
Birth control pills
Cimetidine
Digitalis
Disulfiram
Sedatives
  Barbiturates
  Benzodiazepines
Steroids/ACTH

Endocrine Disorders
Acromegaly
Adrenal
  Addison's disease*
  Cushing's disease
Hyper- and hypoparathyroidism*
Hyper- and hypothyroidism
Insulinoma
Pheochromocytoma
Pituitary

Infections
Encephalitis
Fungal
Meningitis
Neurosyphilis
Tuberculosis

Malignant Disease
Metastases
  Breast
  GI
  Lung
  Pancreas
  Prostate
Remote effect: pancreas

Metabolic Disorders
Electrolyte imbalance
  Hypokalemia
  Hyponatremia
Hepatic encephalopathy
Hypo-oxygenation
  Cerebral arteriosclerosis
  Chronic bronchitis
  Congestive heart failure*
  Emphysema
  Myocardial infarction*
  Paroxysmal dysrhythmias
  Pneumonia*
  Severe anemia*
Uremia*

Neurologic Disorders
Alzheimer's disease
Amyotrophic lateral sclerosis
Creutzfeldt-Jakob disease
Huntington's chorea
Multiple sclerosis
Myasthenia gravis
Normal-pressure hydrocephalus
Parkinson's disease
Pick's disease
Wilson's disease

Trauma
Postconcussion

*Acute life-threatening disorders.
Reproduced with permission from Jenike MA: Depressed in the E.R. *Emerg Med* 16:102–120, 1984.

All severely depressed elderly patients must have a physical examination, mental status examination, and basic laboratory tests including a complete blood count with differential and electrolyte determinations to identify any life-threatening conditions (Jenike, 1984). Once potentially disastrous physical illnesses have been eliminated, the physician's primary concern is deciding who will treat the patient and how the patient will be treated.

SUICIDE RISK ASSESSMENT AND MANAGEMENT

The seriousness of depression in the elderly is shown by the increase in and success of suicidal attempts among this group (Georgotas, 1983). Studies consistently reveal that about 15% of the total deaths of patients with affective disorder are due to suicide (Avery and Winokur, 1976) and the clinician must evaluate the possibility that the depressed or manic patient will commit suicide.

There is a common fear that asking a depressed person about suicide will plant the idea or precipitate an attempt. This is not the case and, in fact, patients are generally relieved when the topic is brought up and are surprisingly open about their thoughts and plans. Not asking about suicidal ideation can be a fatal mistake (Jenike, 1984).

The elderly comprise the age group that is most at risk for suicide, and the rate of suicide among the elderly is 50% higher than the rate for young people. The history can be very helpful. Suicide rates peak for men between the ages of 80 and 90 and for women between the ages of 50 and 65 (Resnick and Cantor, 1967). Schmidt (1974) pointed out that elderly, divorced, and/or separated patients who have made previous suicide attempts represent a high-risk group. In 1983, for example, the United States suicide rate was 12.1 per 100,000 for the nation, 11.9 for those aged 15 to 24 years, and 19.2 for those aged 65 years and older (National Center for Health Statistics, 1985). Compared to younger individuals, older adults communicate their suicidal intent less frequently, use more violent and lethal methods, and less often attempt suicide as a means of manipulation (Osgood, 1988). Miller (1979), noting that the majority of elderly people have significant stress at times during their old age, believed that whether an older person is able to resolve a suicidal crisis or succumbs to self-inflicted death is very much a function of their ability to cope with stress.

Certain demographic factors that increase the risk of suicide among the elderly have been identified. The most at-risk individual is the elderly white man who is widowed and living alone. In addition the "old old" (above the age of 75) are also more at risk than those aged 65 to 74. Although the association of alcohol and suicidality is high for every age group, as Blazer (1982) pointed out, the relationship is known to be greatly increased among the elderly (see chapter 10).

Depression, the most common functional psychiatric disorder of late life,

Table 4–3
Clues and Warning Signs of Suicide in the
Elderly

Verbal clues
- I'm going to kill myself.
- I'm going to commit suicide.
- I'm going to end it all.
- I want to end it all.
- I just want out.
- You would be better off without me.

Behavioral clues
- donating body to a medical school
- purchasing a gun
- stockpiling pills
- putting personal and business affairs in order
- making or changing a will
- taking out insurance or changing beneficiaries
- making funeral plans
- giving away money and/or possessions
- changes in behavior, especially episodes of screaming or hitting, throwing things, or failure to get along with family, friends, or peers
- suspicious behavior, for example, going out at odd times of the day or night, waving or kissing goodbye (if not characteristic)
- sudden interest or disinterest in church and religion
- scheduling of appointment with doctor for no apparent physical cause or very shortly after the last visit to the doctor
- loss of physical skills, general confusion, or loss of understanding, judgment, or memory

Situational clues
- recent move
- death of a spouse
- diagnosis of terminal illness
- flare-up with relative or close friend

underlies two-thirds of the suicides in the elderly (Gurland and Cross, 1983). A sudden calm in a previously depressed suicidal patient may indicate a definite resolve to die. A psychiatric history or previous attempt increases the likelihood of suicide, as does the presence of physical illness. A psychotic depressed patient is at great risk of suicide, especially if he is hearing voices commanding him to hurt himself. All elderly patients who live alone who perceive themselves as without friends or social support systems are more prone to suicide than those who feel loved.

Elderly suicidal patients tend not to contact crisis intervention and hotline workers, but may make contact with physicians or other health and social service providers (Osgood, 1985). In fact, more than 75% of the elderly who commit suicide see a physician shortly before the act (Foster and Burke, 1985). Many give clues to their impending suicidal behavior. Some clues and warning signs of suicide in the elderly are listed in Table 4–3.

Table 4–3 *continued*
**Clues and Warning Signs of Suicide in the
Elderly**

Symptoms of late-life depression
* change in sleep patterns, particularly insomnia
* change in eating patterns, especially loss of appetite
* weight loss
* extreme fatigue
* increased concern with bodily functions (e.g., frequent complaints of constipation, loose bowels, aches and pains, dizziness, increased heart rate)
* change in mood, particularly if listless, apathetic, angry, hostile, nervous, irritable, depressed, sad, or withdrawn
* expression of fears and anxieties without any reason
* low self-esteem or self-concept, feelings of worthlessness, pessimism
Warning signs of alcoholism in the elderly
* increase in amount of alcohol or number of alcoholic drinks taken
* behavioral manifestations of anger, hostility, belligerence
* odor of alcohol on breath, especially in the morning
* flushed face
* trembling and the "shakes"
* blackout periods
* hangovers
* alcoholic hepatitis, cirrhosis, chronic gastritis
* drinking in spite of medical admonitions against alcohol use
* problems with family members, friends, or relatives
* inability to do simple tasks, confusion, slurred speech, or retarded motor skills
* inability to conduct normal everyday tasks without drinking
* financial problems related to alcohol use

Reproduced with permission from Osgood NJ: Suicide in the elderly. Carrier Foundation Letter #133, April 1988.

If there is a serious potential for suicide or if a patient is in a high-risk category, he or she should be hospitalized for protection and further evaluation. Hospitalization is mandatory for a psychotic patient who is talking about suicide, has command hallucinations to hurt himself, or has tried to hurt himself, even if the attempt was trivial; for a survivor of a near-lethal, violent, or premeditated suicide attempt; and for a survivor of a suicide attempt in which there was little chance of rescue. Hospitalization should be considered for a patient who seems unable to care for himself and has no one to care for him, for a survivor of a trivial suicidal attempt who regrets having survived or refuses help, and for a patient who lives alone.

If the patient is intoxicated with drugs or alcohol as well as depressed or suicidal, it is wisest to keep him in a quiet area, with restraints if necessary. His suicide potential and depression can then be evaluated when he is no longer intoxicated. If this is not feasible, a brief hospitalization is necessary. In one study of more than 300 patients (who were seen in an emergency room after an unsuccessful suicide attempt), 67% of the patients went home the same day, 11% either ran away or signed out against medical advice, and only 17% were sent to a psychiatric unit (Guggenheim, 1978). The overwhelming majority of patients discharged after attempting suicide were still alive at the end of one year. Despite these figures, it is best to err on the side of conservatism when dealing with a suicidal patient. As with appendectomy, a certain number of false-positives is to be expected with optimal medical care. Such patients will probably be released within a few days if an extended evaluation indicates that hospitalization is unwarranted.

If the risk of suicide seems low, the patient need not be hospitalized. Many depressed patients are not thinking clearly and need directed assistance. Such patients will feel a sense of hopelessness but the physician should convey a feeling of optimism.

Osgood (1985 and 1988) recommended a number of suggestions for treating the suicidal geriatric patient. Treatment of depression is a major factor in suicide prevention and this chapter later reviews a number of the therapeutic options. In addition to drug treatments, social therapies are very effective. Those working with the depressed or alcoholic older adult should involve the family in treatment (see chapter 10). Therapies that encourage creative, meaningful use of leisure time and socialization with others or that offer group support are the most effective. Family therapy, group psychotherapy, mutual self-help groups such as Alcoholics Anonymous, reminiscence groups, and creative arts groups (drama, dance, music) all encourage older individuals to use their time, knowledge, talents, and skills and to be a part of family, friendship, and community support networks (Osgood, 1988). As noted elsewhere in this chapter, pet therapy may also be effective.

Suicidal elderly patients must be followed carefully for several months after a suicide attempt or serious threat. The most dangerous time is often when things seem to be going very well and the older individual seems to have "recovered" from the depression.

THE DEXAMETHASONE SUPPRESSION TEST
Overview

Not only is depression a common finding in the elderly, but also, as mentioned earlier, it is frequently characterized by atypical presentations which hinder the clinician's ability to make the diagnosis. A few years ago, much was written about the use of the dexamethasone suppression test (DST) as a clinical aid in the evaluation of depressed individuals (Jenike, 1982 and 1983); in fact, for a period of almost a year, about a quarter of the papers in major psychiatric journals involved neuroendocrine tests, of which the DST was the most frequently used. Even though the DST is now used mainly as a research tool, data concerning the DST are seen frequently in papers discussing affective illness in the elderly. A brief review of pertinent details is presented for mainly historical purposes, although the bottom line for clinical usage of such tests is far from conclusive.

Rationale and Procedure for the DST

Normally, plasma cortisol levels fluctuate in a diurnal pattern with maximal levels of as much as $25\mu g/dL$ around 6 AM and minimal levels of less than 8 $\mu g/dL$ around midnight (Martin et al, 1977). Dexamethasone is a potent glucocorticoid, which suppresses endogenous adrenocorticotropic hormone (ACTH) and cortisol production for as long as 24 hours in normal subjects. The DST is often administered as follows: On day 1 at 11 PM, 1 mg of dexamethasone is given orally; on day 2 at 8 AM, 4 PM, and 11 PM, blood is drawn for serum cortisol determinations.The test basically involves serum cortisol sampling after a dose of dexamethasone is administered, to see if cortisol levels have been suppressed. DST results are considered abnormal if any of the serum cortisol levels after administration of dexamethasone exceed 5 $\mu g/dL$ (Carroll et al, 1981). It may not always be possible to draw blood three times on day 2, particularly for outpatients. It has, however, been demonstrated that about 98% of abnormal test results can be obtained from only the 4 PM and 11 PM samples. With the 4 PM sample alone, almost 80% of nonsuppressors (abnormal result on DST) will be detected (Brown, 1981).

Abnormalities on DST imply the existence of hypothalamic imbalance and, in addition, clinical manifestations of depressive illness typically include several symptoms that suggest hypothalamic dysfunction, namely, disturbances of mood, sex drive, appetite, sleep, and autonomic activity with frequent diurnal variation in symptoms. Also, the same neurotransmitters implicated in the chemical pathology of depressive illness, particularly serotonin and norepinephrine, have been shown to regulate the secretion of hypothalamic hormones (Sachar et al, 1980; Maas, 1975).

The physiology of the hypothalamic-pituitary-adrenal axis has been well studied. Plasma cortisol levels reflect limbic, hypothalamic, pituitary, and adrenal gland interactions (Kalin et al, 1981). The hypothalamus secretes corticotropin releasing factor (CRF) in response to limbic commands mediated through stimulatory pathways, which are either cholinergic or serotonergic, and adrenergic inhibitory pathways (Jenike, 1982). CRF is transported via the pituitary portal vasculature to the anterior lobe of the pituitary gland, which stimulates the release of ACTH, which, in turn, causes secretion of cortisol from the adrenal gland. Cortisol regulates the activity of the system by negative feedback on both the pituitary and the hypothalamus (Figure 4–2).

Applications

The DST has been used by endocrinologists for many years to aid in the diagnosis of disorders such as Cushing's syndrome. More recently, however,

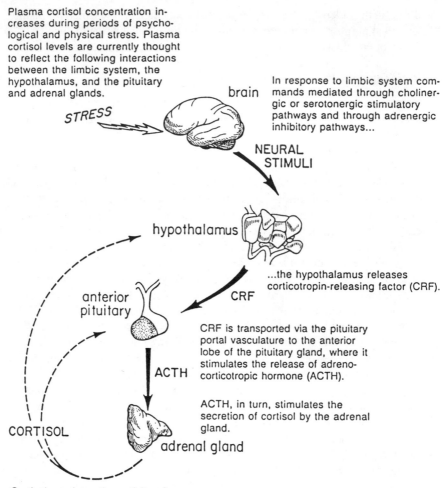

Plasma cortisol concentration increases during periods of psychological and physical stress. Plasma cortisol levels are currently thought to reflect the following interactions between the limbic system, the hypothalamus, and the pituitary and adrenal glands.

STRESS

brain

In response to limbic system commands mediated through cholinergic or serotonergic stimulatory pathways and through adrenergic inhibitory pathways...

NEURAL STIMULI

hypothalamus

...the hypothalamus releases corticotropin-releasing factor (CRF).

CRF

anterior pituitary

CRF is transported via the pituitary portal vasculature to the anterior lobe of the pituitary gland, where it stimulates the release of adrenocorticotropic hormone (ACTH).

ACTH

ACTH, in turn, stimulates the secretion of cortisol by the adrenal gland.

CORTISOL

adrenal gland

Cortisol regulates the activity of this system through negative feedback (----->) to both the pituitary and the hypothalamus.

Figure 4–2 Physiologic basis for the dexamethasone suppression test. Adapted from Jenike MA: Dexamethasone suppression: A biological marker of depression. *Drug Therapy* 9:203–212, 1982.

there has been mounting evidence that the DST is useful as an indicator of hypothalamic-pituitary-adrenal axis abnormalities associated with depressive illness (Carroll et al, 1981). Early researchers noted that cortisol levels were elevated and ACTH secretion disregulated in many depressed patients (see Gelenberg, 1983, for review).

Initially, it appeared that psychiatric disorders other than depression, such as schizophrenia and manic-depressive illness, were not associated with cortisol nonsuppression after dexamethasone administration (Schlesser et al, 1980). More recent reports, however, suggested that a positive result on DST may not be as specific to depression as originally thought. High percentages of abnormalities on DST have been found among manic patients (Graham et al, 1982; Arana et al, 1983) and others found positive results in as many as 30% of apparently nondepressed, nonmelancholic, chronic schizophrenic patients (Dewan et al, 1982). Others reported that patients with primary obsessive-compulsive disorder had an abnormal DST response (Insel et al, 1982). Many of these patients were concomitantly depressed, however, and supporters of the DST would argue that depression produced the abnormal DST results and not primarily the mania, schizophrenia, or obsessive-compulsive disorder (Jenike et al, 1987). However one interprets the data, it is clear that the DST is not a definitive biochemical marker for depression. It may, in fact, turn out to be more analogous to an erythrocyte sedimentation rate (ESR). That is, it could indicate pathology of the neuroendocrine system and must be combined with the entire clinical picture to assist in making the diagnosis. Also, as with the ESR, it may turn out to be a useful marker to follow the course and resolution of psychiatric disease processes.

Certain medical conditions and medication use must be eliminated as a cause of an abnormal DST result in the depressed patient. Some of the conditions that may produce an abnormal result include alcoholism (during and after withdrawal) (Rees et al, 1977; Oxenkrug, 1978), anorexia nervosa (Carroll, 1978), prolonged hemodialysis (McDonald et al, 1979; Wallace et al, 1980), Cushing's syndrome (Kalin et al, 1981), malignancies with ectopic ACTH secretion (mostly small cell bronchogenic carcinoma) (Martin et al, 1977), obesity (Streeten et al, 1969), protein-calorie malnutrition (Smith et al, 1975), renovascular hypertension (Cade et al, 1976), and uncontrolled diabetes mellitus (Carroll et al, 1981). Some medications enhance dexamethasone suppression: high-dose benzodiazepines (Carroll, 1972), corticosteroids (including topical and nasal preparations) (Michael et al, 1967), and dextroamphetamine (Sachar et al, 1981). Other drugs cause a lack of dexamethasone suppression by stimulating hepatic metabolism and decreasing dexamethasone half-life: phenytoin (Carroll et al, 1981; Jukiz et al, 1970), barbiturates (Carroll et al, 1981; Brooks et al, 1972), and meprobamate (Carroll et al, 1981). Alcohol produces an apparent lack of dexamethasone suppression by increasing plasma cortisol (Elias and Gwinup, 1980). L-tryptophan is known to enhance central serotonin but has an uncertain effect on the DST (Nuller and Ostroumova, 1980). Interestingly, most psychotropic drugs, including neuroleptics, tricyclic antidepressants, MAOIs, and lithium carbonate, do not affect the DST (Schlesser et al, 1980; Carroll et al, 1976; Brown et al, 1979; Amsterdam et al, 1982).

The three-sample DST reportedly identifies depressed patients with a sensitivity of 67% and a specificity of 96% (Carroll et al, 1981) and an abnormal DST result may help to confirm the diagnosis of a major depressive disorder. It is of utmost importance, however, to keep in mind that a normal

DST result is not helpful in ruling out such a disorder, as only 40% to 50% of patients known to have a major depressive episode have an abnormal result.

In theory, the DST may be useful to the clinician faced with patients with confusing or mixed clinical pictures. For example, Greden and Carroll (1979) reported a case of a catatonic woman who had an abnormal DST result. Because of this finding, a diagnosis of primary unipolar depression was entertained, and emergency electroconvulsive therapy was begun. She responded rapidly.

There is some preliminary evidence that in nonsuppressing depressed patients, return of normal DST suppression may be a good predictor of when to stop treatment. It is clear that failure to suppress with dexamethasone eventually reverts to a normal dexamethasone response as depression resolves. Some patients, however, may appear clinically to have recovered from their depression but still have an abnormal DST result. Several authors studied this interesting population. Goldberg (1980 and 1980a) looked at ten patients who had abnormal DST results when depressed and whose medication was stopped after they had been clinically free of depression for one month. The DST was repeated immediately prior to the discontinuation of drug therapy. Of the five patients who showed a normal DST result after treatment, none had undergone relapse at seven-month follow-up. On the other hand, all five of the patients who continued to show a failure to suppress plasma cortisol levels with dexamethasone, even though clinically recovered, had significant relapses within two months after medication was stopped. In another study, Greden and colleagues (1980) found similar results, with only two of ten posttreatment DST suppressors undergoing relapse at follow-up, compared with all four of the patients with abnormal DST results, who underwent relapse after treatment was discontinued. These preliminary findings indicate that the DST may be a good predictor of when to stop treatment in those depressed patients who initially have an abnormal DST result; that is, an abnormal DST result in a patient free of symptoms may predict relapse.

The Dexamethasone Suppression Test (DST) and Elderly Patients

To determine the clinical usefulness of the DST in geriatric populations, one must know whether the test result is altered in normal elderly persons. Tourigny-Rivard and associates (1981) compared ten healthy elderly (mean age, 75.3 years) and ten healthy young men (mean age, 29.9 years) and concluded that advanced age alone did not affect the overnight DST result in healthy subjects and should not invalidate its use as a laboratory tool in the diagnosis and investigation of depression.

One of the common clinical dilemmas facing the physician treating elderly patients is to separate the truly demented patient from the patient who has reversible cognitive impairment on the basis of depression (pseudodementia)

(Wells, 1979). If the DST result could be shown to be normal in patients with dementia and abnormal in those with depression, this would be a great aid to the clinician faced with this dilemma. A few case reports suggest that the DST may be useful in some instances. Rudorfer and Clayton (1981) reported the case of a patient with pseudodementia whose abnormal DST normalized after treatment of underlying depressive illness. Also, Greden and Carroll's (1979) patient originally received the diagnosis of dementia but was later thought to have depression-induced catatonia. Her initially abnormal DST result returned to normal following two courses of electroconvulsive therapy. Similarly, McAllister and colleagues (1982) described the cases of two patients for whom the DST appeared to be useful in distinguishing depression with associated severe cognitive deficits from dementia.

These reports are encouraging. On the other hand, however, Spar and Gerner (1982) found abnormal DST results in nine of 17 elderly patients with dementia who did not appear to have major depressive illness and Raskind and co-workers (1982) found that seven of 15 patients with advanced primary degenerative dementia had abnormal DST results. Clearly, these reports dampen enthusiasm for using the DST to differentiate dementia from depression-induced cognitive deficits (pseudodementia), but a few points must be kept in mind when one reviews their findings. First, these patients were severely demented. Spar and Gerner's patients had a mean score of 13.3 out of a possible 30 on the MMSE and an average duration of symptoms of 4.3 years. The patients of Raskind and co-workers were even further advanced. They had a mean duration of illness of 7.4 years and had no correct responses on the Short Portable Mental Status Questionnaire. In addition, each patient had dysphasia severe enough to grossly impair meaningful speech.

It is well documented that dementia is a multisystem illness, and it is not surprising that neuroendocrine abnormalities exist in patients with advanced disease (see chapter 5). Most patients, however, in whom the diagnostic confusion between depression and dementia occur are only mildly demented. Also, it is impossible to say for certain that the patients with abnormal DST results were not depressed without therapeutic trials of electroconvulsive therapy or pharmacotherapy having been made. With this in mind, Jenike and Albert (1984) performed the DST on 18 patients with presenile and senile dementia of the Alzheimer's type. Objective cognitive testing showed that 13 patients were mild to moderately impaired and five were moderate to severely impaired. The patients were nondepressed as determined by the Hamilton Depression Scale and also by clinical interview. The DST was abnormal in only one of the mildly impaired patients, but in four of the five moderately impaired patients. These data suggest that the DST might be a useful clinical and research tool in mildly impaired patients with Alzheimer's disease but is likely to be confounded by disease in moderate to severely impaired patients. These data are consistent with the hypothesis that the DST is not invalidated by early Alzheimer's disease.

Conclusions

In summary, the DST is a potentially useful research tool. In the absence of either medical illness or medication that affects the DST, resistance to dexamethasone suppression suggests the presence of a major depressive disorder. A normal DST result does not, however, rule out such a disorder. As more research is done on the DST, it may turn out that the DST is not as specific as it was thought to be initially. It may be a less specific indicator of psychiatric disease, similar to the ESR for inflammatory disorders, and of value in screening for psychiatric illness and in following the course, treatment, and resolution of such disease.

Normalization of a previously abnormal DST result may be a better guide than the clinical picture to the discontinuation of treatment with antidepressants. Patients who appear to improve clinically but whose DST is still abnormal may be at high risk of experiencing significant relapse if treatment is discontinued.

The utility of the DST as an aid in the diagnosis of depression in patients with severe dementia is unclear at this time, as some data indicate that dementia alone may produce abnormal DST results. Preliminary data, however, indicate that mild-to-moderate dementia may not invalidate the DST as an aid in detecting depression.

COGNITIVE CHANGES ASSOCIATED WITH DEPRESSION (PSEUDODEMENTIA)

When elderly patients appear demented, special care is required to rule out depression. Initially, family members should be asked if they have observed any of the SIG E CAPS symptoms in the patient. Complaints of poor memory may accompany depression and disappear when the depression is treated. Conversely, very early organic brain dysfunction (eg, Alzheimer's disease) with a gradual decline in cognitive functioning may produce a reactive depression which may lead to further cognitive impairment.

The term pseudodementia is often used to describe depression-related cognitive deficits that are reversible with effective treatment of the affective illness. Probably "pseudo" is not a helpful term, because these cognitive changes are real and demonstrable; but this terminology is so ingrained in the medical literature that it will be around for some time. Lack of effort on the part of depressed patients is observed frequently by clinicians, who have noted patients' increased dependency, indecisiveness, and avoidance of responsibility as part of a general picture of motivational change.

Depressed patients perform poorly on a number of motor performance tasks, including tapping, aiming, and circle tracing (Raskin et al, 1982) and are consequently rarely found playing video games. When retested after adequate treatment of depression, their performance often improves strikingly (Cohen et al, 1982). Increasing severity of depression is strongly associated with decrements in motor performance (Stromgren, 1977; Grayson et al, 1987). Byrne (1977) found a significant negative relationship between severity of depression and performance on a signal detection task, suggesting that depressed patients are inattentive, as well.

Patients with depression have also been reported to show deficits in memory (Cronholm and Ottosson, 1961; Breslow et al, 1980; Sternberg and Jarvik, 1976; Henry et al, 1973; Silberman et al, 1983; Raskin et al, 1982; Caine, 1986; Feinberg and Goodman, 1984) and in conceptualization (Raskin et al, 1982). However, some aspects of memory ability are reported to be preserved in depressed patients: recognition of high imagery words (Silberman et al, 1983), recall of related words that have previously been sorted (Weingartner et al, 1981), paired associate learning (Breslow et al, 1980), and rate of forgetting over time (Cronholm and Ottosson, 1961). This suggests that memory tasks that impose structure on the to-be-remembered items are performed relatively well by depressed patients.

Some authors have speculated that it may be unreasonable to hypothesize basic memory deficits in depressive patients and that the most parsimonious explanation of available data would be one based on a single deficit in the central motivational state (Cohen et al, 1982). That is, general deficits in motivation, drive, and attention may account for the clinical and experimental deficits found in patients with depression. Some studies have found, in fact, a negative correlation between intensity of depression and degree of memory impairment (Stromgren, 1977; Byrne, 1977; Cohen et al, 1982).

A number of authors have attempted to identify clues that would separate depressed from demented patients (Grayson et al, 1987). Wells (1979) emphasized the importance of getting a careful history of the disorder. The symptoms of depression usually develop before the onset of cognitive decline (Post, 1975 and 1976). In addition, the cognitive impairments frequently fluctuate along with changes in level of depression. Reports that demented patients are invariably unaware of their cognitive deficits, thus differentiating them from depressed patients, appear to be untrue; many patients with progressive dementia are clearly aware of their impairments and the advancement of their deficits.

Clinically, one may find that depressed patients undergoing cognitive testing with an instrument such as the MMSE (see chapter 2) and other cognitive tests will actually perform better with time; that is, the depressed patient may remember one or none of three items after three minutes, but will remember all three if asked again after 15 minutes. Such an improvement in memory would be very unlikely in patients with a progressive dementing illness.

Miller (1979) discussed difficulties in distinguishing depressive symptoms from a clinically recognizable depressive syndrome in an organically impaired population and called particular attention to problems in the interpretation of vegetative indicators common to both dementia and depression. The rates of depression reported in demented patients vary considerably from study to study and probably reflect differences in the definition of both depression and dementia in each study. In dementing patients, both Reifler and associates (1982) and Reding and colleagues (1985) found a 19% prevalence rate of depression, while Lazarus and associates (1987) found that 40% were depressed, and Knesevich and co-workers (1983) found no significant degree of major depression among mildly demented patients with Alzheimer's disease.

In a careful study in which behavioral data were obtained from a structured interview of caregivers who knew patients well, rather than directly from patient-interviewer interaction, Merriam and associates (1988) found that fully 86% of their sample of 175 cognitively impaired patients met full DSM-III criteria for major depressive episode. With this finding in mind, they questioned the appropriateness of using DSM-III criteria in this population and noted the frequent clinical dilemma that many of the symptoms of depression are present in demented patients who are clearly not depressed. They found that the majority of their "depressed" patients were consistently able to be cheered up or distracted, even when most despondent; thus diagnostic criteria that ignore the capacity for depressed demented patients to be distracted or cheered up may yield false-positive diagnoses of depression. Some researchers are trying to modify standard structured interviews, like the Schedule for Affective Disorders and Schizophrenia (SADS), so that there will be less diagnostic overlap between symptoms of depression and dementia (Albert, Falk, Jenike, Keller, unpublished data).

It was recently suggested that depression in an elderly patient is a red flag, warning of an underlying early dementing illness (Reding et al, 1985). Of 225 patients referred to a dementia clinic over a three-year period, 57% of those initially thought to be depressed and nondemented developed frank dementia. Many of them initially had some sign, often subtle, of neurologic disease. Depressed elderly patients were found to be at high risk for the development of dementia if any of the following were present: cerebrovascular, extrapyramidal, or spinocerebellar disease; a modified Hachinski ischemic score of 4 or greater; a Mental Status Questionnaire score of less than 8; or confusion on low doses of tricyclic antidepressants.

Many patients have both depression and structurally based intellectual impairment and vigorous therapeutic intervention may benefit the affective state, even when there is no rebound in neuropsychological deficits, with resultant improvement in the functional status of the patient. Some reported that depression occurs less frequently as the dementing disease progresses (Reifler et al, 1982) while others (Shuttleworth et al, 1987) reported that the magnitude of depression did not differ as a function of disease severity and they recommended the use of antidepressant therapy at any stage of the disease in appropriate patients.

Ideally, the uncertain clinician will initially consider the depressed, dementing patients to have pseudodementia, where there is hope for recovery, and begin antidepressant therapy (Jenike, 1988 and 1988b). The dangers of assuming that cognitive deficits are secondary to neurologic disease have been outlined by several authors (Kiloh, 1961; Shamoian, 1985; Jenike, 1988a and 1988b).

It is important to guard against fatalistically assuming the cognitively impaired depressed individual as irretrievably demented, and withholding treatment as a result. Therapeutic interventions should be based on the presence of responsive target symptoms and, although diagnosis is important, it may not be essential for initiating effective treatments. The distinction between a psychiatric and neurologic disorder may not be necessary as long as one establishes that the course is nonprogressive and has completed a workup to rule out other treatable causes.

NEUROCHEMICAL CHANGES ASSOCIATED WITH AGING AND DEPRESSION

It is assumed that neurochemical alterations occur in depressed patients (Georgotas, 1983) and hypotheses have arisen concerning the serotonergic (Van Praag et al, 1973) and the noradrenergic (Schildkraut, 1965) transmitter systems. Much recent work has built upon these early ideas. In the elderly, investigators are now finding that specific neurochemical changes occur even without changes in affect and that they have relevance for the clinician who is treating the elderly psychiatric patient.

There appears to be a significant decrease in the dopamine content of parts of the brain (caudate nucleus and putamen) in people over 70 years old as compared to younger subjects (Bertler, 1961; Carlsson and Winblad, 1976). In addition, a decline in brain norepinephrine levels has been reported with age (Robinson et al, 1972; Nies et al, 1973; Robinson, 1975). Based on autopsy studies, MAO activity increases with age in the brain. Similar changes have been documented in platelet and plasma MAO activity (Robinson et al, 1971 and 1972); the relationship between brain and platelet MAO activity is unclear, however, but they may well be similar. These studies suggested that age-associated alterations in monoamine metabolism may predispose to the development of psychiatric disorders such as depression and further might indicate that MAOIs may have a special use in at least a subgroup of geriatric depressed patients (see later section on MAOIs).

As well as neurotransmitters, hormones regulate physiologic activity in the body (Georgotas, 1983) and studies have documented age-related changes in endocrine glands and hormones (Gitman, 1967; Robertson et al, 1972; Fince, 1975; Ganong, 1972 and 1974). For example, diminishing thyroid function and decreased responsiveness of the pituitary to hypothalamic releasing factor have been cited as predisposing to depression (Georgotas, 1983).

TREATMENT OF AFFECTIVE ILLNESS

Psychotherapy

Considerable evidence indicates that antidepressant medication is more effective when used in combination with some type of psychotherapy (Goff and

Jenike, 1986). Psychotherapy is covered in detail in chapter 12 but some of the main points as they pertain to the treatment of depression are reviewed here also.

In 1968, only 2% of patients attending outpatient psychiatric facilities or treated by psychiatrists in private practice were older than 65 years (Steuer, 1982) and this situation has only changed slightly over the last two decades (Vandenbos et al, 1981; General Accounting Office, 1982).

This underutilization of services may reflect a cultural bias where professionals might believe that resources should go to younger clients who have more years of life ahead of them and who are more economically productive. Clinicians may view the elderly as inflexible or consider decline inevitable. Others may believe that special knowledge is required to help the aged. Countertransference issues may surface. Some elderly patients view therapists as they would their children (Grotjahn, 1955) and unresolved conflicts with the therapist's own parents may interfere with objective observation and therapy.

Mental health system factors—such as reimbursement inequities, lack of cooperation among community mental health centers and physicians, discrepant perceptions of the help that is needed, and the lack of referrals from other physicians who have contact with older patients who need mental health services—may be the most important explanations of why so few older adults are seen by mental health professionals (Kahn, 1975).

Despite a bewildering array of psychotherapeutic approaches that are available for use with the elderly, there are no good studies addressing psychotherapy outcome in these age groups. Despite the lack of hard evidence, it has been suggested that four common principles underlie the process of all psychotherapeutic approaches in the elderly: (1) fostering a sense of control, self-efficacy, and hope; (2) establishing a relationship with the caregiver; (3) providing or elucidating a sense of meaning; and (4) establishing constructive contingencies in the environment (Butler, 1975). Butler (1960, 1968, and 1975) also pointed out themes common in old age, such as dysfunctioning of one's body, independence and dependence, and concerns with time, and stereotypes of the young. Concerns about the meaningfulness of life and feelings of uselessness are also common, and therapists may help the aging patient to resolve existential crises through reminiscence and self-evaluation.

Busse and Pfeiffer (1969 and 1977) recommended that the therapist be active in mapping and clarifying the patient's problems and suggested the establishment of limited goals such as symptom relief, support for adaptation to changing life circumstances, acceptance of greater dependency as a normal aspect of the aging process, and renewed or continued involvement in useful activity. They also encouraged social conversation during part of each session to enhance the patient's thoughts of being part of a meaningful relationship. Blume and Tross (1980) pointed out the importance of regularly scheduled sessions as a source of constancy in what may be a life filled with change.

As a means of increasing a patient's sense of self-worth, Burnside (1978) recommended that the therapist consider touching geriatric patients to express caring and gain the patient's attention. Linden (1957) stressed the importance of optimism in the therapist and emphasized that the therapist's personality is a main consideration in psychotherapy outcome.

As the problems of old people are likely to be social as well as intrapsychic, practical interventions are important, and the therapist should have a knowledge of community social agencies and referral sources. A number of agencies and groups are particularly useful in the management of particular types of patients and their families. Support groups and programs involving home visits to frail elderly with the purpose of reducing social isolation have been demonstrated to reduce psychiatric symptoms (Mulligan and Bennett, 1977–1978). Programs that enlist elderly persons as teachers, advisors, and consultants benefit both helpers and the helped (Sherman, 1981). Foster grandparent programs place older adults in positions to help children in various school or hospital settings (Saltz, 1977; Hirschowitz, 1973). Pet therapy, which may afford companionship, demand responsibility in terms of caring for them, and provide physical contact, is reported to improve feelings of isolation, loneliness, and uselessness (Lago et al, 1983).

Tricyclic and Heterocyclic Agents

Choosing a Drug
Pharmacologic strategy for the treatment of depression begins with a choice of antidepressant medication, a decision based on previous responses to treatment and anticipation of which side effects might pose the greatest problems or produce therapeutic benefits for the patient. Since the introduction of imipramine about 30 years ago, tricyclics have been the mainstay of pharmacologic treatment for depression. Because these agents are generally considered to be equally effective, the choice of drug should be based on side effects.

Tertiary amines such as amitriptyline (Elavil) and imipramine (Tofranil) are much more likely to cause orthostatic hypotension than secondary amines such as desipramine (Norpramin), protriptyline (Vivactil), and nortriptyline (Aventyl, Pamelor) (Table 4–4) (Salzman, 1982). However, doxepin, a tertiary amine, is safe in elderly patients in terms of orthostatic changes (Neshkes et al, 1985). As a general rule, tertiary amines also tend to produce more sedation, presumably by blocking synaptic serotonin reuptake or by affecting histamine receptors (Richelson, 1982).

Anticholinergic and noradrenergic side effects are also particularly troublesome in both nondemented and dementing elderly patients. Anticholinergic symptoms may be prominent both centrally (delirium, confusion, and cognitive impairment) and peripherally (tachycardia, urinary retention, constipation, blurred vision, and dry mouth). If desipramine is assigned an anticholinergic potency of 1, amitriptyline would be eight times more anticholinergic. The

Table 4–4
Characteristics of Tricyclic and Heterocyclic Agents in Treatment of Depression

Generic Name	Trade Name	Relative Anticholinergic Effect	Sedative Effect	Inhibition of Reuptake	
				Norepinephrine	Serotonin
Tricyclic Tertiary Amines					
Amitriptyline	Elavil and others	8	High	0	4+
Imipramine	Tofranil and others	2	Moderate	2+	3+
Doxepin	Sinequan, Adapin	2	High	0	4+
Tricyclic Secondary Amines					
Desipramine	Norpramin, Pertofrane	1	Low	4+	0
Protriptyline	Vivactil, Triptil	2	Low	Uncertain	Uncertain
Nortriptyline	Aventyl, Pamelor	2	Moderate	2+	2+
Others					
Amoxapine	Asendin	2	Moderate	4+	1+
Maprotiline	Ludiomil	2	Moderate	4+	0
Trazodone	Desyrel	0	High	0	4+
Fluoxetine	Prozac	0	Low	0	4+

Adapted with permission from Jenike MA: Drug treatment of depression. *Top Geriatr* 2:10, 1983.

other tricyclics lie somewhere in between, with a relative potency of about 2 (Table 4–4).

Amitriptyline is generally regarded as the tricyclic most likely to cause a clinically hazardous tachycardia (Cassem, 1982) and the combination of pronounced anticholinergic activity and danger of orthostatic hypotension makes amitriptyline the least desirable of all the available tricyclics used to treat depression (Jenike, 1988). Based on in vitro comparisons of anticholinergic potency, amitriptyline is about one-twentieth as active as atropine at central and peripheral muscarinic cholinergic receptors, so that a daily dose of 150 mg of amitriptyline corresponds to approximately 7.5 mg of atropine, a dose which would almost never be given (Cassem, 1982). Because of the well-documented abnormalities in the cholinergic system in dementing patients and the effects of anticholinergic drugs on memory even in normal subjects (see chapter 5), any anticholinergic medication given to a dementing patient will worsen cognitive functioning even if it improves affective state.

If a patient has had a prior positive response or if he has a relative who had a good outcome from a particular drug, it may be best to begin treatment with that drug. In general, tertiary amine tricyclics (except doxepin [Sinequan]) and agents with high anticholinergic potency should be avoided in the elderly, especially in those who have dementing illness. Low doses of secondary amine tricyclics with relatively low anticholinergic activity, such as desipramine and nortriptyline, or newer agents, such as trazodone (Desyrel), maprotiline (Ludiomil), or fluoxetine (Prozac), should be the drugs of first choice. If a depressed patient is not sleeping well, trazodone, nortriptyline, maprotiline, doxepin, or trimipramine (Surmontil) given at bedtime may improve insomnia during the early stages of treatment. In hypersomnic or lethargic patients, daytime doses of desipramine, protriptyline, or fluoxetine may help to activate the patient (Jenike, 1988). These so-called "activating agents" may sedate some patients and should then be given around bedtime.

Amoxapine (Asendin) is the demethylated derivative of the antipsychotic loxapine and is comparable in antidepressant efficacy to the standard tricyclic agents (Dominquez, 1983). Hypotension is an uncommon side effect, but several cases of seizures have been reported. Amoxapine inhibits both norepinephrine and serotonin reuptake and also blocks dopamine receptors and produces extrapyramidal side effects typical of neuroleptics. It has been reported to cause acute dystonia, parkinsonism, and akathisia (Lydiard and Gelenberg, 1981; Barton, 1982), and there are reports of tardive dyskinesia associated with amoxapine (Lapierre and Anderson, 1983). Because the elderly are particularly prone to develop tardive dyskinesia, and because the movements associated with it are much less likely to be reversible in older individuals (see chapter 6; Jenike, 1983a), amoxapine should be avoided in elderly patients.

Maprotiline (Ludiomil), introduced in 1981, is a tetracyclic that is very similar to standard tricyclics in action (Dominquez, 1983). It is a specific blocker of norepinephrine reuptake, with apparently no effect on serotonin uptake. It has little anticholinergic effect and does not commonly produce orthostatic hypotension. In addition, it appears to have a lower incidence of cardiovascular side effects (Wells and Gelenberg, 1981). Seizures have been reported and skin rashes occur in as many as 10% of patients (Dominquez, 1983).

Trazodone (Desyrel) has a structure different from other antidepressant agents and is a selective, serotonin uptake blocker. It is similar in efficacy to the standard tricyclics (Murphy and Ankier, 1980), but has a very low incidence of anticholinergic side effects, although clinically some patients complain of dry mouth. The lack of anticholinergic side effects with trazodone is probably responsible for the low incidence of therapy dropouts in comparative studies with tricyclics and other agents (Newton, 1981). As long as they are not oversedated during the day, the elderly seem to tolerate trazodone very well. Clinically, trazodone is sedating and is particularly helpful for depressed patients who cannot sleep. Other common side effects of trazodone include indigestion, nausea, and headaches.

Priapism with trazodone is a rare problem and male patients should be cautioned to discontinue the drug if prolonged or painful erections occur. As of September 1986, approximately 2.4 million patients had received trazodone in the United States and the incidence of all reports of abnormal erectile activity was approximately 1 in 6,000 male patients (personal communication, Mead Johnson Pharmaceutical Company, Evansville, Ill., September 1986). The incidence in elderly men is not known, but appears to be lower than in the general population. In 34 of 123 patients, surgical intervention was performed to achieve detumescence. In at least 60 of the 123 patients, spontaneous detumescence occurred without medical advice or attention. Nonsurgical techniques, such as the intracavernosal injection of epinephrine, metaraminol or norepinephrine, are reportedly of help in relieving the symptom (personal communication, Mead Johnson Pharmaceutical Company, Evansville, Ill., September 1986).

Increased libido, another sexual side effect of trazodone, in women was recently reported by Gartrell (1986) and in men, by Sullivan (1988). Although of interest, further research is needed to explore trazodone's usefulness in treating disorders of sexual desire in the elderly.

Trazodone appears to have a more benign cardiac side effect profile compared with the tricyclics (Himmelhoch, 1981). Caution is still recommended in using trazodone in patients with preexisting cardiac disease. It appears to be particularly nonmalignant when taken in overdose; at this point, there have been no life-threatening complications after trazodone overdose alone such as those frequently associated with overdose of tricyclic antidepressants. The dosing schedule is different from most of the other heterocyclic antidepressants; approximately 400 mg of trazodone is equivalent to 150 mg of amitriptyline or imipramine. Clinicians frequently underdose patients with trazodone (Jenike, 1985 and 1988).

Because of its presumed lack of side effects, trazodone appears particularly suited for use in elderly patients. Since digoxin is frequently prescribed in this population, a possible interaction between trazodone and digoxin should be kept in mind. The following case (Rauch and Jenike, 1984) is reproduced here with permission:

> Case: A 68-year-old woman with a 30-year history of unipolar affective illness was admitted to an inpatient psychiatry service for treatment of severe depression of three weeks' duration. The symptoms, which were characteristic of past depressions, included loss of appetite, lack of energy, disinterest in her appearance, severe anxiety, and refusal to get out of bed. The medical history was significant for congestive heart failure, hypertension, atrial tachyarrhythmia, and impaired renal function presumed secondary to hypertensive nephropathy. Previously, she had undergone a modified radical mastectomy for cancer in the left breast with one positive lymph node and no further evidence of metastatic disease.
>
> On admission, she was medically stable and was receiving digoxin, clonidine, quinidine gluconate, and a triamterene-hydrochlorothiazide combination. The digoxin levels had remained within therapeutic ranges for many months on the same dosage (125 μg/day of digoxin), as did the quinidine levels. The results of laboratory tests on admission were within normal limits except for a slightly elevated creatinine value of 1.3 mg/100 mL with a BUN [blood urea nitrogen] of 24 mg/100 mL. The admission digoxin level was 0.8 ng/mL (therapeutic range 1.2 to 1.7 ng/mL) and the quinidine level was 4.0 μg/mL (therapeutic range 1.5 to 5.0 μg/mL).
>
> Trazodone 50 mg at bedtime was begun (Day 1 of therapy). It was increased by 50 mg every other day until a dose of 300 mg/d was reached (Day 11). On Day 12 she felt less anxious and the staff reported that she was more sociable and attentive to self-care. On Day 14 she complained of nausea and vomiting. The digoxin level was measured in the toxic range at 2.8 ng/mL while the quinidine level was within therapeutic limits at 1.6 μg/mL. Digoxin was temporarily discontinued and the nausea and vomiting resolved over the next three days. On Day 19 of therapy she had a further elevated creatinine value of 1.9 mg/100 mL with a BUN of 30 mg/100 mL, which returned to baseline levels after fluid intake was increased.
>
> She continued on trazodone, 100 mg in the morning and 200 mg at bedtime. After the digoxin level returned to the therapeutic range, she was switched to 125 μg every other day, which produced therapeutic levels. She continued to be free of her depressive symptoms.

This patient not only developed toxic digoxin levels after starting trazodone, but also required only half her previous maintenance dose of digoxin. This case is complicated by the presence of compromised renal function. There was, however, no change in renal function to account for the lowered maintenance dose of digoxin after trazodone was begun. In a canine model, Dec and associates (1984) found no elevation in serum digoxin concentration when trazodone was administered with digoxin. The authors noted that the inability to reproduce a trazodone-digoxin interaction could be due to differences in canine metabolism and excretion of digoxin or trazodone. Canine elimination of digoxin is predominantly renal and more rapid than that observed in humans.

Until more data are available, trazodone should be used cautiously in combination with digoxin. In particular, digoxin levels should be closely monitored when trazodone is used concomitantly.

A new antidepressant, fluoxetine (Prozac) appears to be relatively free of major side effects and may be a useful drug for elderly patients. It is a highly specific, highly potent blocker of serotonin uptake with essentially no ability to block other neurotransmitters and it does not block postsynaptic receptor sites. It has a dosage range of 20 to 80 mg/day and is generally given initially during the day because it may produce insomnia if given at night.

Drug Trials

Prior to starting any antidepressant medication, an electrocardiogram (ECG) should be performed on all elderly patients. Treatment should begin with a very low dose—a maximum of 25 mg for most drugs (except 5 mg for protriptyline, 20 mg for fluoxetine, and 50 mg for trazodone). The dosage can be increased slowly every few days. Subjective response and heart rate are monitored and the clinician must be on the alert for anticholinergic, cardiovascular, or CNS side effects. Dosage increase should be slowed if tachycardia, excessive sedation, or orthostatic hypotension develops. Often the patient is the last to know that he is getting better and family members commonly report that the patient is sleeping and eating better before the dysphoria resolves. An adequate trial takes at least four weeks and probably six weeks at therapeutic levels. Drugs should not be changed until an adequate therapeutic trial is completed; Quitkin and co-workers (1984a), reviewing drug trials in patients who took a representative spectrum of antidepressants, found that 40% of patients who were unresponsive at four weeks responded to treatment if the drug trial was extended to six weeks.

If these agents are not helpful after a reasonable trial, a determination of blood level (when available) will assist the clinician in determining the next step (Table 4–5). Blood levels are well worked out for imipramine and nortriptyline and less so for desipramine (Task Force, 1985). There are rough estimates of therapeutic values for amitriptyline and doxepin. Blood levels for other agents such as trazodone can be available, but it is not known what levels correspond with clinical improvement; such levels are, however, useful occasionally to check on compliance. Blood samples should be drawn in the morning before any morning dose of medication or 10 to 14 hours after the evening dose for patients who are on a once-a-day dosing schedule. Nortriptyline appears to be unique among these agents in that it has a therapeutic window; that is, levels above as well as below the therapeutic range are

Table 4–5
Suggested Blood Levels for Some Tricyclic
Agents (Task Force)

Drug	What Is Measured	Total Therapeutic Level
Imipramine	Imipramine and desipramine	> 200 ng/mL
Desipramine	Desipramine	> 125 ng/mL
Amitriptyline	Amitriptyline and nortriptyline	> 160 ng/mL[†]
Nortriptyline	Nortriptyline	50–150 ng/mL*
Doxepin	Doxepin and desmethyldoxepin	> 100 ng/mL[†]

*Therapeutic window: above or below these levels is associated with decreased response.
[†]Rough estimates.
Reproduced with permission from Jenike MA: *Handbook of Geriatric Psychopharmacology.* Littleton, Mass, PSG Publishing Co, 1985, p 56.

associated with a decreased response (Task Force, 1985). When the level is not in the appropriate range, dosage should be adjusted.

With the same dose, blood levels of antidepressants can vary as much as 30 times among individuals. Even though many elderly patients will respond to very low doses of antidepressant (eg, 10 mg of desipramine or 50 mg of trazodone), others will require the same dosages as younger patients. If patients are not responding and side effects are not a problem, the clinician must be aggressive about increasing the dose. Some clinicians, fearing high dosages of antidepressants in the elderly, chronically underdose their geriatric patients.

Heterocyclic Overdose
Each year in the United States, 5,000 to 10,000 patients try to poison themselves with antidepressants and about 0.7% of them die (Moriarty, 1981). (For a complete review, see Frommer et al, 1987, and Gelenberg, 1984.) Tricyclic antidepressants in therapeutic doses are readily absorbed from the GI tract, circulate in the plasma, and rapidly bind to tissue; their high lipid solubility results in a very large volume of distribution. Large ingestions may be absorbed more slowly because of anticholinergic effects on gastric emptying and peristalsis (Frommer et al, 1987) and the finding of large amounts of tricyclic in autopsied stomachs, including intact pill fragments (Hanzlick, 1984), supports this theory. On the other hand, rapid clinical deterioration within a few hours after an acute overdose indicates that despite these findings, considerable amounts of the medication are absorbed.

Not all body tissues absorb the drug equally as tissue uptake occurs in a preferential fashion; compared to plasma, levels have been found to be roughly five times greater in myocardial cells, 30 times greater in liver cells, and 40 times greater in brain tissue (Frommer et al, 1987). Drugs such as haloperidol, disulfiram, and morphine may prolong tricyclic toxicity by interfering with hydroxylation.

After a significant overdose, symptoms develop within the first few hours. Mild early symptoms and signs of toxic reactions to tricyclics are predominantly anticholinergic, which may include dilated pupils, blurred vision, dry mouth, tachycardia, hyperpyrexia, urinary retention, decreased intestinal peristalsis, and CNS excitation (see chapter 9). More serious features are probably unrelated to anticholinergic effects and may include convulsions, coma, hypotension, arrhythmias, and cardiorespiratory arrest. The progression from being alert with mild symptoms to life-threatening toxic effects may be extremely rapid (Frommer et al, 1987). Increased heart rate is believed to be largely due to an anticholinergic effect, whereas other ECG changes result from the drugs' quinidine-like effects which are thought to be caused by slowing of sodium flux into cells, resulting in altered repolarization and conduction which occurs at the His-ventricular portion of the atrioventricular (AV) node.

ECG changes can be seen within weeks after beginning therapy at even therapeutic dosages. The quinidine-like effects which typically decrease ventricular irritability at therapeutic dosages can also precipitate arrhythmias as levels increase (Frommer et al, 1987). The most common mechanisms of death after overdoses include cardiovascular toxicity with intractable myocardial depression, ventricular tachycardia, or ventricular fibrillation. Hypotension is a serious manifestation of overdose and may be the harbinger of cardiac arrest. However, sinus tachycardia, with a rate of 100 beats/minute or more, is a sensitive indicator of anticholinergic effect, but an insensitive marker for development of serious toxicity.

CNS toxicity with confusion, agitation, hallucinations, coma, myoclonus, and seizures is common after serious overdose. Lethargy may rapidly progress to coma and respiratory arrest.

In one series, more than 50% of serious overdoses resulting in admission to an adult intensive care unit (ICU) involved tricyclic antidepressants (Kathol and Henn, 1983). Reviewing the records of 47 patients who had overdosed on antidepressants, Nicotra et al (1981) found that amitriptyline and doxepin were taken most often. Of the 47 patients, three died: one had cardiopulmonary arrest on admission, the other two had respiratory failure after prolonged courses. Half of the patients required respiratory support, usually for less than 48 hours. Seizures that occurred in the course of hospitalization were all grand mal and abated without treatment. A number of cardiovascular effects were reported. Two patients had cardiac arrests prior to admission but were successfully resuscitated. Tachycardia was common on admission, but usually cleared within a day. Hypotension occurred in over a quarter of the patients. ECG changes included premature atrial and ventricular contractions as well as prolongation of the PR and QT_c intervals.

The relationship between plasma antidepressant levels and clinical evidence of toxicity is unclear. For example, although it has been said that patients with plasma antidepressant levels in excess of 1000 ng/mL usually have QRS complexes of longer than 100 milliseconds, Nicotra and colleagues found that this was not always the case; one patient with a level of 3340 ng/mL had a normal QRS complex. In addition, patients with only modestly elevated plasma levels on hospital admission were not necessarily safe from cardiovascular toxicity. Nicotra and colleagues believed that monitoring the plasma concentration of antidepressants in overdose patients is of limited value and can be misleading. Because the drugs are highly lipophilic and also bind extensively to protein and tissue, plasma levels may reflect only a small portion of the drug available to brain, heart, and other organs. In addition, different organs in different patients may develop tolerance at varying rates.

Pentel and Sioris (1981), noting that dangerous cardiac events have been reported as long as six days after ingestion, attempted to determine how frequently unexpected life-threatening arrhythmias occur after overdose with an antidepressant. This has a bearing on the question of how long patients who take overdoses should undergo cardiac monitoring. To address this question, they reviewed the charts of all adults hospitalized at a medical center over a four-year period after overdoses with tricyclic antidepressants. Amitriptyline, imipramine, and doxepin were the most commonly ingested tricyclic agents in the 129 patients reviewed. Ninety-six patients had also taken some other drug at the same time. Mortality in their series was 5.4% (seven patients), five because of ventricular arrhythmias. Four died within one hour after arrival at the hospital, two were pronounced brain dead several days later following intractable arrhythmias and hypotension, and the seventh patient died of pulmonary emboli 24 hours after ingesting a relatively small amount of antidepressant. All patients in whom arrhythmias or conduction delays on the ECG developed showed these abnormalities within one hour after hospitalization. Furthermore, once a presenting ECG abnormality had resolved, no patient experienced further cardiac difficulties. In no patient did an arrhythmia develop after the patient was alert and had a normal ECG for one hour.

Pentel and Sioris noted that in the previously reported cases of arrhythmias or sudden deaths occurring as long as six days after an antidepressant overdose, patients were never free from CNS or cardiac toxicity prior to the event. Rather, their courses were characterized by major complications such as severe ECG abnormalities, hypotension, and coma. The authors concluded that whereas arrhythmias and death can follow antidepressant ingestion by a number of days, life-threatening events appear to result from serious ongoing complications of overdose, rather than appearing unexpectedly after a benign interval. On the basis of their review, the authors recommended the following: after an antidepressant overdose, if (1) a patient is clinically normal, and (2) the ECG is stable for 24 hours, and (3) no contra-active or supportive therapy is required, and (4) the patient does not have a preexisting cardiac problem, then intensive monitoring may be discontinued.

In a comprehensive review of the treatment of patients after an overdose with tricyclic antidepressants, Jackson and Bressler (1982) highlighted a number of important aspects of diagnosis and management. For one, they emphasized the importance of other drugs that might be ingested along with the antidepressant. These other drugs, as well as ancillary medical problems, can complicate a clinical picture. For example, seizures that follow a tricyclic overdose could be attributed to the antidepressant, yet they may reflect hypoxia or hypoglycemia. Therefore, the authors recommended the intravenous administration of naloxone (Narcan) and glucose to patients with seizures and, for that matter, to all comatose or obtunded patients—in case opiates or hypoglycemia may be present.

Similar to the findings of the Nicotra group, Jackson and Bressler reported the most common cardiovascular findings in patients after a tricyclic overdose as sinus tachycardia, hypotension, prolonged QRS complexes, and prolonged PR and QT intervals. Less frequent, but more ominous, are other supraventricular tachycardias, intraventricular conduction defects, AV block, bradycardia, nodal rhythms, and ventricular irritability.

As a general therapeutic measure, the authors stressed the importance of maintaining adequate ventilation—via mechanical means, if necessary. Once vital functions are stabilized, any unabsorbed drug should be removed from the GI tract. As noted earlier, because of their anticholinergic activity, antidepressants (and other psychotropic compounds) may be present in the stomach for many hours after an overdose. Ipecac, which can be of some use at home immediately after ingestion, should not be administered to a patient with ileus or to a stuporous or unresponsive patient. Rather, gastric lavage should be performed with a large (34 F or larger) orogastric tube (small nasogastric tubes cannot remove concretions of tablets). Administration of a cathartic, such as castor oil, and activated charcoal, 50 to 100 g, should follow. Because of enterohepatic recirculation of active antidepressant metabolites, castor oil and charcoal should be repeated every 8 to 12 hours. The authors noted that late occurring toxicity following an overdose could be related to delayed absorption of drugs that have remained in the GI tract—which underscores the importance of prompt and complete removal.

When seizures occur following an antidepressant overdose, physostigmine (Antilirium) can be administered. However, the authors were extremely wary of this approach, noting the paradoxical possibility of increased seizures, as well as enhanced overall mortality. Among standard anticonvulsants, diazepam (Valium) is probably the most effective; phenytoin (Dilantin and others) seems relatively ineffective in these circumstances.

In four reported patients who had an overdose with amoxapine severe, multiple seizures developed. Physostigmine, 2 to 8 mg, was ineffective in treating the seizures. In one particularly severe case, seizures were similarly refractory to treatment with diazepam, 300 mg, and thiopental sodium (Pentothal) 1,200 mg (Krenzelok and North, 1981). Goldberg and Spector (1982) reported two cases of amoxapine overdose, which resulted in severe and persistent impairment of the CNS. The first was that of a 24-year-old, previously healthy woman, who took approximately 4 g of amoxapine (the maximum dose recommended by the manufacturer is 600 mg daily in divided doses). At the hospital, she was treated with gastric lavage, then activated charcoal and a saline cathartic and, because of an elevated body temperature, a cooling blanket. Soon after, she had a tonic-clonic seizure, followed by severe metabolic acidosis and hypokalemia. Recurrent seizures developed and the patient fell into a deep coma, requiring endotracheal intubation and mechanical ventilation. Seizures persisted for about eight hours and were refractory through intravenous administration of phenytoin, diazepam, pheno-barbital, and physostigmine. However, she never became hypotensive, hyper-tensive, hypoxemic, or oliguric, and her vital signs, blood gases, and urine output remained stable. Her neurologic condition improved gradually over seven months, but at three months after the overdose she could speak only in short phrases with dysarthria, had severe memory deficits and poor judgement, and required ongoing nursing care. The same authors saw an almost identical case of a 29-year-old woman who had taken at least 2 g of amoxapine, and in whom multiple seizures and severe metabolic acidosis also developed, and she remained comatose for two weeks. Four weeks after the overdose, the patient was still hospitalized with neurologic symptoms similar to those in the other woman.

Kulig and collaborators (1982) described an additional five cases of amoxapine overdoses, noting seizures in each, but again relatively benign cardiovascular effects. The patients were a 6-year-old boy, a 51-year-old woman, and two women and a man in their 30s. Each of these patients went through a period of coma, and two required endotracheal intubation. All patients recovered fully, although the course of one patient was complicated by rhabdomyolysis, myoglobinuria, and renal failure. In particular, cardiovas-cular reactions to the overdose were surprisingly mild—little more than sinus tachycardia—which the authors contrasted with the complications often ob-served with tricyclic antidepressant overdoses. The possibility that amoxapine overdose may cause a greater incidence of seizures, but a lower incidence of cardiotoxicity, is worth considering, although it remains unproved.

Amoxapine has shown a remarkable lack of cardiotoxicity, even in pa-tients after extremely large overdose, and, as the just mentioned data point out, the main toxicity involves the CNS (Frommer et al, 1987). A more recent report on overdose toxicity by Litovitz and Trautman (1983) reviewed all ingestions reported to poison centers in Washington, DC, and New Mexico over an 18-month period between 1980 and 1982. Of all reported overdoses, 479 included heterocyclic antidepressants, 33 of which were amoxapine. "Sub-stantial toxic conditions" developed in fifteen of the amoxapine overdose patients. Eight (24%) became comatose. Thirteen (9%) had supraventricular tachycardia. Twelve (36%) had seizures. Hyperthermia developed in three patients (9%), all of whom sustained prolonged convulsions. In two patients (6%) a coagulopathy developed, and one of them had profuse hemorrhage. Five patients (15.2%) died. By contrast, of 446 patients who took excessive amounts of other antidepressants, 19 (4%) had seizures and three (less than 1%) died. Previous reports had noted the high frequency of seizures in patients after amoxapine overdose; the general impression, however, had been that amoxapine was less likely than other heterocyclic compounds to produce fatalities. Against this background, Litovitz and Trautman's report is most worrisome. Cases reported to regional poison centers are not all inclusive and are therefore open to possible bias; however, the number of cases reported by these authors is impressive. Appropriate caution should be exercised in prescribing any antidepressant to patients with a seizure diathesis, but confirming whether some of the newer antidepressants may be more hazardous in this regard must await additional information.

Maprotiline, a tetracyclic antidepressant, was initially advertised as being less cardiotoxic than the tricyclics, but it has shown similar CNS and cardiac toxicity after overdose (Knudsen and Heath, 1984).

Overdose-induced cardiac arrhythmias often respond well to alkalinization with intravenously administered sodium bicarbonate, may respond to phenytoin, and might possibly be decreased with beta-blockers such as propranolol (Inderal). It is important to avoid type I antiarrhythmic agents— quinidine, procainamide hydrochloride (Pronestyl), and disopyramide phosphate (Norpace)— which tend to aggravate the effects of a tricyclic on the cardiac conduction system and myocardium.

If antidepressant-induced impairment of cardiac rhythm results in diminished (or absent) hemoperfusion, external support of ventilation and cardiac output (ie, cardiopulmonary resuscitation) should be continued for a longer period—hours, if necessary. In previously healthy patients, this support can allow metabolism and distribution of the offending agent, with the possibility of full recovery (Orr and Bramble, 1981).

As new antidepressant agents become available, the problem of serious toxicity from overdoses may diminish. For example, trazodone (Desyrel) is said to be much less toxic when taken in excess. At this point there are no reported fatalities when trazodone has been taken alone in overdose. But while the more toxic antidepressants remain with us, the risk of overdose will still be present. And for that reason, physicians should be careful to assess the suicide potential of patients to whom they prescribe these drugs. Furthermore, patients should be seen frequently during the early days of therapy, both to increase clinical monitoring and to diminish the amount of antidepressants that must be prescribed at each visit. Since elderly patients are at high risk for suicide and are particularly vulnerable to the malignant side effects of these agents when taken in overdose, these issues are of the utmost importance.

Monoamine Oxidase Inhibitors (MAOIs)

Overview
Among the somatic treatments available for treating depressed elderly patients, the MAOIs are the least used (Table 4–6). It is now well documented through

Table 4–6
MAOIs

Generic Name	Trade Name	Initial Dose	Maintenance Dose
Phenelzine	Nardil	15 mg daily	15–90 mg daily
Tranylcypromine	Parnate	10 mg daily	10–60 mg daily
Isocarboxazid	Marplan	10 mg daily	10–50 mg daily
Pargyline	Eutonyl	25 mg daily	25–200 mg daily

studies of human platelets, plasma, and brain, that there is a positive correlation between MAO activity and age (Robinson et al, 1971 and 1975; Mann, 1979; Mann et al, 1984; Robinson et al, 1982). Many clinicians avoid the use of MAOIs in elderly patients because of fears of adverse reactions. In fact, many textbooks of geriatrics make no mention of the use of MAOIs for the elderly, even though it is now known that these agents can be safely used for the elderly when certain precautions are taken (Jenike, 1984). Many patients who do not respond to tricyclics or some of the newer antidepressants will improve with MAOIs. Also, MAOIs may be especially effective in treating depression related to dementia (Ashford and Ford, 1979; Jenike, 1985). Dementing patients have higher levels of MAO than age-matched control subjects and this may account for the improvement in some depressions in dementing patients who take MAOIs (Jenike, 1984a). The following is an example of a not uncommon case:

Mr A, a 72-year-old retired laborer, was brought to a geriatric psychiatry clinic with a one-year history of worsening memory. In addition, the patient's wife told us that he had become increasingly withdrawn and was losing interest in his hobbies. Previously an avid traveler, he now wanted to just sit at home, often alone and in the dark. He was refusing to drive, had lost his appetite, with a resultant weight loss of 12 pounds, and seemed frequently confused and unable to concentrate. He denied suicidal ideation but admitted to feeling very depressed and hopeless. He had a strong family history of depression and his mother had received electroconvulsive therapy (ECT) on one occasion, with good result.

Results from Mr A's workup were entirely negative, and neuropsychiatric testing results were consistent with the initial impression that Mr A had an affective illness with secondary memory impairment (pseudodementia).

Mr A was started on desipramine, 25 mg each morning, and the dose was increased slowly to 200 mg daily. He had no side effects but also got no better over the next eight weeks, despite measured blood levels of the drug in the therapeutic range. Desipramine eventually was discontinued and nortriptyline was begun, starting with a low dosage. Once again he failed to respond despite blood levels in therapeutic range.

Because Mr A had not improved after trials of two tricyclic antidepressants and the family feared ECT, treatment with a MAOI was begun. After a ten-day drug-free period, tranylcypromine was started at 10 mg twice a day and slowly increased to 20 mg twice a day. After two weeks, Mr A was much improved, and within eight weeks he was "back to his former self." He continued on tranylcypromine and, at a return visit to the clinic three months later, was observed to be doing well. Repeat clinical testing at that time showed that his cognitive disturbances had resolved.

Atypical Depression and Hysteroid Dysphoria
Patients with typical depressions, as described already, often respond to MAOIs; in addition, a group of patients with symptoms fitting a particular picture have been reported to respond especially well to MAOIs. Patients meeting criteria for this depressive subgroup have been referred to as suffering from atypical depression (Quitkin et al, 1984; Liebowitz et al, 1984). These MAOI-responsive patients exhibit reactivity of mood, as well as two of four associated features which include hypersomnia, overeating, lethargy, and rejection sensitivity.

Klein (1969) earlier referred to a similar group of patients as hysteroid dysphorics who, when rejected or criticized, particularly in a romantic context, developed depressive episodes characterized by oversleeping and overeating, and preferentially responded to MAOIs over tricyclic antidepressants. There are no data on the response to MAOIs in the elderly who have atypical depressions, but a trial of MAOI is indicated in those who fail to improve with heterocyclic agents.

Nies (1984) suggested that MAOIs are particularly useful for patients who have symptoms that include panic and/or generalized anxiety with or without supervening atypical depression.

Effects of Monoamine Oxidase Inhibitors
Most MAOIs act by inhibiting the enzyme MAO which serves the function of oxidative deamination within the outer membrane of neuronal mitochondria (Tollefson, 1983). This is one of two major routes for the inactivation of nonmethylated biogenic amines (the other is extracellular and involves catechol-o-transferase). Two MAO subtypes have been identified by their respective substrate and inhibitor specificities. Type A preferentially deaminates norepinephrine, cortical dopamine, and serotonin and is selectively inhibited by clorgyline. Type B, which degrades phenylethylamine, dopamine, and benzylamine, is sensitive to deprenyl (at least at low dosages) or pargyline inhibition. Disorders that preferentially respond to clorgyline would be more likely to involve a disturbance of norepinephrine, serotonin, or dopamine while those responding to low-dose deprenyl should involve a disorder of either dopamine or phenylethylamine (Mann et al, 1984).

Commonly used MAOIs, such as tranylcypromine (Parnate) and phenelzine (Nardil), are nonselective inhibitors which affect both Types A and B. Nonselective MAOIs have been found to be highly effective for the treatment of panic disorder and some subgroups of depressive disorders (Mann et al, 1984). The differentiation between the two types of MAOI will become more important as new MAOIs which are selective for one or the other type of enzyme become clinically available. Ideally, if a particular MAOI were selective, one might produce antidepressant effects (eg, inhibit MAO Type B inhibition in the brain) without the danger of the tyramine reaction (eg, from MAO Type A inhibition in the gut) (to be described).

Not all of the effects of MAOIs can be attributed directly to MAO inhibition alone since a number of different neuronal effects of MAO inhibition have been described (see Murphy et al, 1984, for full discussion). The most prominent consequence of MAO inhibition is a rapid increase in the intracellular concentrations of monoamines. Brain concentrations of serotonin are raised to a greater extent than are those of norepinephrine and dopamine. After these amine concentrations rise, secondary adaptive consequences begin to occur. These include a reduction in amine synthesis via an apparent feedback mechanism which has been most clearly demonstrated for the noradrenergic system. Shortly after the neuron-specific amine concentrations have increased, other amines accumulating in the cytoplasm begin to enter amine storage vesicles, from which they may displace the endogenous amines or from where they may be released as cotransmitters or partial false transmitters. A resultant slowing of neuronal firing rates has been demonstrated in both serotonin-containing neurons in the median raphe and in norepinephrine-containing neurons in the locus ceruleus. After several weeks of MAOI treatment, reductions in beta-adrenoreceptor numbers and in beta-receptor functional activity as well as in alpha$_2$-adrenergic binding sites and serotonin binding sites are noted.

Precautions and Side Effects of Monoamine
Oxidase Inhibitors

Because MAOIs have essentially no anticholinergic effects, they are useful for patients who are sensitive to these side effects such as patients with dementing illnesses. Also, the elderly patient who has urinary retention with only a 10-mg dosage of desipramine may do very well with a MAOI. Some women taking MAOIs are unable to achieve orgasm (The Medical Letter, 1980). Serious hepatic toxicity, which used to occur frequently in patients who took MAOIs, is rare with those currently available.

The side effects of MAOIs that cause the most problems for the elderly are hypotension and insomnia. Higher doses of the MAOIs cause rapid eye movement (REM) suppression and frequent nocturnal awakenings (Walker et al, 1984) that can be minimized by giving the last daily dose no later than 4 PM. Some patients, however, feel drowsy while taking these agents, particularly phenelzine, and can be given the drug at bedtime. It is best to start with a daytime dosing schedule and switch to evenings only if the patient complains of drowsiness.

Orthostatic hypotension is a dangerous side effect for geriatric patients, because they tolerate falls poorly. It had been thought that if MAOI-induced orthostatic hypotension occurred early in the course of treatment and if patients could tolerate the first few days of medication, hypotension would rarely necessitate discontinuing the drug (Mielke, 1976; Robinson et al, 1978). Recently, however, Kronig and associates (1983) carefully followed a small group of patients (n = 14; average age, 52 years) and reported that orthostatic hypotension increased with time and peaked between three and four weeks after MAOIs were begun. Their data imply that clinicians should continue to watch for orthostatic changes at least throughout the first month of treatment. During the first few weeks of treatment patients may complain of mild light-headedness and unsteadiness secondary to the postural hypotension. Drinking small amounts of coffee or tea results in a minor rise in blood pressure sufficient to control this in many patients (Walker et al, 1984). If the symptoms are severe, the MAOI should be discontinued because the elderly tolerate falls poorly. We generally do not discontinue MAOIs if patients exhibit asymptomatic orthostatic drops in blood pressure but will stop them immediately if dizziness or unsteadiness occurs upon arising. In young patients, large doses of sodium chloride (500 to 650 mg twice daily) have been used to counteract orthostatic hypotension induced by both tricyclic drugs and MAOIs (Kranzler and Cardoni, 1988), but this tactic should not be tried in frail elderly patients because of the risk of intravascular overload.

Rarely a disinhibition syndrome, characterized by talkativeness, extroversion, antisocial behavior, and hypomania occurs (Walker et al, 1984) which is often exacerbated by alcohol or benzodiazepines and can be treated with lithium carbonate or by lowering or stopping the medication. Occasionally this progresses into a full-blown manic attack or paranoid psychosis (Jenike et al, 1981; Walker et al, 1984).

Less common side effects occur (Walker et al, 1984). Neuropathy secondary to vitamin B_6 deficiency occurs rarely and can be treated with 100 mg of pyridoxine daily. Occasional generalized edema occurs, but this usually subsides within a week without specialized intervention; electrolytes, however, should be monitored if the edema persists because of the possibility of inappropriate antidiuretic hormone secretion. Weight gain, often associated with carbohydrate craving, can be significant during the first few months of treatment. We have seen occasional patients who almost double their weight while taking MAOIs.

A reversible lupus-like reaction (positive result on lupus erythematosus preparation), hyper-prolactinemia (in absence of plasma cortisol change), and exacerbation of centrencephalic changes on the electroencephalogram (EEG) (Tollefson, 1983) have been reported in association with the use of MAOIs. MAOI treatment may retard phenothiazine metabolism and potentiate hypotension or extrapyramidal reactions or prolong the effects of anticholinergics, barbiturates, narcotics, and ethanol on the CNS. In addition, a paradoxical pressor response has been reported with the use of centrally active antihypertensives and thiazide diuretics (Tollefson, 1983). A summary of such potential drug interactions has been collected by Gaultieri and Powell (1978).

Hepatocellular damage (with 25% fatality rate) occurred in about 1 of every 5000 patients treated with iproniazid, a MAOI that is no longer on the market, and led to concern that other MAOIs may be associated with this potential problem (Davidson et al, 1984). In one survey of liver functions of patients taking MAOIs, Zisook (1984) found marked elevations of liver enzymes in only 1 of 48 patients who received isocarboxazid for six weeks. In this patient, levels of serum glutamic-oxaloacetic transaminase (SGOT) and serum glutamic-pyruvic transaminase (SGPT) were markedly elevated, while levels of bilirubin and alkaline phosphatase remained normal. Borderline elevation of enzyme levels is not in itself sufficient justification for the discontinuation of a MAOI, but such changes need to be carefully monitored and the dose perhaps reduced. Overall, it appears that liver damage is very rare and most clinicians do not measure routine liver function tests in patients who are taking MAOIs (Davidson et al, 1984).

When patients have hypertension and depression, MAOIs are likely to control the blood pressure, and usually other antihypertensive medication can be stopped or dosage lowered (Oates et al, 1965; Gibbs, 1966; Tollefson, 1983). Once the depression had been treated it is important to remember to restart antihypertensive medication when MAOI is discontinued, or dangerously high blood pressure may result. A note on the cover of the patients chart should be considered, as it may be difficult to remember that an individual patient had hypertension before MAOI treatment.

The most important adverse effect associated with MAOIs is the uncommon, but frightening, occurrence of a hypertensive crisis caused by a toxic interaction with certain drugs or tyramine-containing foods, especially aged cheese which has been involved in virtually all fatal reactions (McCabe and Tsuang, 1982; Walker et al, 1984). This reaction is a hyperadrenergic state characterized not only by hypertension but also by headache, diaphoresis, mydriasis, neuromuscular excitation, and potential cardiac dysrhythmia (Tollefson, 1983). In the presence of MAOI, tyramine is not inactivated in the GI tract and liver, and enters the bloodstream and releases norepinephrine from intracellular vesicles in the sympathetic nerve terminals, producing a three-stage symptom pattern of increasing severity of illness: (1) sudden onset of intensely painful, throbbing headaches; (2) severe hypertension with profuse sweating, pallor, and headache; and (3) hypertension, palpitation, chest pain, and, occasionally, death (Walker et al, 1984; The Medical Letter, 1980). The elderly patient who has fragile atherosclerotic blood vessels could easily have a stroke during such a hypertensive episode. Intravenously administered phentolamine (5 mg as needed), an alpha-adrenergic blocker, is recommended for treatment of severe hypertensive reactions. This produces a short-lived response, and treatment may need to be repeated after several hours (Davidson et al, 1984). Because fluid retention may be a complication of phentolamine, 40 mg of furosemide may be added. An alternative approach, and one that produces a more sustained response, is to administer diazoxide, 300 mg, intravenously over 15 seconds, or sodium nitroprusside, 50 to 100 mg in 500 mL of 5% dextrose and water. Still another option is to use chlorpromazine, which also has alpha-adrenergic blocking activity and can be given by the intramuscular route or by rectal suppository. A recent report suggested that intravenous administration of labetalol (20 mg given over five minutes) may also be effective in treating tyramine-induced hypertensive crises (Abrams et al, 1985).

It is essential that all patients taking MAOIs receive dietary and drug precautions (Tables 4–7 and 4–8) (Jenike, 1984a and 1988; Sheehan et al, 1980–1981). Elderly patients comply well and rarely complain about such restrictions. A low tyramine diet is required, necessitating avoidance of foods such as fermented cheese, yogurt, beer, red wine, and excessive amounts of caffeine and chocolate. The tyramine content of cheese varies considerably; in general, aged cheeses have a high content while fresh yogurt, sour cream, and processed American cheese have lower amounts. Cottage and cream cheese have no detectable amounts of tyramine.

Any food exposed to microbial degradation is likely to contain tyramine. Pickled herring, smoked fish, chicken and beef liver, and dry, fermented sausage have been implicated. Fresh poultry, game, and fish are safe. The pods of Italian green beans, also called fava beans or broad beans, can produce a hypertensive crisis secondary to the pressor effects of dopamine found in the pods of this vegetable (Walker et al, 1984). The pods of the Italian green bean are one-half inch in width and should not be confused with the usual green bean or lima bean. Chocolate has been implicated as the cause of a hypertensive crisis in a single case report, in which there were mitigating circumstances; the lack of additional reports indicates that dietary exclusion of chocolate is unwarranted (Walker et al, 1984). Excess intake of caffeine, while responsible for CNS stimulation, has not been implicated in hypertensive crisis secondary to combination with a MAOI (Walker et al, 1984). Patients can safely drink white wine, vodka, gin, and whiskey, and a blanket instruction to avoid all alcohol not only is unwarranted but also may decrease compliance dramatically (Jenike, 1983b). Chianti wine, with approximately 700 mg of tyramine per ounce of wine, should definitely be restricted (Walker et al, 1984). Combination cold tablets, nasal decongestants, appetite suppressors, and amphetamines must be avoided. Pure antihistamines, such as chlorpheniramine, however, can safely be used to treat patients who have rhinitis (Jenike, 1983b and 1984a).

There is a poorly understood potentially fatal toxic interaction between MAOIs and meperidine hydrochloride, which was first described in 1955 (Mitchell, 1955) and has been reported occasionally since that time (Meyer and Halfin, 1981). Clinically, patients appear agitated, disoriented, cyanotic, hyperthermic, hypertensive, and tachycardic. Should this occur, chlorpromazine has been used as an effective treatment (Papp and Benaim, 1958; Jenike, 1984a). There have been no clinical reports of the same severe toxic interactions with other narcotics, although increased potency has been noted experimentally in animals (Meyer and Halfin, 1981). Novocaine and xylocaine, used during minor surgery or dental work, are safe if they do not contain sympathomimetic vasoconstrictors. Should narcotics be needed for a patient who takes a MAOI, a prudent course would be to begin with half the usual dosage and titrate the dosage slowly on the basis of symptomatic response, bearing in mind that increased potency will be more pronounced if the narcotic is given close to the time that the MAOI was taken that day (Meyer and Halfin, 1981).

If possible, MAOIs should be discontinued two weeks prior to elective surgery because inhalation anesthesia can cause hypotensive reactions in patients taking MAOIs and also it may be difficult to control pressor overshoot of some drugs used in hypovolemic states. If hypotension develops during surgery, intravenously administered hydrocortisone may be of help (Davidson et al, 1984). Succinylcholine has led to prolonged apnea in patients receiving electroconvulsive therapy (ECT) and concomitant phenelzine therapy (Bodley et al, 1969).

Some of the newer drugs on the market, such as buspirone (Buspar) and fluoxetine (Prozac), have been associated with toxic reactions when used concomitantly with MAOIs. Clomipramine (Anafranil), an antidepressant also used to treat obsessive-compulsive disorder, which is available in Europe, Mexico, and Canada (should be released on US market in 1990) is also very toxic in combination with MAOIs. At least five weeks should intervene between stoppage of either clomipramine or fluoxetine and beginning any MAOI.

One systematic study of dietary noncompliance showed that although nearly 40% of 98 patients taking tranylcypromine acknowledged "cheating" on their restrictions, no serious complications ensued (Neil et al, 1979). A number of factors, including the amount of tyramine ingested, determine the likelihood of a hypertensive reaction. At least 6 mg is required to produce a moderate rise in blood pressure, which becomes progressively more severe as the amount of tyramine increases to 10 mg (Davidson et al, 1984). Quantities of more than 20 mg will produce a severe hypertensive reaction.

Little is gained by measuring platelet MAO activity while patients take these agents. The assay is generally not readily available and some researchers have found no significant relationships between clinical response and platelet MAO inhibition (Davidson and White, 1983). Also, White and colleagues (1983) found that MAO inhibition levels were not consistent and could vary with assay methodology, laboratory technique, and gender unmatched comparison groups.

For a number of years, physicians at the Massachusetts General Hospital have routinely used MAOIs as maintenance therapy for elderly patients who have received ECT for severe depressive disorders. Most of these patients are older than 60 years. To our knowledge, a hypertensive episode has not developed in a single patient; the overwhelming majority tolerate these agents very well. Tranylcypromine is our preferred MAOI for elderly patients because it is shorter-acting and, when discontinued, will be out of the patient's system

Table 4–7
Dietary and Drug Precautions for Patients Taking Monoamine Oxidase Inhibitors

Danger of Rise in Blood Pressure	Food and Drink	Drugs
Very dangerous	All cheese All foods containing cheese (eg, pizza, fondue, many Italian dishes, salad dressings) Broad bean pods (English, Chinese pea pods)	Cold medications (eg, Dristan, Contact) Nasal decongestants, sinus medicine Asthma inhalants Meperidine (Demerol) Amphetamines Indirect-acting sympathomimetic amines (eg, amphetamines, methylphenidate, phenylpropanolamine, ephedrine, cyclopentamine, pseudoephedrine, tyramine) Direct- and indirect-acting sympathomimetic amines (eg, metaraminol, phenylephrine) Buspirone (Buspar) Serotonergic antidepressants (fluoxetine, clomipramine)
Moderately dangerous	Sour cream All fermented or aged foods, especially aged meats or aged fish (eg, corned beef, salami, fermented sausage [pepperoni, summer sausage], pickled herring) Liver (chicken, beef, or pork) Liverwurst Meat or yeast extracts (eg, Bovril or Marmite) Spoiled or dry fruit (eg, spoiled bananas, figs, raisins) Red wine, sherry, vermouth, cognac Beer and ale	Allergy and hay fever medications Antiappetite (diet) medicine Direct-acting sympathomimetic amines (eg, epinephrine, isoproterenol, methoxamine, norepinephrine) Local anesthetics with epinephrine Levodopa for parkinsonism Dopamine

Minimally dangerous	Chocolate, anchovies, caviar, coffee, colas, sauerkraut, mushrooms, beet root (beets), rhubarb, curry powder, junket, Worcestershire sauce, soy sauce, licorice, snails*	Pure steroid asthma inhalants (eg, beclomethasone diproprionate [Vanceril]) Pure antihistamines (chlorpheniramine, brompheniramine) Other narcotics (eg, codeine) in lowered doses Local anesthetics without epinephrine (eg, mepivacaine [Carbocaine]) Diabetics taking insulin may have increased hypoglycemia requiring a decreased dose of insulin, but insulin is otherwise safe Patients on hypotensive agents for high blood pressure may have more hypotension, requiring a decrease in their use of hypotensive agent, which otherwise is safe
Safe	Fresh cottage cheese, cream cheese, yogurt in moderate amounts Baked products raised with yeast (eg, bread) Yeast Fresh fruits, except pineapple and avocados Other alcoholic drinks (eg, gin, vodka, whiskey, in true moderation)	

*These foods rarely have been reported to cause hypertensive reactions with MAOIs. The evidence supporting these claims is weak and often based on a single isolated case. Warnings based on such evidence have been uncritically perpetuated, especially in view of the large number of patients taking MAOIs who have eaten these foods with no problem. In practice, a blanket prohibition of these foods seems unjustified, unless they are clearly spoiled or decayed, except for specific patients in whom they have already caused symptoms.

Reproduced with permission from Jenike MA: Assessment and treatment of affective illness in the elderly. *J Geriatr Psychiatr Neurol* 1:89–107, 1988.

Table 4–8
Instructions for Patients Taking Monoamine Oxidase Inhibitors

Avoid all the food and drugs mentioned on the dietary restrictions list. Be particularly careful to avoid those foods and drugs that are considered moderately and very dangerous.

In general, avoid all foods that are decayed, fermented, or aged in some way. Avoid any aged food even if it is not on the list.

If you get a cold or flu, you may use aspirin or acetaminophen (Tylenol). For a cough, glycerin cough drops or *plain* Robitussin may be used.

All laxatives or stool softeners may be used for constipation.

All antibiotics, eg, penicillin, tetracycline, and erythromycin, may be safely used to treat infections.

Do not take other medications without first checking with me. This includes any over-the-counter medicines bought without prescription, eg, cold tablets, nose drops, cough medicines, diet pills.

Eating one of the restricted foods may cause a sudden elevation of your blood pressure. When this occurs, you get an explosive headache, particularly in the back of your head and temples. Your head and face will feel flushed and full, your heart may pound, and you may perspire heavily and feel nauseated.

If you need medical or dental care while on this medication, show these restrictions and instructions to the doctor. Have the doctor call my office if they have any questions or need further clarification or information.

Side effects such as postural lightheadedness, constipation, delay in urination, delay in ejaculation and orgasm, muscle twitching, sedation, fluid retention, insomnia, and excess sweating are quite common. Many of these side effects lessen considerably after the third week.

Lightheadedness may occur following sudden changes in position. This can be avoided by getting up slowly. If tablets are taken with meals, lightheadedness and the other side effects are lessened.

The medication is rarely effective in less than three weeks.

Care should be taken while operating any machinery or while driving, since some patients have episodes of sleepiness in the early phases of treatment with MAO inhibitors.

Take the medication precisely as directed. Do not regulate the number of pills without first consulting me.

In spite of the side effects and special dietary restrictions, your medication, an MAO inhibitor, is safe and effective when taken as directed.

If any special problems arise, call me at my office.

Reproduced with permission from Jenike MA: *Handbook of Geriatric Psychopharmacology.* Littleton, Mass, PSG Publishing Co, 1985, p 66.

within 24 hours. In contradistinction, phenelzine's effects may persist for over a week when discontinued (Goodman and Gilman, 1975). The usual starting dose of tranylcypromine is 10 mg twice daily and most elderly patients can be treated effectively on this dose, but some may require gradual increase to as much as 60 mg daily. Phenelzine should be started at 15 mg once daily and may need to be increased slowly to as high as 90 mg for some patients. One study with isocarboxazid (Marplan) demonstrated that depressed patients were more likely to improve on a daily dose of 50 mg when compared to 30 mg per day (Davidson and Turnbull, 1984); these were not elderly patients, however, so probably only patients who fail to improve at lower dosages should be increased to the higher range. There are no known long-term adverse effects of MAOIs, such as the tardive dyskinesia that occurs with chronic use of neuroleptics.

Clinicians frequently find that positive antidepressant effects of MAOIs begin to decrease over a few weeks. Full antidepressant effect can usually be regained by increasing the dose or, if the patient is already at the maximum dose, by stopping the medication completely for one or two weeks and restarting it.

Monoamine Oxidase Inhibitor Overdose

Mortality has been reported with large doses of tranylcypromine (170–650 mg), phenelzine (375–1,500 mg), and nialamide (5,000 mg) (Tollefson, 1983). After ingestion, there may be as much as a 12-hour lag period before clinical symptoms occur, and observation may be required for several days.

Clinically, patients become weak and may progress to agitation, confusion, tachypnea, hypertension, tachycardia, hyperthermia, miosis, increased deep tendon reflexes, involuntary movements, convulsions, headache, dizziness, chest pain, or coma and to a state of circulatory collapse. Because MAOIs may slow gut motility, gastric lavage may be helpful up to several hours after ingestion. Acidification of urine to pH 5 has been shown to markedly increase tranylcypromine excretion by as much as seven times. In contradistinction to heterocyclic agents, with which significant tissue stores and protein binding occur, hemodialysis has been associated with rapid recovery following intoxications with tranylcypromine or phenelzine (Tollefson, 1983).

Conclusions

The following conclusions may be drawn with regard to MAOIs:

(1) MAOIs are safe and effective for the elderly when certain simple precautions are taken;

(2) Give patients a list of foods to avoid (Table 4–7) and an instruction sheet (Table 4–8)—advise them not to take any medications that are not listed as safe on the instruction sheet unless they check with a physician;

(3) To lessen chances of insomnia, give the last dose of medication before 4 PM;

(4) Reasonable starting doses are 10 mg twice daily for tranylcypromine or 15 mg once daily for phenelzine—maintain elderly patients on this dose for at least one week and increase the dose slowly;

(5) Monitor blood pressure for orthostatic changes for at least six weeks, as recent evidence indicates that such changes may not be present

initially. Stop MAOI if symptoms of orthostatic changes (eg, dizziness, unsteadiness) develop; if the patient remains asymptomatic, MAOI does not have to be discontinued despite measured changes in blood pressure and pulse upon arising;

(6) If a hypertensive crisis develops, phentolamine, chlorpromazine, or labetalol can be used for rapid blood pressure control;

(7) Do not administer meperidine for pain relief to patients taking MAOIs—other narcotics can be used safely, but should be started at a lower than usual dosage.

Combined Heterocyclic–Monoamine Oxidase Inhibitor Treatment

For many years clinical wisdom dictated that heterocyclic agents and MAOIs should not be coadministered; but the results of contemporary studies suggested that the overall incidence and severity of side effects of combined use is no greater than that with either agent used alone (Tollefson, 1983). Ananth and Luchins (1977) reported combination therapy to be useful in refractory patients. In a large series, Gander (1965) reported that 62% of 157 depressed outpatients improved considerably when taking the combination, after all had proved unresponsive to one or more previous antidepressant trials (not detailed in the report). Others reported similar responses (Winston, 1971; Sethna, 1974; Halle, 1965; Zetin, 1982; White and Simpson, 1984). It has been suggested (Goldberg and Thornton, 1978) that MAOIs may increase levels of biogenic amines and that heterocyclics may alter receptor sensitivity and block amine reuptake, thus working in a synergistic manner to improve refractory depressions. There are little data on the use of combination treatments in the elderly, but we have had a few patients who responded well and did not have complications.

Current general guidelines for combined therapy include: proper dietary restrictions; avoidance of concurrent CNS stimulating agents; and preferential use of amitriptyline, trimipramine, or doxepin (White and Simpson, 1984) over imipramine, fluoxetine, or clomipramine. In addition, the heterocyclic agent should be started first or both drugs should be started together at low dosages and raised gradually over a matter of weeks (White and Simpson, 1984). Isolated fatalities have occurred when MAOI was started as the initial drug. If the patient is currently receiving a MAOI, at least a week without medication should precede introduction of the heterocyclic (Tollefson, 1983). Initial therapy should be started at lower dosages of both agents and maximal doses are often less than the routinely accepted upper therapeutic limits of either individual drug.

Three drugs (imipramine, clomipramine, and fluoxetine) have been associated with severe and sometimes fatal reactions when they were given in combination with MAOIs and their concomitant use should be strictly avoided until more information is available. One point of confusion about these danger-ous adverse reactions arises in distinguishing them from hypertensive crises. Rather than the striking elevations of blood pressure and complications of cerebrovascular accidents seen in those situations, the MAOI-heterocyclic interactions have primarily caused hyperthermia, agitation, delirium, convul-sions, and coma (White and Simpson, 1984). There is, in fact, accumulating evidence that patients receiving combined treatment may be less vulnerable to tyramine-mediated hypertensive crises than patients taking MAOIs alone, as suggested in theory by the ability of heterocyclics to inhibit neuronal uptake of monoamines such as tyramine and thus inhibit the tyramine pressor effect (White and Simpson, 1984).

As White and Simpson (1984) pointed out, alternatives for heterocyclic-resistant depression include ECT, MAOI alone, lithium, psychostimulants, or other antidepressants that belong to a class different than the failed drug. In addition, there is a large array of other promising combinations such as MAOI or heterocyclic with lithium, MAOI with L-tryptophan, tricyclic with thyroid medication, tricyclic with methylphenidate, etc. Also, other treatments such as sleep deprivation or phase shifting of sleep and photother-apy may prove to have a role in treating depressions in the elderly. The role of psychotherapy alone or in combination with medication is under study. The final niche for MAOI-heterocyclic combinations is yet to be determined, but it appears to have a place in the treatment of elderly patients with severe refractory depression.

Lithium

Therapeutic Uses

It is unusual for mania to occur initially after the age of 65 years, and most elderly patients who present in a manic state have a history of manic episodes (Jefferson, 1983). Only about 5% of patients admitted to psychogeriatric wards have manic episodes and of those elderly patients admitted for affective disorders, Roth (1955) found that 13% had predominantly manic symptoms.

The median age of onset for bipolar illness is 30 years; the risk of illness remains fairly high until the age of 50 and then decreases sharply. Almost 90% of all patients have onset before the age of 50 years (Angst et al, 1973). Early-onset bipolar disorder is an illness that usually continues into later life; so even though the initial onset of bipolar disorder may be rare after the age of 65, the bipolar population that eventually reaches old age will be substantial. The New York State Psychiatric Institute Lithium Clinic reported that about 20% of 200 active patients were older than 65 years (Dunner et al, 1979). As in younger patients, the primary uses of lithium in the elderly are to treat acute mania and prevent recurrent episodes in those with bipolar disorder. Lithium has also been used with some success for schizoaffective disorder and recurrent unipolar depression (Jefferson, 1983). The utility of lithium in treating acute depression is not well established although occasional lithium-responsive bipolar and unipolar depressives are reported (Jefferson, 1983). Lithium is not the drug of first choice for depression in elderly patients, but may be a useful adjuvant in tricyclic antidepressant-resistant unipolar depressed patients (see later section).

Based on little data, it appears that lithium is just as effective in the elderly as it is in younger patients. In patients with coexisting dementia, however, lithium is reportedly less effective and is associated with increased risk (Jefferson, 1983).

Special Precautions in the Elderly

The glomerular filtration rate (GFR) decreases with age (Rowe et al, 1976) and because lithium is almost exclusively excreted by the kidneys, dosage modification will be routinely required and in patients with renal disease, drastic reductions in dose will be needed. While the mean half-life of lithium is 18 hours in a 20-year-old person, it rises to 36 hours in a healthy 70 year old; with any renal disease the half-life may be markedly increased.

Compared to the young, elderly patients tend to have more acute and chronic diseases that can complicate lithium use. For example, superimposed renal disease not only impairs lithium excretion, but also may increase chances of lithium-induced nephrotoxicity. Dementing illnesses may sensitize a patient to lithium-induced neurotoxicity and also decrease ability to comply with dosing schedules (Himmelhoch et al, 1980). Cardiovascular disease may make patients vulnerable to fluid and electrolyte alterations and may increase risk of cardiotoxicity (Jefferson, 1983).

Elderly patients with more disease will be taking multiple medications. Not only will there be an increased incidence of side effects, but also it will be harder to establish which drug is responsible for which side effect. Also, compliance problems will increase and there will be an increased likelihood of adverse drug interactions.

Common Drug Interactions with Lithium

Because many elderly patients have idiopathic hypertension, thiazide diuretics are frequently taken in combination with lithium. They consistently cause decreased renal clearance of lithium and raise serum lithium levels. If a thiazide is added to ongoing lithium therapy, dosage will generally have to be lowered. Conversely, to avoid subtherapeutic levels, dosage may have to be increased when a thiazide is discontinued.

Nonsteroidal antiinflammatory drugs, such as indomethacin and phenylbutazone, have been reported to reduce lithium clearance and raise serum lithium levels by 25% to 60% (Jefferson and Marshall, 1981; Reimann and Frolich, 1981). It is unknown if other prostaglandin synthesis inhibitors cause a similar action.

Cases of patients with rare and probably idiosyncratic interactions have been reported with neuroleptics, neuromuscular blocking agents, antibiotics, methyldopa, and digitalis (Jefferson and Marshall, 1981). Definite recommendations await further data.

Before Lithium Is Started

It is important to consider causes of secondary mania. Onset at a late age and the absence of a family history of affective illness should make one suspicious of a medical cause for mania (Table 4–9). Medical causes that have been reported to produce the picture of mania include drugs (eg, levodopa and steroids), metabolic abnormalities, infection, neoplasm, and temporal lobe epilepsy (Krauthammer and Klerman, 1978).

Mania is also occasionally seen in previously depressed individuals who are being treated with tricyclic antidepressants or MAOIs. Some researchers believe that this represents the uncovering of an underlying bipolar disorder while others suggest that it is simply a true drug-induced side effect.

To rule out secondary mania, a detailed medical history should be supplemented by a physical examination and appropriate laboratory testing. Because of the potential pitfalls involved in treating the manic elderly patient, hospitalization for evaluation and treatment should be strongly considered—particularly if the patient lives alone or has concurrent medical illnesses.

Renal function must be evaluated prior to initiating lithium treatment. Because of the insensitivity of the serum creatinine test in the elderly, a determination of 24-hour creatinine clearance is a better test for evaluating GFR.

Table 4–9
Reported Cases of Secondary Mania

General Category	Specific Agent
Drugs	Corticosteroids
	Isoniazid
	Procarbazine
	Levodopa
	Bromide
Metabolic disturbance	Hemodialysis
	Postoperative state
Infection	Influenza
	Q Fever
	Post-St. Louis type A encephalitis
Neoplasm	Parasagittal meningioma
	Diencephalic glioma
	Suprasellar diencephalic tumor
	Benign speno-occipital tumor
Epilepsy	Right temporal focus

Adapted with permission from Krauthammer C, Klerman GL: Secondary mania. *Arch Gen Psychiatry* 35:1335, 1978.

Thyroid function should be evaluated by measuring serum levels of thyroxine (T4), L-triiodothyronine (T3), and thyroid-stimulating hormone (TSH). A baseline ECG is mandatory in all elderly patients. Without focal neurologic signs, there is no need to perform an EEG or computed tomography (CT) scan (Jefferson, 1983).

Starting Lithium Treatment

In the elderly it is important to initiate lithium therapy with a low dose and increase dosage slowly. Liptzin (1984) recommended beginning with a dose of 75 to 300 mg per day while Dunner and associates (1979) began with a 300-mg daily dose of lithium carbonate in all their healthy elderly manics. Doses of 75 mg can be obtained by using lithium citrate and doses of 150 mg, by breaking a 300-mg tablet in half.

The elimination half-life of lithium is prolonged with normal aging to as long as 36 hours or more (Jefferson, 1983). In patients with renal disease, lithium half-life may be greatly increased. In elderly manics, more frequent determinations of serum lithium levels are generally indicated to minimize the likelihood of toxicity but the clinician should remember that it may take more than a week after a dosage change to reach a steady-state plasma level (eg, four to five times a mean half-life of 36). To appropriately interpret serum lithium levels, they should be drawn 12 hours after the last dose. Unlike most other medications used in psychiatry, the oral dose of lithium is not an adequate guideline and blood levels are crucial for proper management. Therapeutic levels are still not clearly defined in the elderly. In general, they may respond to lower levels than those that are generally effective in younger patients. Foster and Rosenthal (1980) sought blood levels that were in the range of 0.4 to 0.7 mmol/L and did not exceed 0.7 mmol/L unless a very classic manic picture was present clinically.

Maintenance of Lithium

Serum lithium levels and clinical evaluations should be performed more frequently in the elderly as compared to a younger population. If the patient is compliant or is closely watched, he or she can be evaluated on a monthly basis for the first year of therapy. It is important that the patient and family be aware of the proper use and toxic side effects and that they are encouraged to contact the physician whenever questions arise. Psychiatrists should have a good working relationship with the patient's internist or general physician.

Side Effects and Toxicity

Some side effects of lithium are listed in Table 4–10. Patients with therapeutic levels may complain of tremor, urinary frequency, mild nausea, and a subjective feeling of "being medicated." Early signs of intoxication include increasing tremor, ataxia, weakness, slurred speech, blurred vision,

Table 4–10
Side Effects of Lithium

Neuromuscular	Nausea
General muscle weakness or	Vomiting
hyperexcitability	Diarrhea
Ataxia	Constipation
Tremor	Dry mouth
Choreoathetotic movements	Metallic taste
Hyperactive reflexes	
	Cardiovascular
Central nervous system	Irregular pulse
Incontinence of urine and feces	Decreased blood pressure
Slurred speech	ECG changes
Blurred vision	Bradycardia
Dizziness	Circulatory collapse
Vertigo	
Seizures	Miscellaneous
Difficulty concentrating	Polyuria
Confusion	Polydipsia
Somnolence or restlessness	Glycosuria
Stupor or coma	Dehydration
	Skin rash
Gastrointestinal	Weight loss or gain
Anorexia	Alopecia

Reproduced with permission from Jenike MA: *Handbook of Geriatric Psychopharmacology.* Littleton, Mass, PSG Publishing Co, 1985, p 72.

tinnitus, and drowsiness or excitement. Severe intoxication produces increased deep tendon reflexes, nystagmus, confusion, lethargy, and stupor which may progress to seizures and coma.

Bradyarrhythmia secondary to sinus node dysfunction occurs uncommonly with lithium therapy (Cassem, 1982). Measuring pulse routinely and asking about typical symptoms such as dizziness or fainting are necessary.

Extrapyramidal effects, particularly parkinsonian movements, have been reported with lithium use and the elderly may be more sensitive to such complications (Jefferson, 1983).

Lithium produces subtle cognitive changes in healthy young volunteers that may be more marked in the elderly. These can progress to the point where early senile dementia may be suspected (Judd et al, 1977).

There have been reports of acute worsening of eye lens opacification after lithium was started (Makeeva et al, 1974). The number of patients is small and this does not seem to be a common effect. Jefferson stated that lithium use in the elderly is not generally considered reason for periodic eye evaluation (Jefferson, 1983).

The elderly are prone to lithium intoxication because of reduced lithium clearance secondary to reduced renal function and because of increased sensitivity to the drug, more associated illnesses, multiple medications, poor compliance, decreased food and fluid intake, and lack of social supports. The presence of coexisting neurologic illness is the most critical predisposing factor, according to Himmelhoch and colleagues (1980).

Polyuria and polydipsia are so common that they can be considered routine. Thiazide diuretics can be used to decrease these symptoms when they are severe but the mechanism of this paradoxical response to diuretics remains unclear.

Propranolol hydrochloride in small doses (10–30 mg/day) may be used to treat lithium-induced tremor. Because propranolol may worsen cardiovascular status and induce depression, it should be used at the lowest possible dose (Liptzin, 1984).

Psychostimulants

Overview
Psychostimulants were used briefly as antidepressants until the advent of the tricyclics, at which time the latter became the first line of drugs in the treatment of depression (Myerson, 1936). Nonetheless, results of recent studies advocating their use in medically ill depressed patients (Kayton and Raskind, 1980; Hackett, 1978; Kaufmann et al, 1984; Woods et al, 1986), as adjuvants to morphine in the treatment of postoperative pain (Forest, 1977), and for adjustment reactions in patients recovering from chronic illnesses or surgical procedures (Hackett, 1978), have rekindled interest in the investigation of these agents. Silberman (1981), in a double-blind study of 18 endogenously depressed patients, demonstrated superiority of amphetamine over placebo in improving mood and psychomotor activity. Two studies have shown the effectiveness of methylphenidate in treating depressive symptoms in patients with concurrent dementia. In the first study (Holliday and Joffe, 1965), depressed patients with dementia responded better to methylphenidate than to the tricyclic antidepressant protriptyline. In the second (Kaplitz, 1975), methylphenidate was clearly superior to placebo in a double-blind eight-week study; and the methylphenidate group was free of significant side effects. Kaufmann and colleagues (Kaufmann et al, 1982 and 1984; Kaufmann, 1982) reported a number of patients with neurologic or medical disease who responded to psychostimulants.

Indications for Stimulants
Some indications for stimulants are listed in Table 4–11 (Kaufmann et al, 1982; Kaufmann, 1982). At Massachusetts General Hospital, stimulants such as methylphenidate or dextroamphetamine are frequently used to treat medically ill patients or elderly patients after surgery who are apathetic, withdrawn, or depressed. The following case is illustrative.

Table 4–11
Indications for Psychostimulants

---

1. Medically ill, apathetic, weakened patients, in whom depression may be easily masked by their concomitant illness
2. To facilitate the rehabilitation process in elderly patients with chronic illnesses, in whom poor compliance with ambulation requirements is frequently due to fatigue, lack of motivation, or anergia
3. Patients with dementia and coexistent retarded/depressive and/or abulic features
4. When electroconvulsive therapy is contraindicated or administratively difficult to perform; eg, if the patient is living in a nursing home
5. Depression with symptoms such as apathy, withdrawn behavior, dysphoria, decreased energy, loss of interest, and poor appetite

---

Adapted from Kaufmann MW, Cassem NH, Murray GB, et al: Use of psychostimulants in medically ill patients with neurological disease and major depression. *Can J Psychiatry* 26:46–49, 1984.

Mrs A is a 78-year-old woman who became profoundly psychomotorically retarded after gallbladder surgery. She was uncooperative, refused to eat or drink, and stated that she wanted to be left alone to die. A psychiatric consultant recommended treatment with methylphenidate, 10 mg twice daily. The day after this was begun she brightened considerably, ate and drank on her own, and even walked the corridor a few times. Methylphenidate was discontinued six days later and she was discharged from the hospital 12 days after her operation, in good spirits.

We also frequently find that stimulants are helpful for patients with abulia (lack of initiative) secondary to frontal lobe disease or in demented patients with coexistent retarded-depressive features. The following is an example of such a case (Kaufmann et al, 1984).

Mr B, a 70-year-old retired man who lived with his three sisters, was admitted to our inpatient psychiatric service because of increasing depression. He had no psychiatric history. During the year prior to admission, he stayed in bed most of the time with lack of interest in all activities. Approximately three months prior to admission, he began to experience dysphoria, but was not aware of any precipitating events. He denied suicidal ideation, but complained of anorexia with a 20-lb weight loss and noted a need for more sleep. He also had persistent fatigue, decreased energy, and constipation. About one month prior to admission, he started to urinate and have bowel movements in bed. For the two weeks before hospitalization, he refused to move or get out of bed. His sisters arranged for admission to a neurology service where findings of a complete neurologic and metabolic workup were negative except for clinical signs of recent memory impairment, poor concentration, episodic disorientation, and the CT scan which revealed marked frontal and temporal lobe atrophy. He was treated with doxepin, up to 200 mg daily, and transferred to our psychiatric unit with diagnoses of organic brain disease and retarded depression. After lack of significant improvement on doxepin, concurrent with some further deterioration of cognitive function as the dose was being raised, the medication was discontinued. He was then given a full course of ECT which normalized his eating and sleeping patterns. However, he remained dysphoric and abulic, and refused to get out of bed or even to wash and care for himself. A trial of low-dose haloperidol produced no improvement. While nursing home placement was being considered, a trial of methylphenidate, 5 mg three times a day, was started. Results were dramatic. The morning after methylphenidate was started, he got out of bed and washed and shaved himself. For the first time since admission, he started several conversations with patients, his mood became brighter, and he approached his ward physician with questions about discharge. This improvement persisted throughout the remainder of his hospitalization. However, impairment in his cognitive functioning, associated with chronic organic brain disease, did not improve. Nonetheless, he was discharged to his home. On six-month follow-up, there had been no relapse of depression, and he continued to take methylphenidate, 5 mg three times a day, with no side effects.

Alternatives to tricyclic antidepressants may be necessary in the treatment of depression in medically ill patients. The development of confusional states secondary to anticholinergic side effects and excessive sedation of some antidepressants has been discussed. Depressed patients with structurally compromised brain function who are undergoing treatment with tricyclic antidepressants may have a deficit of acetylcholine, and therefore may be especially vulnerable to these adverse reactions (Crook and Cohen, 1981).

Hackett described the usefulness of psychostimulants in diagnosing and effectively treating medically ill apathetic weakened patients in whom depression might be easily masked by their concomitant illness (Hackett, 1978). The rapid improvement in the physical and psychological symptomatology speeds up recovery, in some patients dramatically. This rapid response to treatment, usually within 24 to 48 hours, is of additional benefit for this type of patient, because concurrent medical illness makes it more of a hazard to wait 10 to 14 days for the tricyclic antidepressants to become clinically effective.

Psychostimulants may exert their antidepressant effects by blocking reuptake of catecholamines, thus prolonging the effects of synaptically released dopamine and norepinephrine (Brown, 1977).

The therapeutic use of amphetamine and methylphenidate for depression may not be legal in some jurisdictions and not considered acceptable in others. It is tempting to speculate from previous studies (Forest, 1977; Holliday and Joffe, 1965; Kaplitz, 1975; Myerson, 1936; Kayton and Raskind, 1980; Woods et al, 1986) that there is a wide margin of safety between therapeutic and toxic doses in patients in whom unwanted physical and psychologic side effects may appear. Further well-designed clinical studies are warranted to confirm these observations.

Dosage and Monitoring
Dextroamphetamine is roughly twice as potent as methylphenidate. Therapeutic effects are usually achieved with daily doses of 20 to 40 mg of methylphenidate or 10 to 20 mg of dextroamphetamine given orally in two divided doses, preferably 30 minutes before meals (Kaufmann, 1982). It is best to administer the last dose before 4 PM in order to avoid insomnia. If there is no therapeutic

response in 48 to 72 hours, the medication should be discontinued. Occasionally, some emotional lability may develop, at which point the dose may be reduced to 10 mg daily.

The duration of treatment is usually empirical and individualized to the clinical situation (Kaufmann, 1982; Kaufmann et al, 1984). For example, if the onset of depressive symptoms is recent, is of moderate intensity, and is associated with a concurrent medical illness, the stimulant might be needed for only one or two weeks. In other cases, if the symptoms are progressing in severity or there has been a relapse, treatment may be necessary for a few months.

Although no clinically significant alterations in blood, serum, or urinary parameters occur at therapeutic dosages, during prolonged therapy it is recommended that routine laboratory tests be performed on a regular basis. Vital signs, especially blood pressure, should be monitored in hypertensive patients (Kaufmann, 1982). Common drug interactions are listed in Table 4-12.

The response to methylphenidate in many patients illustrates three important issues: (1) the quick remission of symptoms following a small dose of stimulant, (2) the lack of toxic side effects, and (3) no recurrence of symptoms after stimulant was discontinued. Although stimulants are not a panacea, there are specific indications for their short-term use and they may be helpful on a chronic basis for abulic patients.

Potentiation by Lithium or Thyroid Hormone

As noted earlier, lithium may be a useful adjuvant in tricyclic antidepressant-resistant unipolar depression. DeMontigny and associates (1981) reported that eight such patients (aged 33 to 64) responded within 48 hours after low-dose lithium was added to the tricyclic regimen. In addition, Louie and Meltzer (1984) reported the cases of nine patients who were unresponsive to antidepressants alone and who were given lithium carbonate to potentiate the antidepressant.

Table 4–12
Drug Interactions with Stimulants

Drug	Effect
Guanethidine	Decreases hypotensive effects
Vasopressors	Increase pressor effect
Oral anticoagulants	Increase prothrombin time (methylphenidate only)
Phenobarbital, phenytoin, primidone	Increases anticonvulsant blood levels
Imipramine, desipramine	Increases antidepressant blood levels

Reproduced with permission from Jenike MA: *Handbook of Geriatric Psychopharmacology.* Littleton, Mass, PSG Publishing Co, 1985, p 76.

Two patients showed sustained improvement, two showed transient improvement but then relapsed, two others with a history of bipolar disorder became manic, and three did not respond. In their study, the time between the addition of lithium and improvement of depressive symptoms was frequently longer than what deMontigny and associates reported and ranged from 2 to 12 days. Kushnir (1986) reported successful lithium augmentation of an antidepressant in five elderly patients (mean age, 81 years; range 65–93 years). No significant complications were noted.

L-Triiodothyronine (T3) has also been reported to potentiate the effect of the tricyclics. Goodwin et al (1982) reported on six women and six men who were treated in a double-blind fashion for major depressive illness which did not respond to imipramine or amitriptyline, 150 to 300 mg/day, during periods ranging from 26 to 112 days. After the addition of 25 µg/day (ten patients) or 50 µg/day (two patients) of T3, nine patients showed statistically significant improvement in depression scores; in eight the response was marked. Improvement generally began within one to three days and was noted in all aspects of the depressive syndrome. Side effects were minimal and T3 did not change plasma levels of imipramine or desipramine or their ratio but did suppress thyroxine. The work of Goodwin and associates followed earlier uncontrolled reports of T3 acceleration of response to tricyclic antidepressants; results of five studies suggested that some depressed patients who were not responsive to tricyclics became responders when T3 was added (Earle, 1970; Ogura et al, 1974; Banki, 1975 and 1977; Tsutsui et al, 1979).

These adjuvants may be particularly helpful in treatment-resistant patients. Despite the well-established efficacy of tricyclic antidepressant agents (Baldessarini, 1977), results of controlled studies indicated that the rate of nonresponse or partial response is in the range of 20% to 35% (Goodwin et al, 1982; Klein and Davis, 1969). Goodwin and colleagues went so far in their report to suggest that a trial of a tricyclic antidepressant in a depressed patient should not be considered a failure until T3 potentiation has been tried.

Duration of Antidepressant Treatment

There are few available data on length of required treatment for the depressed patient who has been successfully treated with medication. A major difficulty for the practitioner has been the lack of satisfactory guidelines as to how long continuation drug treatment of depressive episodes must be maintained to ensure that the episode is over. Continuation of drug therapy after the acute symptoms are relieved is based on the assumption that antidepressant drugs can suppress depressive symptoms without immediately correcting the biological process or pathophysiology underlying the disorder. It is analogous to continuing antibiotic therapy for a number of days after acute signs of infection have resolved, to prevent a relapse. With depression, there may be a gap of several weeks or even months between the initial control of symptoms and the actual end of the episode. During this time, the patient may relapse if medication is discontinued.

The confusion about duration of drug continuation therapy often leads to either premature withdrawal of the drug and subsequent relapse or unnecessarily prolonged treatment. Results from a collaborative project of the National Institute of Mental Health (NIMH) provided the first study-derived guidelines on the optimal length of continuation therapy (Prien and Kupfer, 1986). The authors of this report noted that the need for continuation therapy is supported by a number of studies and they described six studies in particular: in each, an antidepressant was used to control acute symptoms, after which about half of the patients were switched to placebo and the other half continued to receive antidepressant medication. Patients were then observed for 2 to 8 months. A high relapse rate for patients receiving placebo demonstrated their continued vulnerability for months following apparent recovery. They noted that it is possible that some of the patients who relapsed after they were switched to placebo had a new episode rather than a continuation of the old episode, but they doubted that this was usually the case as most of the relapses occurred relatively rapidly, within 1 week to 2 months following discontinuation of active medication. Also, reemergence of symptoms after withdrawal of medication apparently was independent of the frequency of prior episodes.

The decision to continue medication is complicated by the fact that it is not known whether drugs eventually correct the postulated underlying disorder, thereby shortening the episode, or merely suppress symptoms until the episode runs its natural course. When continuation therapy is effective, it may be difficult to determine when the episode is over on the basis of symptoms alone. Decisions about the length of continuation treatment must take into account the risks and consequences of a relapse as well as the risks and side effects associated with long-term pharmacotherapy.

In an attempt to answer some of the above questions, the NIMH coordinated a five-center study of patients with primary major depressive or manic disorder. The study consisted of two phases, the preliminary phase (to control acute symptoms) and the long-term preventive phase (to evaluate the need for long-term treatment). The preventive phase was the major experimental phase of the study and consisted of a two-year double-blind comparison of three drug treatments and a placebo. Initially, acute symptoms were treated with the psychiatrist's choice of medication. After acute symptoms were controlled, the patient received continuation treatment with maintenance doses of the combination of imipramine and lithium. The maintenance dose of imipramine ranged from 75 mg to 150 mg/day, depending on patient tolerance, and the serum lithium level was targeted at 0.6 to 0.9 mEq/L.

Once patients had been stable while taking imipramine and lithium for at least two consecutive months and had returned to baseline functioning, they were assigned to long-term preventive treatments consisting of continuation of the imipramine-lithium combination, imipramine alone, lithium alone, or placebo. Placebo was used only with patients who had unipolar disorder because it was considered to be an unethical long-term treatment for those with bipolar disorder. Relapses were treated ad lib by a psychiatrist who was not involved in the study and, after recovery from relapse, subjects were reassigned to their original double-blind medication regimen.

This NIMH study found that 17 (23%) of 72 patients relapsed within the first eight weeks of double-blind treatment. Relapse occurred in 13 (38%) of the 34 placebo-treated patients as compared with 4 (11%) of the 38 patients who continued to receive the imipramine-lithium combination, a significant difference. Of interest was the finding that the patients receiving imipramine only did not have significantly different relapse rates from those patients receiving the imipramine-lithium combination. In the group that received lithium only, however, the relapse rate (38%) was identical to that for the placebo-treated group. These results indicated that imipramine was the critical drug in the imipramine-lithium combination for controlling the episode and preventing relapse and was equally as effective as the lithium-imipramine combination. For the placebo-treated group, relapse was related to the length of time the patient was symptom-free before assignment to double-blind treatment; patients who were symptom-free for at least 16 weeks before receiving placebo had a significantly lower rate of relapse (18%) than patients who were free of symptoms for less than 16 weeks (59%). Patients who were symptom-free for 16 weeks or more before double-blind assignment did no worse with placebo than with the combination treatment.

The results of this multicenter study supported the hypothesis that antidepressant medication can control overt symptoms without immediately curing the episode. Substitution of placebo for active medication resulted in a rapid return of symptoms in a significant number of patients who had no symptoms on the day of withdrawal from active drug. Results of this study suggested that patients should be free of significant symptoms for 16 to 20 weeks before treatment is discontinued. In addition, the first eight weeks following discontinuation of active medication constitutes the period of highest risk for relapse; 71% of those who relapsed during the two years following withdrawal of active therapy did so during this period.

Antidepressant medication should be continued for four or five months after resolution of acute depressive symptoms and clinicians should have frequent contact with the patient during the first two months after discontinuing antidepressant medication because of the chance of relapse.

Electroconvulsive Therapy

Overview
ECT, as practiced today, is the electrical induction of a series of grand mal seizures, usually six to ten, in patients with susceptible psychiatric disorders,

primarily severe depression. The seizure itself, rather than the electrical stimulus, is the therapeutic agent. The technique of ECT has been refined over the past few decades, and today the use of anticholinergic premedication, short-acting barbiturates for anesthesia, muscle relaxants, oxygenation, low-energy stimulus wave forms, and unilateral stimulus electrode placement have all acted to decrease the risks and side effects without diminishing its therapeutic efficacy (Jenike, 1984b; Weiner, 1982).

ECT is typically given every other day, three times a week, in order to minimize brain dysfunction. If there is significant confusion, memory loss, or behavior change, all of which tend to increase with the number of treatments, the interval between treatments may be extended.

When it was initially introduced in 1938, ECT represented the first line of treatment, not only for depression but also for schizophrenia (Weiner, 1982). With the advent of antidepressant medication in the 1950s, the use of ECT began to decline. Although these drugs are not as effective as ECT, they are more convenient and do not involve a procedure whose mere mention can be frightening to many patients and their families. During the last decade, the use of ECT has stabilized at approximately 80,000 patients per year in this country (Electroconvulsive Therapy, American Psychiatric Association Task Force on ECT, 1978).

ECT may be the only choice of treatment in the elderly depressed patient whose illness is accompanied by self-destructive behavior, such as suicide attempts or refusal to eat, or in patients who have become catatonic or stuporous from severe depression when a drug trial lasting four to six weeks may be associated with significant risk. In these patients, ECT, which characteristically begins to exert significant beneficial effects within the first week, may be dramatically lifesaving.

Depression is common in all age groups, but ECT is used to a greater extent in the elderly. This is because depression is more likely to be severe in the older patient, and also because the elderly are more likely to have concurrent chronic diseases for which antidepressant drugs may be less desirable due to their anticholinergic, cardiotoxic, and hypotensive effects (Weiner, 1982).

ECT is both more effective and faster-acting than drugs in the treatment of depression. Many depressed elderly patients, especially those with psychotic symptoms, do not respond to drugs but do respond to ECT. In one study, for example, remission occurred in 80% to 85% of drug nonresponders (Scovern and Kilmann, 1980). ECT has consistently outperformed tricyclic antidepressants and MAOIs with 10% to 20% more patients showing improvement. Not only is ECT more effective than pharmacologic agents, but also it may be safer for those patients with serious illness, particularly that involving cardiac dysfunction.

During the ECT itself, a number of physiologic events occur in the body centrally and peripherally (Banazak et al, 1989). In addition to simultaneous parasympathetic and sympathetic discharge resulting in elevation of blood pressure and tachycardia, ECT also alters the neurotransmitter and neuroendocrine systems. Results of animal studies demonstrated that ECT decreases the number of rat cerebral cortex beta-adrenergic receptors and increases brain norepinephrine (Bergstron and Kellar, 1979). In contrast, ECT increases rat mesolimbic, striatal, pituitary, and hypothalamic postsynaptic dopamine responsiveness (Modigh et al, 1984); serotonin-type 2 receptor density (Kellar et al, 1981); and rat brain acetylcholine and gamma-aminobutyric acid (GABA) (Atterwill, 1984).

Efficacy Studies in the Elderly
Banazak and colleagues (1989) reviewed the small number of studies of the use of ECT in the elderly.

Karlinsky and Shulman (1984) reported that 14 (42%) of 33 depressed older patients had immediate remission of all symptoms while 12 patients (36%) showed partial relief. At follow-up of six months 23 patients (69%) had not required rehospitalization and 11 (33%) of them remained free of symptoms.

Avery and Winokur (1977) found that in patients over the age of 60, 45% had symptom alleviation with ECT while 57% had marked improvement with ECT plus antidepressant treatment.

Glassman and associates (1975) used ECT to treat psychotic depression in ten imipramine nonresponders, nine of whom showed total symptom remission after ECT.

Gaspar and Samarasinghe (1982) found that 26 (79%) of 33 elderly patients were able to return home free of depressive symptoms after ECT and Burke and colleagues (1987) reported complete resolution of depression using ECT in 30 (75%) of 40 depressed patients.

The bulk of the data as well as our anecdotal experience indicates that ECT is both safe and effective for the treatment of affective illness in the elderly.

Risks and Side Effects
The mortality with the use of ECT has been estimated at around 1/25,000 patients. According to a review of available literature (Banazak et al, 1989), elderly patients experiencing ECT-related deaths most frequently expire as a result of cardiac complications such as myocardial infarction or cardiac vessel thrombosis. These cardiac deaths appear to be associated with preexisting atherosclerotic heart disease, congestive heart failure, left ventricular hypertrophy, and left bundle branch block. Besides cardiac complications, Ehrenberg and Gullingsrud (1955) described the cases of two patients in their series of possible ECT-related deaths who died of pneumonia eight days to two weeks after ECT. Fatal cerebral hemorrhage and fat embolism have been described in elderly patients treated with ECT (MacClay, 1952; Barker and Baker, 1959). Overall mortality with ECT is probably considerably less than that associated

with any of the drugs indicated in the treatment of depression (Fink, 1979; Weiner, 1982).

Of nonfatal complications of ECT, cardiovascular events are most frequently reported (Feldman et al, 1946). Feldman and colleagues (1946) found that although 33 patients had preexisting cardiovascular pathology, only one patient had worsening of congestive failure and atrial fibrillation and Gaspar and Samarasinghe (1982) found no instances of cardiac or respiratory arrest or hypotension in 384 treatments. One patient, with apparently normal cardiac parameters, had a nonfatal myocardial infarction after the third ECT (Mielke et al, 1984). Alexopoulos and associates (1984) compared 199 geriatric patients to 94 younger controls and found that cardiovascular side effects developed in 18 (9%) of the elderly patients compared to none of the controls. Most complications remitted with medication treatment.

Summarizing seven studies of ECT in the elderly, which included the ones just mentioned, Banazak et al (1989) found that in nearly 10% of 407 elderly patients who received ECT some type of nonlethal cardiac complication developed and about half of the complications were arrhythmias (atrial fibrillation, tachycardia, premature ventricular contraction—bigeminy and trigeminy). Transient hypertension constituted about 25% of cardiac difficulties while hypotension was problematic in 10%. In their collective sample of 407 patients, four patients evidenced ECT-related myocardial ischemia and one had a myocardial infarction during ECT. Congestive heart failure developed in two patients. These data point out the importance of identifying cardiac disease prior to ECT and also the need for skilled medical personnel during and after the ECT procedures.

Clinically, ECT is commonly associated with confusion and temporary amnesia, and physiologically, by slowing on EEG. Even though some patients complain of mild memory loss for months or even years after receiving ECT, objective memory testing in such patients does not appear to bear out the presence of an organic defect. No studies have documented any significant irreversible pathologic changes in the brain (Weiner, 1982). Most ECT patients do not consider themselves affected by persistent memory deficits, and they tend to view their treatments as no more upsetting than a visit to the dentist (Hughes et al, 1981).

Insulin-dependent diabetes mellitus is reportedly more difficult to control when diabetic patients are concomitantly depressed (Kronfol et al, 1981; Crammer and Gillies, 1981). If insulin levels are adjusted upward while a patient is depressed, sugars should be carefully monitored during and after treatment of the depression. The following case report describes an elderly insulin-dependent diabetic woman who had significantly lowered blood sugars after ECT (Normand and Jenike, 1984, reproduced with permission).

A 73-year-old woman with a 20-year history of insulin-dependent diabetes mellitus was admitted to our inpatient psychiatric service for treatment of a psychotic depression. She was suffering from insomnia, decreased appetite with a 10 pound weight loss in the last few months, agitation, and paranoia. She believed that her food was being poisoned and that she was being punished for past sins. She had recently been treated with maprotiline, thiothixene, and lithium citrate without effect. Her history included three episodes of depression (the last one three years prior to this admission) which were clinically similar to the present episode and did not respond to medication but did resolve completely after ECT.

On this admission she refused ECT and thus guardianship proceedings were begun. She consumed a 1,500-calorie diet (American Diabetic Association) throughout this hospitalization. Blood sugar levels remained above 80 mg/dL for the next two weeks prior to starting ECT, on 15 to 30 units of NPH insulin each morning. Two weeks after admission, ECT was begun and administered at most every other day until six treatments had been given. She received 20 units NPH and 5 units regular insulin on each day that she did not receive ECT. Since she was given nothing by mouth on ECT mornings, the insulin dose was lowered to 10 units NPH in the morning with 5 units in the afternoon on days she received ECT.

Her mood improved markedly and delusions abated; however, she was intermittently confused and disoriented. The confusion was initially attributed to ECT, but two blood sugar levels measured between the fourth and fifth ECT treatments were at 78 and 58 mg/dL—lower than any pre-ECT levels at our hospital. Insulin was discontinued and over the next three days sugar levels remained between 100 to 200 mg/dL with only 5 units of regular insulin each afternoon. Her confusion resolved despite another ECT treatment. Over the next week, the sugar levels gradually rose to almost 400 mg/dL and insulin was restarted. A few weeks later she was discharged euthymic on 15 units NPH insulin each morning with well-controlled sugar levels.

There are earlier reports of elderly depressed patients whose blood sugars fell after ECT and one group (Fakhri et al, 1980; Fakhri, 1966) even suggested that ECT may be a cure for diabetes mellitus. In all of the diabetics that responded to ECT, however, the diabetes was of recent onset and noninsulin-dependent. All of the patients were depressed clinically and the primary indication for ECT was treatment of the depression. It is now well documented (Carroll et al, 1981; Jenike, 1982a) that many endogenously depressed nondiabetic patients have abnormally high plasma cortisol concentrations 24 hours after a dose of dexamethasone. These patients also have high concentrations of ACTH and corticosteroids (Butler and Besser, 1968; Sachar et al, 1973). Perhaps Fakhri's "diabetics" who responded to ECT were actually endogenously depressed and their hyperglycemia and glycosuria were secondary to the diabetogenic effects of increased ACTH and corticosteroids (Jenike, 1982a).

It has been shown that after ECT, the ACTH and corticosteroid levels return to normal, which may in time bring the blood glucose level back to normal and could account for the amelioration of the apparent diabetes. Kronfol and associates (1981) alternatively suggested that the blood sugar level may be driven up in depression by elevated levels of growth hormone, an insulin antagonist. Baldessarini (1981), however, described conflicting results from different studies on growth hormone levels during depression. The Kronfol group also wondered if increased epinephrine secretion during depression could account for insulin resistance; however, Crammer and Gillies (1981) measured urinary vanillylmandelic acid excretion (a measure of peripheral epinephrine turnover) on two occasions in one patient and it was normal. Even though mechanisms remain speculative, the weight of the evidence indicates that blood sugar levels and insulin requirements of depressed insulin-dependent diabetics are lowered after a course of ECT. If blood sugar levels are not carefully monitored and insulin dosage reduced accordingly, levels may become dangerously low, producing a clinical picture that may resemble the mental status changes occasionally occurring after ECT.

In ECT therapy, it is the electrical stimulus, not the seizure itself, that is the component most responsible for the side effects of confusion and transient loss of memory. One study involving 29 patients (mean age, 73 years) showed that electrical stimuli given only over the nondominant hemisphere produced therapeutic results comparable to bilateral stimulation (Fraser and Glass, 1978 and 1980). The degree of postictal confusion, however, was much greater for those receiving bilateral ECT, indicating that the acute cerebral impairment was less in those patients who received unilateral, nondominant stimulation.

Even though there are really no absolute contraindications to ECT, there are certain conditions in which a marked increase in associated morbidity and mortality may be seen (Electroconvulsive Therapy, American Psychiatric Association Task Force on ECT,. 1978; Fink, 1979). These include recent myocardial infarction or stroke, severe hypertension, and the presence of an intracerebral mass. In these patients, ECT should generally be delayed until effective medical management has been initiated or until adequate recovery time has elapsed. If ECT is urgently indicated, however, appropriate premedication and close monitoring can help to minimize risk.

PSYCHOTIC DEPRESSION

Disability

It is estimated that depressed patients account for 30% to 40% of the admissions to acute care psychiatric hospitals in the United States, and that patients who are delusionally depressed account for at least 5% of the admissions to such hospitals (Spiker et al, 1985). Patients who are psychotically depressed have much longer lengths of hospitalization with an average of about 50 to 60 days (Brown et al, 1982; Frances et al, 1981). Spiker and colleagues (1985), in a retrospective chart review at one psychiatric institution, found that delusionally depressed patients were unable to perform their usual daily activities for an average duration of 47.6 weeks before they were admitted to the hospital. These patients also had a higher risk of suicide than nonpsychotically depressed patients. Thus, psychotic depression has major social and economic implications for patients, their families, and society in general.

Treatment

There is some controversy about how delusionally depressed patients should be treated. Current dogma is that these patients should be treated with both neuroleptic and antidepressant medication. However, occasional studies have shown that some delusionally depressed patients improve with antipsychotic medication alone and others with a tricyclic alone. In most of the studies, response rates were less than 50% and some of them have been criticized because not enough medication was given and patients were not treated for a sufficiently long period of time.

In an effort to clarify this issue, Spiker and colleagues (1985) investigated the pharmacological treatment of delusional depression by assigning patients, in a random double-blind trial, to the antidepressant amitriptyline (Elavil) alone, to the antipsychotic agent perphenazine (Trilafon) alone, or to a combination of the two. They found that 14 (78%) of the 18 patients assigned to both amitriptyline and perphenazine were responders, compared to 7 (41%) of 17 patients treated with amitriptyline alone and 3 (19%) of the 16 patients treated with perphenazine alone. Their study demonstrated that the combination of amitriptyline and perphenazine was superior to the use of either drug alone.

Spiker and colleagues also noted that it is known that phenothiazines raise the plasma level of tricyclic antidepressants and found, in fact, that their patients who were also taking perphenazine had higher levels of amitriptyline plus nortriptyline, the metabolite of amitriptyline. However, analysis of variance (ANOVA) controlling for amitriptyline plus nortriptyline plasma levels as a covariate showed that amitriptyline plus perphenazine was still the superior treatment, independent of the increased amitriptyline plus nortriptyline plasma levels seen in the patients taking the combination treatment. In reference to comments in the literature suggesting that tricyclic antidepressants should not be given to depressed patients who were delusional, they found that none of their amitriptyline nonresponders became more psychotic as measured on a number of rating scales.

The study of Spiker and colleagues (1985) demonstrated that although there were clearly some patients who responded to amitriptyline alone or to perphenazine alone, the combination was the treatment of choice. Whether the efficacy of combining an antidepressant and antipsychotic drug to treat patients with a delusional depression holds only for these two drugs or whether it applies equally to other medications remains to be determined. Clearly, as noted earlier in this chapter, amitriptyline would be a poor choice of medication in the elderly because of its high level of anticholinergic potency and also its tendency to induce orthostatic hypotension. It is likely that other antidepressants combined with neuroleptics would have similar effects in delusionally depressed elderly patients. This, in fact, has been our clinical experience over the past ten years.

Many patients with extremely disabling delusional depression are begun immediately on a course of ECT.

Hallucinations

Hallucinations occur in all sensory modalities, with auditory hallucinations by far the most common. Hallucinations, among other perceptual disturbances, may be very hard to evaluate for there are few objective signs associated with them; the presence of other associated signs and symptoms is usually required to establish a specific diagnosis. Common clinical wisdom suggests that the less formed the hallucinations are, the more likely they are due to biochemical or neurologic causes, while the more formed, describable and prolonged hallucinations probably denote a functional psychiatric disorder (Ludwig, 1980). This in not invariably the case, however.

There are a few case reports of elderly patients identified by the clinical association of musical hallucinations and acquired hearing loss (Ross et al, 1975; Hammeke et al, 1983; Miller and Crosby, 1979; Aizenberg et al, 1987). The hallmark of this group is the lack of psychopathology and advanced age. In two such patients, Aizenberg and associates (1987) recently found regional brain atrophy on CT scan and a degree of hearing loss. The association of hearing loss and musical hallucinations to dysphoria (Eastwood et al, 1985; Gilhome-Herbst and Humphrey, 1980) and nonpsychotic depression (Aizenberg et al, 1986) have been described. Salicylate-induced musical hallucinations in an elderly woman with otosclerosis is an example of the clinical constellation of hearing loss and drug effect in an elderly patient (Allen, 1985). These cases would suggest that formal musical hallucinations associated with deafness and/or depression are more common than generally appreciated (Aizenberg et al, 1986).

CHOLINERGIC ALTERATIONS IN ALZHEIMER'S DISEASE

When treating affective illness in patients with Alzheimer's disease and probably many other dementing illnesses, abnormalities of the cholinergic system must be considered (Jenike, 1988a). Involvement of the cholinergic system with memory is based on a number of findings:

(1) Anticholinergic drugs, such as scopolamine, induce memory deficits in healthy young subjects similar to those observed in nondemented elderly subjects;

(2) These deficits are reversed by physostigmine, a cholinomimetic agent that potentiates synaptic acetylcholine;

(3) Cholinergic drugs such as tetrahydroaminoacridine (THA), arecho-line, and physostigmine improve aspects of learning and memory in normal subjects;

(4) Cholinergic neurons (in nucleus basalis of Meynert) are found to be selectively destroyed early in the course of the illness in the brains of patients with Alzheimer's disease;

(5) The activity of choline acetyltransferase, which catalyzes the synthesis of acetylcholine, is reduced in brain tissue obtained from patients with Alzheimer's disease (Bartus et al, 1982; see chapter 5).

In normal subjects, experimental manipulations of the cholinergic system have supported the idea that it is involved in memory. Drachman and Leavitt (1974) used an anticholinergic agent, scopolamine, to produce measurable memory deficits in young normal subjects and demonstrated that these deficits could be reversed by intravenously administered physostigmine, a cholinomimetic agent, but not by the nonspecific activation of amphetamine. Drachman and Sahakian (1980) later demonstrated that a single subcutaneous injection of physostigmine improved memory and other cognitive functions in normal elderly subjects. Also, Davis and colleagues (1978) demonstrated improvement after the administration of physostigmine in long-term memory processes in normal humans. Agnoli and associates (1983) showed a correlation among the degree of memory loss, intellectual impairment, the quantity of senile plaques, and a decrease in choline acetyltransferase and acetylcholinesterase activity in patients affected by Alzheimer's disease. In this study, patients were subjected to a series of computerized EEG recordings and neuropsychological evaluations after acute administration of a number of cholinergic drugs, including physostigmine, and anticholinergic drugs (scopolamine and orphenadrine). Their results showed that the acute administration of some cholinergic drugs improved memory and also attention performances, whereas anticholinergic drugs induced opposite effects. In addition, the cholinergic drugs exhibited a tendency to shift the EEG spectrum analysis into more normal patterns compatible with the patient's age. Results of this study further supported the view that the cholinergic system plays an important role in the memory and attention disturbances found in patients with Alzheimer's disease.

Francis and co-workers (1985) studied acetylcholine synthesis by measuring the incorporation of radiolabeled glucose into the transmitter in temporal-cortex specimens obtained at diagnostic craniotomy in 17 young patients with Alzheimer's disease (mean age, 59; SD = ±5). They found that synthesis of acetylcholine was significantly negatively correlated with cognitive impairment and they believed that these results were consistent with the view that the deficit in the presynaptic cholinergic system is a relatively early change in the development of clinical features of the disease.

The loss of cholinergic markers is consistently found in patients with

Alzheimer's disease, whereas other neurochemical markers are usually decreased to a lesser extent and not as consistently (Terry and Davies, 1980; Davies, 1979; Cross et al, 1981), especially early in the course of the illness. In addition, quantitative measurements of cholinergic cell loss correlate with an increase in the number of senile plaques and a reduction in memory function (Perry et al, 1978).

These alterations in the cholinergic system help to explain why some dementing patients are exquisitely sensitive to the anticholinergic side effects of medications. Such patients should be treated with the least anticholinergic drugs available.

CARDIAC PATIENTS

Physicians probably allow many moderately severe depressions to go untreated because of unwarranted fears about cardiac side effects of antidepressants. Cassem (1982) reviewed relevant issues in detail and concluded that when certain precautions are taken, antidepressants can generally be safely used even in very ill cardiac patients.

There are four main side effects that are of particular concern in using antidepressants in cardiac patients: (1) orthostatic hypotension, (2) anticholinergic effects, (3) cardiac conduction effects, and (4) decreased cardiac contractility. These will be reviewed individually.

Orthostatic Hypotension

Postural changes in blood pressure occur commonly with antidepressant agents. Tertiary amine tricyclics (eg, amitriptyline, imipramine), with the exception of doxepin (Neshkes et al, 1986), tend to cause more severe hypotensive effects than secondary amines (eg, nortriptyline, desipramine). With tricyclics, the best clinical predictor of drug-induced postural hypotension is orthostatic fall in blood pressure before drug administration. Cassem (1982) estimated that in patients with a mean decrease in lying-to-standing systolic blood pressure of 10 mm Hg before drug administration, the mean orthostatic change in patients taking imipramine will be about 25 mm Hg. It is not known whether such conclusions can be drawn for the newer nontricyclic antidepressants or for the MAOIs.

Newer agents such as amoxapine, maprotiline, and trazodone appear to offer no advantage in avoiding orthostatic hypotension (Cassem, 1982). Roose and colleagues (1987) found that orthostatic hypotension not only occurred significantly more frequently with imipramine than with nortriptyline but also was more common in patients with heart disease.

Orthostatic hypotension is one of the primary side effects of MAOIs. It is not believed to be dose-dependent and has usually been described as an early side effect. That is, it was thought that if patients tolerated the first few days of medication, then hypotension would rarely necessitate stopping the drug. As noted earlier, however, these concepts are not correct. Kronig and associates (1983) studied 14 patients (mean age, 52 years) who were treated with phenelzine and found that the mean orthostatic drop increased with time in a generally linear fashion and that the maximum mean orthostatic drop was 12 mm Hg at week 4. It also appeared, from their data, that the elderly were no more likely to have severe orthostatic changes than were younger patients. The consequences, however, of a decrease in blood pressure in an old person are much more likely to be serious.

Lithium therapy is not associated with orthostatic hypotension.

Anticholinergic Effects

Anticholinergic potency can be quantified (Table 4–13) (Snyder and Yamamura, 1977; Richelson, 1982). The cardiac effect of most concern is tachycardia. In general, tertiary amines are more potent anticholinergic agents than secondary amines, with amitriptyline significantly exceeding all other tricyclics (Cassem, 1982). Those cardiac patients with ischemic disease are least able to tolerate an increase in heart rate.

Amoxapine and maprotiline offer little improvement over earlier tricyclics in terms of anticholinergic properties. Trazodone, however, has no anticholinergic effects and may be useful in patients who are at risk from tachycardia.

Table 4–13
Anticholinergic Potency of Some Psychotropic Agents

Agent	Richelson (1982)*	Snyder and Yamamura (1977)†
Atropine	55	0.4
Trihexyphenidyl (Artane)	—	0.6
Benztropine (Cogentin)	—	1.5
Amitriptyline (Elavil)	5.5	10
Protriptyline (Vivactil)	4.0	—
Doxepin (Sinequan)	1.3	44
Imipramine (Tofranil)	1.1	78
Nortriptyline (Aventyl)	0.7	—
Desipramine (Norpramin)	0.5	170
Maprotiline (Ludiomil)	0.2	—
Amoxapine (Asendin)	0.1	—
Trazodone (Desyrel)	0.003	—
Phenelzine (Nardil)	—	100,000

*The larger the number, the greater the anticholingeric effect.
†The smaller the number, the greater the anticholinergic effect.
Reproduced with permission from Jenike MA: *Handbook of Geriatric Psychopharmacology.* Littleton, Mass, PSG Publishing Co, 1985, p 79.

One great advantage of the MAOIs is their essential lack of anticholinergic side effects (Table 4–13) (Jenike, 1984a). No regular changes in cardiac rhythm have been associated with the MAOIs, even in overdose patients.

Lithium also has no anticholinergic effects and does not produce tachycardia (Cassem, 1982).

Decreased Contractility

It is a frequent fear that tricyclics may induce congestive heart failure because of their negative ionotropic effect. In reviewing the data, Cassem (1982) noted that most early studies employed indirect measurements of cardiac function, such as systolic time intervals, which could have reflected slowing of AV conduction commonly produced by tricyclics rather than decreased contractility. Veith et al (1982), using radionuclide ventriculograms to measure ejection fractions in vivo before and during maximum exercise in depressed patients with heart disease who were taking therapeutic doses of imipramine and doxepin, demonstrated no adverse effects on left ventricular function.

Glassman and colleagues (1983) also studied a group of depressed patients with clinically significant preexisting left ventricular dysfunction by means of radionuclide angiography. Of 15 patients in their study, 13 had ejection fraction values that were more than two standard deviations below normal control values. They found that therapeutic levels of imipramine did not further impair left ventricular performance and that ejection fraction was unchanged during treatment.

There is also no evidence that the newer nontricyclic agents, lithium, or the MAOIs affect cardiac contractility.

Cardiac Conduction Effects

Tricyclics slow conduction in the His bundle and Purkinje fibers with ECG manifestations including increased PR, QRS, and QT_c intervals as well as a decrease in T-wave amplitude (Cassem, 1982; Moss, 1986). This effect appears to be correlated with anticholinergic activity with trazodone causing the least slowing (Gomoll and Byrne, 1979; Hayes et al, 1983). This can exacerbate preexisting ventricular conduction deficits (Rudorfer and Young, 1980).

At one time it was thought that there was no relationship between the initial PR and QRS intervals and drug-related change after starting imipramine (Giardina et al, 1979). That is, patients with preexisting prolonged PR or QRS interval were not thought to have any greater likelihood of cardiac changes than those with an initially short PR or QRS interval. Results of a recent study (Roose et al, 1987), however, indicated that there may be an increased risk and that these patients should be followed carefully with serial ECGs. In this study, the prevalence of second-degree AV block was significantly greater in patients with preexisting bundle-branch block (9%) than in patients with normal electrocardiograms (0.7%).

Prolongation of the QT interval is associated with an increased likelihood of drug-induced malignant ventricular arrhythmias (Moss, 1986). Although this is rare with tricyclic-induced prolongation, caution is required if the corrected QT interval exceeds 0.44 milliseconds. The QT interval is measured from the earliest onset of the QRS complex to the terminal portion of the T wave, where it meets the isoelectric baseline. A consensus regarding the optimal lead for QT measurement does not exist, but it is usually measured in lead II. Since the QT interval is influenced by autonomic tone and heart rate, measurement should be made during a resting state. The QT interval bears an inverse relationship with heart rate, and several formulas are available for correcting the QT interval for heart rate (Moss, 1986); the most widely used algorithm is the Bazett equation, in which the corrected QT interval is calculated by dividing the measured QT interval by the square root of the preceding R-R interval in seconds. In patients with normal QRS durations, QT values longer than 0.44 milliseconds are prolonged. Heterocyclic agents should be used with extreme caution, if at all, in patients with pretreatment corrected QT intervals of longer than 0.44 milliseconds. It is imperative that a pretreatment ECG be obtained in any elderly patient about to begin antidepressant medication.

Clinical problems associated with slowed conduction are rare. Giardina and associates (1979) found that second-degree heart block developed in none of 14 patients with conduction abnormalities. Of the 14 patients, five had first-degree heart block and five had right bundle-branch block. Of those patients who overdosed on tricyclics, only 6% to 20% had significant clinical problems with conduction abnormalities (Biggs et al, 1977; Callahan, 1979).

It has been demonstrated that increases in PR and QRS intervals are directly related to tricyclic plasma levels (Giardina et al, 1979), and ECGs can provide a reliable guide to the cardiac effects of the tricyclic as dose is increased. In patients with severe conduction abnormalities, such as sick sinus syndrome, Cassem (1982) recommended pacemaker protection from complete heart block.

The risk of worsening cardiac arrhythmias with antidepressant therapy has been overemphasized in the past because imipramine and nortriptyline and probably the other tricyclic antidepressants are actually effective antiarrhythmic agents, similar in action to group I agents like quinidine and procainamide (Giardina et al, 1979). In fact, patients taking quinidine or procainamide should be followed carefully, and their antiarrhythmic medication may need to be reduced or stopped when a tricyclic antidepressant is added. Results of studies documenting the antiarrhythmic efficacy of imipramine (Raskind et al, 1982a) and nortriptyline (Giardina et al, 1981) can be shared with colleagues who may be reluctant to use antidepressants in patients with arrhythmias (Goff and Jenike, 1986).

There are case reports associating both amoxapine and maprotiline with arrhythmias (Cassem, 1982; Zavodnick, 1981). Trazodone generally does not result in clinical conduction problems in healthy individuals, but has been associated with arrhythmias in patients with preexisting cardiac illness. There are no consistent changes in cardiac rhythm associated with the MAOIs, even in cases of overdosage (Cassem, 1982).

Lithium regularly produces T-wave flattening in about 50% of the ECGs of patients with drug levels over 0.5 mmol/L (Jefferson and Greist, 1977). These changes may be secondary to altered ionic equilibrium with intracellular hypokalemia; serum potassium levels are normal in these patients. Toxic cardiac effects are uncommon, but reversible sinus node abnormalities and other conduction disturbances have been reported (Wellens et al, 1975; Wilson et al, 1976; Jaffe, 1977). Cassem (1982) recommended that patients with preexisting cardiac conduction abnormalities be given continuous cardiac monitoring during the initiation of lithium therapy.

Conclusions

Patients with heart disease can generally be managed with antidepressant medication. All elderly patients with heart disease, however, should be followed with occasional ECGs. Inquiry about cardiac symptoms such as ankle edema, dyspnea on exertion, orthopnea, and paroxysmal nocturnal dyspnea should be done at each visit. The patients should be examined for rales and the presence of changing heart sounds.

PSYCHIATRIC SYMPTOMS ASSOCIATED WITH COMMON NEUROLOGIC ILLNESSES

Many patients with neurologic illnesses have affective symptoms as well as cognitive difficulties (Jenike, 1985 and 1988a). Even though the underlying neurologic illness may not be treatable, the resolution of concomitant psychiatric symptoms will often improve the quality of both the patient's and the caregiver's life.

Alzheimer's Disease

Some dementing patients have treatable depressive symptoms; estimates of the prevalence of clinical depression among such patients have been reported to be from 0% to 57% (Kral, 1983; Ron et al, 1979; Liston, 1978; Cummings et al, 1987; Knesevich et al, 1983); our experience would indicate that major depression seems to be relatively uncommon in Alzheimer's patients. Cummings and associates (1987) found that only 5 (17%) of 30 Alzheimer's patients manifested depressive symptoms and none had major depression. Knesevich and co-workers (1983) found no evidence of depression in a group of Alzheimer's patients when first seen or even when reexamined one year later.

Psychosis (Caine and Shoulson, 1983; Cummings et al, 1987) with delusions of persecution, infidelity, and theft occur at some time in the course of the illness in 50% of patients (Cummings et al, 1987). Psychosis may occur alone or in the context of a depressive illness.

Personality changes in Alzheimer's patients occur but are usually not as troubling as those observed in patients with subcortical dementias such as Huntington's chorea (see chapter 5 for discussion of cortical and subcortical dementias) (Cummings and Benson, 1988). Alzheimer's patients tend to maintain a facade of acceptable social behaviors despite intellectual deterioration and occasional emotional indifference.

One problem with using scales like the Hamilton Depression Rating Scale (Hamilton, 1960) in an attempt to diagnose depression in a demented patient is that some items assess impairment in work and daily activities as well as psychomotor retardation, weight loss, fatigue, decreased libido, and insomnia—items that may be secondary to dementia alone. This overlap of symptoms in dementia and depression may account for elevated scores on the depression rating scale in patients with primary degenerative dementia (Alzheimer's disease), leading to an overestimation of the prevalence of depression in dementing patients (Miller, 1980). Lazarus and associates (1987) studied the frequency and severity of depressive symptoms among elderly patients who had a DSM-III presumptive diagnosis of primary degenerative dementia (definitive diagnosis can be made only at autopsy) as compared with normal, age-matched, community-dwelling control subjects. They attempted to identify specific depressive symptoms in the demented patients to ascertain whether there are specific signs and symptoms that provide a reliable basis for accurately diagnosing concomitant depression. They found that 18 (40%) of the dementing patients compared with 5 (12%) of the control subjects exhibited evidence of at least mild depression and that within the dementia group, there was no relationship between degree of cognitive impairment and extent of depressive symptoms. To determine which symptoms of depression predominate in dementia, they performed an item analysis of the Hamilton scale and found significant differences between patients and control subjects on 11 of the 24 items. In the depressed patients with dementia significant elevations of scores were found on the Hamilton items that assess signs and symptoms reflecting inner feeling states of depression and despair, rather than somatic or vegetative symptoms of depression. For example, scores for depressed mood, anxiety, and feelings of helplessness, hopelessness, and worthlessness were significantly greater in the depressed patients than in the control subjects. In contrast, the dementing patients did not score significantly higher than control subjects on the majority of items assessing vegetative symptoms, such as sleep disturbance, weight loss, and insomnia.

This study demonstrated that the evaluation of possibly depressed demented patients should focus more on symptoms reflective of an intrapsychic state of depression, such as depressed mood, anxiety, and feelings of helplessness, hopelessness, and worthlessness, rather than on vegetative signs of depression which may be the result of the dementing process alone.

Stroke

In contrast to Alzheimer's disease, depression occurs commonly in stroke patients and these depressions can and should be treated aggressively. Each year roughly 440,000 people have thromboembolic strokes in the United States (Wolf et al, 1977) and between 30% and 60% become clinically depressed with the period of high risk lasting for two years after the stroke (Robinson, 1981; Lipsey et al, 1984).

Statistically, patients with left frontal lobe damage are most likely to have severe depression (Robinson et al, 1983). Robinson and colleagues concluded from animal studies that brain catecholamines are depleted in patients who had cerebrovascular accidents and suggested that antidepressant medications might be used to treat these conditions (Robinson et al, 1983; Robinson and Szetela, 1981).

Information from close friends, family members, or caregivers will be helpful in diagnosing depression in the stroke patient. In general, cognitive impairment in stroke patients does not prevent them from giving accurate responses concerning depressive symptoms, although this is not invariably so. Patients with right-side brain damage (for right-handed and most left-handed individuals) may have aprosodias and impaired ability either to receive the emotional meaning of words and situations or to communicate emotional distress or depression.

Recent evidence indicated that half the depressions occurring in the acute period after stroke fulfill DSM-III diagnostic criteria for major depression (Robinson et al, 1983) and that untreated, these disorders last more than six months (Robinson, 1981). Patients with affective illness after stroke and patients with functional major depression have very similar depressive symptoms (Lipsey et al, 1986).

There are case reports that psychostimulants, which may exert their effects by blocking the reuptake of depleted catecholamines, may be useful in treating stroke-induced depressions (Kaufmann et al, 1984; Robinson, 1981; Woods et al, 1986).

In one study, the tricyclic nortriptyline, compared to placebo in a double-blind manner, significantly improved depression after stroke (Lipsey et al, 1984), with successfully treated patients having nortriptyline levels in the therapeutic range (50–150 ng/mL). Because the number of patients in this study was small (n = 34) the authors were unable to determine the relationship between location of the lesion and response to medication. Another controlled trial demonstrated the safety and efficacy of trazodone in treating depressed stroke patients (Reding et al, 1986).

Stroke patients have many difficulties dealing with rehabilitation and loss of function and should not be forced to suffer concomitant depression when clinicians have the tools at hand to effectively treat such symptoms.

Parkinson's Disease

Cummings (1988) in a review of 27 studies representing 4,336 patients with Parkinson's disease found that the prevalence of overt dementia was 39.9%. The studies reporting the highest incidence of intellectual impairment (69.9%) used psychologic assessment techniques, whereas studies identifying the lowest prevalence of dementia (30.2%) depended on nonstandardized clinical examinations. Neuropsychologic investigations revealed that parkinsonian patients manifested impairment in memory, visuospatial skills, and set aptitude while language function was largely spared. Intellectual deterioration correlated with age, akinesia, duration, and treatment status. Neuropathologic and neurochemical observations demonstrated that Parkinson's disease is a heterogeneous disorder: the classic subcortical pathology with dopamine deficiency may be complicated by atrophy of the nucleus basalis and superimposed cortical cholinergic deficits, with a few patients having the histopathologic hallmarks of Alzheimer's disease. Mild intellectual impairment also occurs with the classic pathology, and the more severe dementia syndromes have cholinergic alterations or Alzheimer's disease. Cummings concluded that Parkinson's disease includes several syndromes of intellectual impairment with variable pathologic and neurochemical correlates.

Parkinson's disease is complicated by depression in one-quarter to one-half of the patients (Mayeux, 1982). Depressive symptoms have been reported in as many as 34% of patients even prior to onset of motor manifestations (Patrick and Levy, 1922). Most studies in which severity of symptoms was recorded found depression to be of mild-to-moderate intensity (Celesia and Wanamaker, 1972; Mayeux et al, 1981; Warburton, 1967); suicidal thoughts were common, but actual attempts rare (Mjones, 1949). Some patients may experience depression as a reaction to the knowledge of the disease or its disability, but in others affective symptoms develop prior to obvious indications of the disease. Most investigators concur that neither the presence nor the intensity of depression can be consistently related to any factor such as age, sex, degree of disability, or type of treatment (Mayeux, 1982; Horn, 1974; Mayeux et al, 1981).

L-Dopa, the drug most commonly used to treat Parkinson's disease, may also provoke depression, sometimes with suicidal tendencies (Raft et al, 1972). It may also induce other mental symptoms, such as paranoid ideation and psychotic episodes (Adams and Victor, 1981). Patients with a history of depression prior to onset of motor symptoms may be particularly prone to L-dopa–induced depression (Mayeux, 1982).

There are a number of reports of favorable responses to tricyclic antidepressants in depressed parkinsonian patients (Andersen et al, 1980; Laitinen, 1969; Strang, 1965). Imipramine and its major metabolite desipramine have been effective in placebo-controlled trials (Laitinen, 1969; Strang, 1965) in reducing depression and fatigue. Improvement in mood (as well as in bradykinesia and rigidity) following ECT has been reported (Asnis, 1977; Lebensohn and Jenkins, 1975; Yudofsky, 1979) and is a reasonable option in depressed parkinsonian patients for whom medication trials fail.

Psychosis, even in the setting of depression, is uncommon in untreated idiopathic Parkinson's disease (Cummings and Benson, 1988).

When the clinician is faced with a parkinsonian patient, it is likely that cognitive and/or psychiatric symptoms will complicate the clinical picture.

Huntington's Disease

Personality changes may occur early in the course of Huntington's chorea and may be of two general types (McHugh and Folstein, 1975). In one, the patient becomes generally apathetic, may appear depressed, and tends to neglect himself or herself, his or her job, and his or her former interests. In the other, the patient becomes increasingly irritable and oversensitive with a tendency toward angry outbursts and violence.

Psychiatric symptoms occur commonly in patients with Huntington's chorea. Episodes of depression can last from weeks to months and may persist for several years. When Huntington patients with disease-related affective symptomatology were examined with the Schedule for Affective Disorders and Schizophrenia (SADS) (Endicott and Spitzer, 1978), 20% received a diagnosis of dysthymic syndrome and 17% were diagnosed as having a major depressive syndrome. Caine and Shoulson (1983) found that approximately 50% of patients with Huntington's disease exhibited significant affective disturbances (major depressive episodes or dysthymic disorders). If the mood disorders precede the motor disturbances or dementia, it may be impossible to differentiate them from functional disorders without the family history of Huntington's chorea.

Depression occasionally can reverse into a manic state, which can last for weeks and may resolve spontaneously, in which the patient is elated, expansive, and grandiose, and may overeat and talk incessantly. Psychosis is also common in patients with Huntington's disease (Caine and Shoulson, 1983; Cummings et al, 1987). Schizophrenia-like symptoms may also precede motor abnormalities and may consist of feelings of unreality, delusions of influence and control, and hallucinations and illusions. Patients typically are convinced of the reality of these hallucinations and delusions and may act on them.

Depression in Huntington's patients appears to be responsive to antidepressant agents as well as ECT (McHugh and Folstein, 1975; Brothers and Meadows, 1955) and may occasionally resolve spontaneously. Suicide rates in at-risk individuals are significantly greater than those for the general population (Schoenfeld et al, 1984) and suicide is the cause of death in as many as 7% of nonhospitalized patients with Huntington's disease (Reed and Chandler, 1958).

Treatment Decisions

If there is any doubt whether a patient with a neurologic illness is depressed, he or she should be treated. Many patients are both demented and depressed and the only way to clearly separate the two is by response to treatment. Depression, even in a patient with an underlying dementing process, can usually be resolved. Cognition may not improve, but patients will become less negative and more interested in hobbies, social activities, and sex.

GRIEF

A recent large scale study and accompanying editorial discussed the health consequences of losing a family member (Levav et al, 1988; Rogers and Reich, 1988). Levav and colleagues from Jerusalem found a surprisingly small effect of loss of a child on subsequent mortality of the surviving parents. Rogers and Reich (1988) noted that the death of a spouse or of a child is widely viewed as the most stressful of all human experiences, and that such stresses have adverse effects on health is so embedded in folklore that the relative lack of scientific support for such a belief has often been overlooked.

Reviewing previous studies, Rogers and Reich noted several clinically relevant trends; that is, the literature on conjugal bereavement suggested a brief increase in mortality among both widows and widowers after bereavement and then a later slight increase in mortality among men. These effects are certainly less dramatic than had previously been hypothesized. Parkes and associates (1969) described increased number of deaths among widowers within the first six months after bereavement, with nearly half being the result of coronary heart disease. A Finnish study (Kaprio et al, 1987) showed mortality that was two times the expected rate in the week after the death of a spouse, again from heart disease. Another large study found no excess mortality among bereaved spouses during the first year of bereavement; however, starting in the second year and continuing for as many as 10 years, there was a small but significant increase in mortality among men, especially those who did not remarry.

Rogers and Reich's discussion reflected Freud's observations that normal grief is not generally associated with the morbid sense of worthlessness or prolonged functional impairment that is common in clinical depression. Uncomplicated mourning may last as long as a year, although vestiges of grief may continue longer, often triggered by anniversaries, losses, or other reminders of the loved one. They believe that the loss of a loved one is never fully resolved, but on the other hand, the stresses of bereavement may strengthen persons and families, refocusing their energies and deepening other attachments.

Sometimes grief can reach pathologic depths and can merge with depression requiring treatment (Clayton, 1974; Clayton et al, 1974). Rogers and Reich suggested that physicians and other health care providers should be watchful and supportive in times of bereavement, without overemphasizing the possibility of adverse effects—listening, reassuring, reaffirming, referring survivors when appropriate to specific self-help groups such as the Widow-to-Widow program, and sometimes sharing directly in the grief. They recommended special vigilance for unusually vulnerable subgroups such as those with mental disorders, alcoholism, or limited social support. Men appear to be more vulnerable, for unknown reasons.

In one small open trial, 7 of 10 bereaved, depressed spouses had moderate-to-marked improvement of depressive symptoms during a four-week trial of the tricyclic antidepressant desipramine (Jacobs et al, 1987). Antidepressants may facilitate improvement in grieving patients whose symptoms are prolonged and merge into depression.

SUMMARY

Depression is a common debilitating and often life-threatening illness in the elderly patient. Diagnosis and medical assessment have been reviewed. Tertiary amines, such as imipramine and amitriptyline (with the exception of doxepin), cause significant orthostatic hypotension and should be avoided as agents of first choice in the elderly. Amitriptyline is also extremely anticholinergic. Amoxapine is essentially a neuroleptic with antidepressant properties and may induce neurologic sequelae, including tardive dyskinesia.

If a patient has had a prior positive response or if he has a relative who had a good outcome from a particular drug, it may be best to begin treatment with this drug. The initial choice of antidepressant can be based largely on the clinical picture. For example, if a depressed patient is sleeping much more than usual and is lethargic during the day, potentially activating agents like desipramine, fluoxetine, or protriptyline would be good drugs to try initially. If, on the other hand, the patient is unable to sleep, a more sedating agent like nortriptyline or trazodone should be given before bedtime. Risks and side effects, as well as use in cardiac patients, are reviewed in detail.

Many clinicians avoid the use of MAOIs in the elderly patient because of fears of adverse reactions. Precautions, side effects, and specific recommendations are outlined. Dietary restrictions imposed by these drugs are not burdensome and there are patients who respond promptly to MAOIs who fail to respond to any other medication. A clear explanation of the action, onset, duration, and side effects of these medications will aid in the patient's recovery.

Using lithium in the elderly requires special precautions because of decreased GFR and potential interactions with concomitantly used drugs. Side effects and toxicity are discussed.

The use of psychostimulants, such as methylphenidate and amphetamine, to treat medically ill depressed patients is reviewed. These agents are also sometimes useful in demented individuals or in patients with abulic frontal lobe syndromes.

Depressions are common after a stroke and recent evidence indicates that they can be adequately treated. Stroke patients have many difficulties dealing with issues of rehabilitation and should not be forced to suffer concomitant depression when clinicians have the tools at hand to effectively treat such symptoms.

Recent data on the potentiation of antidepressant effects by lithium or T3 indicate that they may be useful in some heterocyclic-resistant patients.

Risks, side effects, and recent procedural advances in the use of ECT are reviewed. ECT is both more effective and faster-acting than drugs in the treatment of depression and many depressed elderly patients, especially those with psychotic symptoms, do not respond to drugs but improve dramatically with ECT.

REFERENCES

Abrams JH, Schulman P, White WB: Successful treatment of a monoamine oxidase inhibitor-tyramine hypertensive emergency with intravenous labetalol. *N Engl J Med* 313:52, 1985.

Achte KA, Vauhkonen JL: Cancer and the psyche. *Omega* 2:46–56, 1971.

Adams RD, Victor M (eds): *Principles of Neurology*. New York, McGraw-Hill, 1981.

Agnoli A, Martucci N, Manna L, et al: Effect of cholinergic and anticholinergic drugs on short-term memory in Alzheimer's dementia: A neuropsychological and computerized electroencephalographic study. *Clin Neuropharmacol* 6:311–323, 1983.

Aizenberg D, Modai I, Roitman M, et al: Musical hallucinations, depression and old age. *Psychopathology* 20:220–223, 1987.

Aizenberg D, Schwartz B, Modai I: Musical hallucinations, acquired deafness and depression. *J Nerv Ment Dis* 174:309–311, 1986.

Alexopolous G, Shamoian C, Lucas J, et al: Medical problems of geriatric patients and younger controls during ECT. *J Am Geriatr Soc* 32:651–654, 1984.

Allen JR: Salicylate-induced musical perceptions. *N Engl J Med* 313:642–643, 1985.

Amsterdam JD, Winokur A, Caroff SN, et al: The dexamethasone suppression test in outpatients with primary affective disorder and healthy control subjects. *Am J Psychiatry* 139(3):287–291, 1982.

Ananth J, Luchins D: A review of combined tricyclic and MAOI therapy. *Compr Psychiatry* 18:221–272, 1977.

Andersen J, Aabro E, Gulmann N, et al: Antidepressive treatment of Parkinson's disease. *Acta Neurol Scand* 62:210–219, 1980.

Anderson WH: Depression, in Lazare A (ed): *Outpatient Psychiatry*. Baltimore, Williams and Wilkins, 1979, pp 257–260.

Angst J, Baastrup P, Grof P, et al: The course of monopolar depression and bipolar psychoses. *Psychiatr Neurol Neurochir* 76:489–500, 1973.

Anonymous: Psychiatric illness among medical patients. *Lancet* 1:479, 1979.

Arana GW, Barreira PJ, Cohen BJ, et al: The dexamethasone suppression test in mania, schizophrenia, and other psychotic disorders. *Am J Psychiatry* 140:1521–1523, 1983.

Ashford W, Ford CV: Use of MAO inhibitors in elderly patients. *Am J Psychiatry* 136:1466, 1979.

Asnis G: Parkinson's disease, depression and ECT: A review and case study. *Am J Psychiatry* 134:191–195, 1977.

Atterwill CK: The effects of ECT on central cholinergic and interrelated neurotransmitter systems in ECT, in Lerer B, Weiner RD, Belmaker RH (eds): *ECT: Basic Mechanisms*. Washington, DC, American Psychiatric Association Press, 1984.

Avery D, Winokur G: Mortality in depressed patients treated with electroconvulsive therapy and antidepressants. *Arch Gen Psychiatry* 33:1029–1037, 1976.

Avery D, Winokur G: The efficacy of electroconvulsive therapy and antidepressants in depression. *Biol Psychiatry* 32:507–523, 1977.

Baldessarini RJ: A summary of biomedical aspects of mood disorders. *McLean Hosp J* 6:1–34, 1981.

Baldessarini RJ: *Chemotherapy in Psychiatry*. Cambridge, Mass, Harvard University Press, 1977.

Banazak DA, Teri L, Boroson S: The use of ECT in older adults: A review. Submitted for publication.

Banki CM: Cerebrospinal fluid amine metabolites after combined amitriptyline-triiodothyronine treatment of depressed women. *Eur J Pharmacol* 11:311–315, 1977.

Banki CM: Triiodothyronine in the treatment of depression. *Orv Hetil* 116:2543–2546, 1975.

Barker JC, Baker AA: Deaths associated with electroplexy. *J Ment Sci* 105:339–348, 1959.

Barton JL: Amoxapine-induced agitation among bipolar depressed patients. *Am J Psychiatry* 139:387, 1982.

Bartus RT, Dean RL, Beer R, et al: The cholinergic hypothesis of geriatric memory dysfunction. *Science* 217:408–416, 1982.

Bergstron DA, Kellar KJ: Effect of electroconvulsive shock on monoaminargic receptor binding sites in rat brain. *Nature* 278:464–466, 1979.

Bertler A: Occurrence and localization of catecholamines in the human brain. *Acta Physiol Scand* 51:97, 1961.

Biggs JT, Spiker DG, Petit JM, et al: Tricyclic antidepressant overdose. *JAMA* 238:135–138, 1977.

Blazer D: *Depression in Late Life*. St Louis, CV Mosby, 1982.

Blume JE, Tross S: Psychodynamic treatment of the elderly: A review of issues in theory and practice, in Eisdorfer D (ed): *Annual Review of Gerontology and Geriatrics*. New York, Springer, 1980, vol 1.

Bodley PO, Potts L, Halwax K: Low serum pseudocholinesterase levels complicating treatment with phenelzine. *Br Med J* 3:510–512, 1969.

Breslow R, Kocsis J, Belkin B: Memory deficits in depression: Evidence using the Wechsler Memory Scale. *Percept Mot Skills* 51:541–542, 1980.

Brooks SM, Werk EE, Ackerman SJ, et al: Adverse effects of phenobarbital on corticosteroid metabolism in patients with bronchial asthma. *N Engl J Med* 286:1125–1128, 1972.

114

Brothers CRD, Meadows AW: An investigation of Huntington's chorea in Victoria. *Ment Sci* 101:548–563, 1955.

Brown JH, Henteleff P, Barakat S, et al: Is it normal for terminally ill patients to desire death? *Am J Psychiatry* 143:208–211, 1986.

Brown RP, Frances A, Kocsis JH, et al: Psychotic versus nonpsychotic depression: Comparison of treatment response. *J Nerv Ment Dis* 170:635–637, 1982.

Brown WA, Johnson R, Mayfield D: The 24-hour dexamethasone suppression test in a clinical setting: Relationship to diagnosis, symptoms, and response to treatment. *Am J Psychiatry* 136:543–547, 1979.

Brown WA: Psychologic and neuroendocrine responses to methylphenidate. *Arch Gen Psychiatry* 34:1103–1108, 1977.

Brown WA: The dexamethasone suppression test: Clinical applications. *Psychosomatics* 22:951–955, 1981.

Burke W, Rubin E, Zorumski C, et al: The safety of ECT in geriatric psychiatry. *J Am Geriatr Soc* 35:516–521, 1987.

Burnside IM: Principles from Yalom, in Burnside IM (ed): *Working with the Elderly: Group Process and Techniques*. North Scituate, Mass, Duxbury Press, 1978.

Busse EW, Pfeiffer E: *Behavior and Adaptation in Late Life*, ed 2. Boston, Little, Brown, 1977.

Busse EW, Pfeiffer E: Functional psychiatric disorders in old age, in Busse EW, Pfeiffer E (eds): *Behaviour and Adaptation*. Boston, Little, Brown, 1969.

Butler PW, Besser GM: Pituitary-adrenal function in severe depressive illness. *Lancet* 1:1234–1236, 1968.

Butler R: Intensive psychotherapy for the hospitalized aged. *Geriatrics* 15:644, 1960.

Butler RN: Psychiatry and the elderly: an overview. *Am J Psychiatry* 132:893, 1975a.

Butler RN: Psychotherapy in old age, in Arieti S (ed): *American Handbook of Psychiatry*, ed 2. New York, Basic Books, 1975, vol 5.

Butler RN: Toward a psychiatry of the life-cycle: Implications of sociopsychologic studies of the aging process for the psychotherapeutic situation. *Psychiatric Res Rep* 23:233, 1968.

Byrne DC: Affect and vigilance performance in depressive illness. *J Psychiatr Res* 13:185–191, 1977.

Cade R, Shires DL, Barrow NV, et al: Abnormal diurnal variation of plasma cortisol in patients with renovascular hypertension. *J Clin Endocrinol Metab* 27:800–806, 1976.

Caine ED, Shoulson I: Psychiatric syndromes in Huntington's disease. *Am J Psychiatry* 140:728–733, 1983.

Caine ED: The neuropsychology of depression: The pseudodementia syndrome, in Grant I, Adams KM (eds): *Neuropsychological Assessment of Neuropsychiatric Disorders*. New York, Oxford, 1986, pp 221–243.

Callahan M: Tricyclic antidepressant overdose. *JACEP* 8:413–425, 1979.

Carlsson A, Winblad B: Influence of age and time interval between death and autopsy in dopamine and 3-methyoxytyramine levels in human basal ganglia. *J Neural Trans* 38:271, 1976.

Carroll BJ, Curtis GC, Mendels J: Neuroendocrine regulation in depression: Discrimination of depressed from nondepressed patients. *Arch Gen Psychiatry* 33:1051–1058, 1976.

Carroll BJ, Feinberg M, Greden JF, et al: A specific laboratory test for the diagnosis of melancholia. *Arch Gen Psychiatry* 38:15–22, 1981.

Carroll BJ: Neuroendocrine function in psychiatric disorders, in Lipton MA, DiMascio A, Killam DR (eds): *Psychopharmacology: A Generation of Progress*. New York, Raven Press, 1978, pp 487–496.

Carroll BJ: The hypothalamic-pituitary-adrenal axis in depression, in Davies B, Carroll

BJ, Mowbray RM (eds): *Depressive Illness, Some Research Studies*. Springfield, Ill, Charles C Thomas, 1972.

Cassem NH: Cardiovascular effects of antidepressants. *J Clin Psychiatry* 43(11 [sect 2]):22–28, 1982.

Celesia GG, Wanamaker WM: Psychiatric disturbances in Parkinson's disease. *Dis Nerv Sys* 33:577–583, 1972.

Clayton PJ, Herjanic M, Murphy et al: Mourning and depression: their similarities and differences. *Can Psychiatr Assoc J* 19:309–312, 1974.

Clayton PJ: Mortality and morbidity in the first year of widowhood. *Arch Gen Psychiatry* 30: 747–750, 1974.

Cohen RM, Weingartner H, Smallberg SA, et al: Effort and cognition in depression. *Arch Gen Psychiatry* 39:593–597,1982.

Cole JO, Branconnier R, Salomon M, et al: Tricyclic use in the cognitively impaired elderly. *J Clin Psychiatry* September (sect 2):14–19, 1983.

Crammer J, Gillis C: Psychiatric aspects of diabetes mellitus: Diabetes and depression. *Br J Psychiatry* 139:171–172, 1981.

Cronholm G, Ottosson J: Memory functions in endogenous depression. *Arch Gen Psychiatry* 5:193–197, 1961.

Crook T, Cohen GD (eds): *Physicians' Handbook on Psychotherapeutic Drug Use in the Aged*. New Canaan, Conn, Mark Powley Associates, 1981.

Cross AJ, Crow TJ, Perry EK, et al: Reduced dopamine beta-hydroxylase activity in Alzheimer's disease. *Br Med J* 282:93–94, 1981.

Cummings JL, Benson DR: Psychological dysfunction accompanying subcortical dementias. *Ann Rev Med* 39:53–61, 1988.

Cummings JL, Miller BL, Hill M, et al: Neuropsychiatric aspects of multi-infarct dementia and dementia of the Alzheimer type. *Arch Neurol* 44:389–393, 1987.

Cummings JL: Intellectual impairment in Parkinson's disease: Clinical, pathologic, and biochemical correlates. *J Geriatric Psychiatr Neurol* 1:24–36, 1988.

Davidson J, Turnbull C: The importance of dose in isocarboxazid therapy. *J Clin Psychiatry* 45(7, Sec. 2):49–52, 1984.

Davidson J, White H: The effect of isocarboxazid on platelet MAO activity. *Biol Psychiatry* 18:1075–1079, 1983.

Davidson J, Zung WWK, Walker JI: Practical aspects of MAO inhibitor therapy. *J Clin Psychiatry* 45(7, Sec. 2):81–84, 1984.

Davies P: Neurotransmitter-related enzymes in senile dementia of the Alzheimer type. *Brain Res* 171:319–327, 1979.

Davis KL, Mohs RC, Tinklenberg JR, et al: Physostigmine: Improvement of long-term memory processes in normal humans. *Science* 201:272–274, 1978.

Dec GW, Jenike MA, Stern TA: Trazodone-digoxin interaction in an animal model. *J Clin Psychopharmacol* 4:153–155, 1984.

deMontigny C, Grunberg F, Mayer A, et al: Lithium induces rapid relief of depression in tricyclic antidepressant drug non-responders. *Br J Psychiatry* 138:252–256, 1981.

Dewan M, Pandurangi AK, Boucher ML, et al: Abnormal dexamethasone suppression test results in chronic schizophrenic patients. *Am J Psychiatry* 139:1501–1503, 1982.

Dominquez RA: Evaluating the effectiveness of the new antidepressants. *Hosp Community Psychiatry* 34:405–407, 1983.

Drachman DA, Leavitt J: Human memory and the cholinergic system. *Arch Neurol* 30:113–121, 1974.

Drachman DA, Sahakian BJ: Memory and cognitive function in the elderly: A preliminary trial of physostigmine. *Arch Neurol* 37:674–675, 1980.

Dunner DL, Roose SP, Bone S: Complications of lithium treatment in older patients, in Geshon S, Kline NS, Shou M (eds): *Lithium Controversies and Unresolved Issues*. Amsterdam, Excerpta Medica, 1979, pp 427–431.

116

Earle BV: Thyroid hormone and tricyclic antidepressants in resistant depressions. *Am J Psychiatry* 126:1667–1669, 1970.

Eastwood MR, Corbin SL, Reed M, et al: Acquired hearing loss and psychiatric illness: an estimate of prevalence and co-morbidity in a geriatric setting. *Br J Psychiatry* 147:552–556, 1985.

Ehrenberg R, Gullingsrud M: Electroconvulsive therapy in elderly patients. *Am J Psychiatry* 4:743–747, 1955.

Electroconvulsive Therapy, American Psychiatric Association Task Force on ECT: *Task Force Report No. 14.* Washington, DC, American Psychiatric Association, 1978.

Elias AN, Gwinup G: Effects of some clinically encountered drugs on steroid and degradation. *Metabolism* 29:582–595, 1980.

Endicott J, Spitzer RL: A diagnostic interview: The schedule for affective disorders and schizophrenia. *Arch Gen Psychiatry* 35:837–844, 1978.

Essen-Moller E, Larsson H, Uddenberg EC, et al: Individual traits and morbidity in a Swedish rural population. *Acta Psychiatr Scand* Suppl 100, 1956.

Fakhri O, Fadhl AA, el Rawdi RM: Effective electroconvulsive therapy on diabetes mellitus. *Lancet* 11:775–777, 1980.

Fakhri O: Blood sugar after electroplexy. *Lancet* 1:587, 1966.

Feinberg T, Goodman B: Affective illness, dementia, and pseudodementia. *J Clin Psychiatry* 45:99–103, 1984.

Feldman F, Susselman S, Lipetz B, et al: Electric shock therapy of elderly patients. *Arch Neurol Psychiatry* 56:158–170, 1946.

Fince CE: Neuroendocrinology of aging: as view of an emerging area. *Bioscience* 25:645, 1975.

Fink M: *Convulsive Therapy: Theory and Practice.* New York, Raven Press, 1979.

Fogel BS, Kroessler D: Treating late-life depression on a medical-psychiatric unit. *Hosp Community Psychiatry* 38:829–831, 1987.

Forest WH: Dextroamphetamine with morphine for the treatment of postoperative pain. *N Engl J Med* 296:712–715, 1977.

Foster BG, Burke WJ: Assessing and treating the suicidal elderly. *Fam Pract Recertification* 7(11):33–45, 1985.

Foster JR, Rosenthal JS: Lithium treatment of the elderly, in Johnson FN (ed): *Handbook of Lithium Therapy.* Lancaster, England, MTP Press, 1980, pp 414–420.

Frances A, Brown RP, Kocsis JH, et al: Psychotic depression: A separate entity? *Am J Psychiatry* 138:831–833, 1981.

Francis PT, Palmer AM, Sims NR, et al: Neurochemical studies of early-onset Alzheimer's disease: Possible influence of treatment. *N Engl J Med* 313:7–11, 1985.

Fraser RM, Glass IB: Recovery from ECT in elderly patients. *Br J Psychiatry* 133:524, 1978.

Fraser RM, Glass IB: Unilateral and bilateral ECT in elderly patients. *Acta Psychiatr Scand* 62:13, 1980.

Frommer DA, Kulig KW, Marx JA, et al: Tricyclic antidepressant overdose. *JAMA* 257:521–526, 1987.

Gander DR: Combining the antidepressant drugs. *Br Med J* 1:521, 1965.

Ganong WF: Brain mechanisms regulating the secretion of the pituitary gland, in Schmitt FO, Worden FG (eds): *The Neurosciences: Third Study Program.* Cambridge, Mass, MIT Press, 1974, pp 549–564.

Ganong WF: Evidence for a central noradrenergic system that inhibits ACTH secretion, in Knigge EM, Scott DE, Weindl A (eds): *Brain Endocrine Interaction.* Basel, Karger, 1972, pp 254–266.

Gartrell N: Increased libido in women receiving trazodone. *Am J Psychiatry* 143:781–782, 1986.

Gaspar D, Samarasinghe LA: ECT in psychogeriatric practice—a study of risk factors and outcome. *Compr Psychiatry* 23:170–175, 1982.

Gaultieri CT, Powell SF: Psychoactive drug interactions. *J Clin Psychiatry* 39:62–71, 1978.

Gelenberg AJ: Heterocyclic antidepressant overdose. *Mass Gen Hosp Topics Geriatr* 2:33–34,36, 1984.

Gelenberg AJ: The DST in perspective. *Biol Ther Psychiatry* 6:1–2, 1983.

Georgotas A: Affective disorders in the elderly: Diagnostic and research considerations. *Age Ageing* 12:1–10, 1983.

Giardina EGV, Bigger JT, Glassman AH, et al: The electrocardiographic and antiarrhythmic effects of imipramine hydrochloride at therapeutic plasma concentrations. *Circulation* 60:1045–1052, 1979.

Giardina EGV, Bigger JT, Johnson LL: The effect of imipramine and nortriptyline on ventricular premature depolarizations and left ventricular function. *Circulation* 64:316, 1981.

Gibbs RHS: Essential hypertension in general practice. An evaluation of pargyline hydrochloride. *Practitioner* 196:426–430, 1966.

Gilhome-Herbst K, Humphrey C: Hearing impairment and mental state in the elderly living at home. *Br Med J* 281:903–905, 1980.

Gitman L: *Endocrines and Aging.* Springfield, Ill, Charles C Thomas, 1967.

Glassman A, Kantor S, Shostak M: Depression, delusions and drug response. *Am J Psychiatry* 132:716–719, 1975.

Glassman AH, Johnson LL, Giardina EGV, et al: The use of imipramine in depressed patients with congestive heart failure. *JAMA* 250:1997–2001, 1983.

Goff DC, Jenike MA: Treatment-resistant depression in the elderly. *J Am Geriatr Soc* 34:63–70, 1986.

Goldberg LK: Dexamethasone suppression test as indicator of safe withdrawal of antidepressant therapy. *Lancet* 2:376, 1980.

Goldberg LK: Dexamethasone suppression tests in depression and response to treatment. *Lancet* 2:92, 1980a.

Goldberg MJ, Spector R: Amoxapine overdose: Report of two patients with severe neurologic damage. *Ann Intern Med* 96:463–464, 1982.

Goldberg RS, Thornton WE: Combined tricyclic-MAOI therapy for refractory depression: A review with guidelines for appropriate usage. *J Clin Pharmacol* 18:143–146, 1978.

Gomoll AW, Byrne JE: Trazodone and imipramine: Comparative effects on canine cardiac conduction. *Eur J Pharmacol* 57:335–342, 1979.

Goodman LS, Gilman A: *The Pharmacological Basis of Therapeutics.* New York, MacMillan Publishing Co, 1975.

Goodwin FK, Prange AJ, Post RM, et al: Potentiation of antidepressant effects of L-triiodothyronine in tricyclic nonresponders. *Am J Psychiatry* 139:34–38, 1982.

Graham PM, Booth J, Boranga E, et al: The dexamethasone suppression in mania. *J Affective Disord* 4:201–211, 1982.

Grayson DA, Henderson AS, Kay DWK: Diagnoses of dementia and depression: a latent trait analysis of their performance. *Psychol Med* 17:667–675, 1987.

Greden JF, Albala AA, Haskett RF, et al: Normalization of dexamethasone suppression test: A laboratory index of recovery from endogenous depression. *Biol Psychiatry* 15:449–458, 1980.

Greden JF, Carroll BJ: The dexamethasone suppression test as a diagnostic aid in catatonia. *Am J Psychiatry* 136:1199–1200, 1979.

Green RL, McAllister TW, Bernat JL: A study of crying in medically and surgically hospitalized patients. *Am J Psychiatry* 144:443–447, 1987.

Grotjahn M: Analytic psychotherapy with the elderly. *Psychoanal Rev* 42:419, 1955.

118

Guggenheim FG: Suicide, in Hackett TP, Cassem NH (eds): *Massachusetts General Hospital Handbook of General Hospital Psychiatry*. St. Louis, CV Mosby, 1978, pp 250–263.

Gurland BJ: The comparative frequency of depression in various adult age groups. *J Gerontol* 31:283–292, 1976.

Gurland BJ, Cross PS: Suicide among the elderly, in Aronson MK, Bennett R, Gurland BJ (eds): *The Acting-Out Elderly*. New York, Haworth Press, 1983, pp 456–465.

Hackett TP: *The Use of Stimulant Drugs in General Hospital Psychiatry* (tape). Glendale Cal, Audio-Digest Foundation, 1978, vol 7(12).

Halle HM: Combining the antidepressant drugs. *Br Med J* 1:384, 1965.

Hamilton M: A rating scale for depression. *J Neurol Neurosurg Psychiatry* 23:56–62, 1960.

Hammeke TA, McQuillen MP, Cohen BA: Musical hallucinations associated with acquired deafness. *J Neurol Neurosurg Psychiatry* 46:570–572, 1983.

Hanzlick RL: Postmortem blood concentrations of parent tricyclic antidepressant (TCA) drugs in 11 cases of suicide. *Am J Forensic Med Pathol* 5:11–13, 1984.

Hayes RL, Gerner RH, Fairbanks L, et al: EKG findings in geriatric depressives given trazodone, placebo or imipramine. *J Clin Psychiatry* 44:180–183, 1983.

Henry A, Weingartner H, Murphy DL: Influence of affective states and psychoactive drugs on verbal learning and memory. *Am J Psychiatry* 130:966–971, 1973.

Himmelhoch JM, Neil JF, May SJ, et al: Age, dementia, dyskinesias, and lithium response. *Am J Psychiatry* 137:941–945, 1980.

Himmelhoch JM: Cardiovascular effects of trazodone in humans. *J Clin Psychopharmacol* 1(65):765–815, 1981.

Hirschowitz RG: Foster grandparents program: Preventive intervention with the elderly poor. *Hosp Community Psychiatry* 24:418–420, 1973.

Holliday AR, Joffe JR: A controlled evaluation of protriptyline compared to placebo and to methylphenidate hydrochloride. *J New Drugs* 5:257, 1965.

Horn: The psychological factors in parkinsonism. *J Neurol Neurosurg Psychiatr* 37:27–31, 1974.

Hughes J, Barraclough BM, Reeve W: Are patients shocked by ECT? *J Roy Soc Med* 74:283, 1981.

Insel TR, Kalin NH, Guttmacher LB, et al: The DST in patients with primary obsessive-compulsive disorder. *Psychiatry Res* 6:153–160, 1982.

Jackson JE, Bressler R: Prescribing tricyclic antidepressant: Part III: Management of overdose. *Drug Ther* 12(2):175–189, 1982.

Jacobs SC, Nelson C, Zisook S: Treating depressions of bereavement with antidepressants: A pilot study. *Psychiatr Clin North Am* 10:501–510, 1987.

Jaffe CM: First-degree atrioventricular block during lithium carbonate treatment. *Am J Psychiatry* 134:88–89, 1977.

Jefferson JW, Greist JH: *Primer of Lithium Therapy*. Baltimore, Williams and Wilkins Co, 1977.

Jefferson JW, Marshall JR: *Neuropsychiatric Features of Medical Disorders*. New York, Plenum Press, 1981.

Jefferson JW: Lithium and affective disorder in the elderly. *Compr Psychiatry* 24:166–178, 1983.

Jenike MA, Albert MS: The dexamethasone suppression test in patients with presenile and senile dementia of the Alzheimer's type. *J Am Geriatr Soc* 32:441–444, 1984.

Jenike MA, Anderson WH: Depression: Emergency assessment and differential diagnosis, in Manschreck TC, Murray GB (eds): *Psychiatric Medicine Update*. New York, Elsevier, 1984, pp 55–71.

Jenike MA, Baer L, Brotman AW, et al: Obsessive-compulsive disorder and the dexamethasone suppression test. *J Clin Psychopharmacol* 7:182–184, 1987.

Jenike MA: Alcohol and antihistamines not contraindicated with MAOIs? *Am J Psychiatry* 140:1107, 1983b.

Jenike MA: Alzheimer's disease—What the practicing clinician needs to know. *J Geriatr Psychiatr Neurol* 1:37–46, 1988a.

Jenike MA: Assessment and treatment of affective illness in the elderly. *J Geriatr Psychiatr Neurol* 1:89–107, 1988.

Jenike MA: Depressed in the ER. *Emerg Med* 16:102–120, 1984.

Jenike MA: Depression and other psychiatric disorders, in Albert MS, Moss M (eds): *Geriatric Neuropsychology*. New York, Guildford Press, 1988b, pp 115–144.

Jenike MA: Dexamethasone suppression test as a clinical aid in elderly depressed patients. *J Am Geriatr Soc* 31:45–48, 1983.

Jenike MA: Dexamethasone suppression: A biological marker of depression. *Drug Ther* 12(9):203–212, 1982.

Jenike MA: ECT and diabetes mellitus. *Am J Psychiatry* 139:136, 1982a.

Jenike MA: Electroconvulsive therapy: What are the facts? *Geriatrics* 38:33–38, 1984b.

Jenike MA: *Handbook of Geriatric Psychopharmacology*. Littleton, Mass, PSG Publishing Co, 1985.

Jenike MA: MAO inhibitors as treatment for depressed patients with primary degenerative dementia (Alzheimer's disease). *Am J Psychiatry* 142:763–764, 1985.

Jenike MA: Rapid response of severe obsessive-compulsive disorder to tranylcypromine. *Am J Psychiatry* 138:1249–1250, 1981.

Jenike MA: Tardive dyskinesia: Special risk in the elderly. *J Am Geriatr Soc* 31:71–73, 1983a.

Jenike MA: The use of monoamine oxidase inhibitors in elderly depressed patients. *J Am Geriatr Soc* 32:571–575, 1984a.

Judd LL, Hubbard B, Janowsky DS, et al: The effect of lithium carbonate on the cognitive functions of normal subjects. *Arch Gen Psychiatry* 34:355–357, 1977.

Jukiz W, Meilke AW, Levinson RA, et al: Effect of diphenylhydantoin on the metabolism of dexamethasone: Mechanism of abnormal dexamethasone suppression in humans. *N Engl J Med* 283:11–14, 1970.

Kahn RL: The mental health system and the future aged. *Gerontologist* 15(Part II):24–31, 1975.

Kalin NH, Risch SC, Janowsky DS, et al: Use of the dexamethasone suppression test in clinical psychiatry. *J Clin Psychopharmacol* 1(2):64–69, 1981.

Kaplitz SE: Withdrawn, apathetic geriatric patients responsive to methylphenidate. *J Am Geriatr Soc* 23:271–276, 1975.

Kaprio J, Koskenvuo M, Rita H: Mortality after bereavement: a prospective study of 95,647 widowed persons. *Am J Public Health* 77:283–287, 1987.

Karlinsky H, Shulman K: The clinical use of electroconvulsive therapy in old age. *J Am Geriatr Soc* 32:180–182, 1984.

Kathol RG, Henn FA: Tricyclics: The most common agent used in potentially lethal overdoses. *J Nerv Ment Dis* 171:250–252, 1983.

Kaufmann MW, Cassem NH, Murray GB, et al: Use of psychostimulants in medically ill patients with neurological disease and major depression. *Can J Psychiatry* 29:46–49, 1984.

Kaufmann MW, Murray GB, Cassem NH: Use of psychostimulants in medically ill depressed patients. *Psychosomatics* 23:817–819, 1982.

Kaufmann MW: Use of methylphenidate in the elderly. *Mass Gen Hosp Top Geriatr* 1:3–4, 1982.

Kay DWK, Bergman K: Physical disability and mental health in old age. *J Psychosom Res* 10:3–12, 1966.

Kayton W, Raskind M: Treatment of depression in the medically ill elderly with methylphenidate. *Am J Psychiatry* 137:963–965, 1980.

Kellar KJ, Cascio CS, Butler JA, et al: Differential effects of electroconvulsive shock and antidepressant drugs on serotonin–2 receptors in rat brain. *Eur J Pharmacol* 69:515–518, 1981.

Kiloh LG: Pseudodementia. *Acta Psychiatr Scand* 37:336–361, 1961.

Klein DF, Davis JM: *Diagnosis and Drug Treatment of Psychiatric Disorders*. Baltimore, Williams and Wilkins Co, 1969.

Klerman GL: Age and clinical depression: today's youth in the twenty-first century. *J Gerontol* 31:318–323, 1976.

Knesevich JW, Martin RL, Berg L, et al: Preliminary report on affective symptoms in the early stages of senile dementia of the Alzheimer type. *Am J Psychiatry* 140:233–235, 1983.

Knudsen K, Heath A: Effects of self poisoning with maprotiline. *Br Med J* 288:601–603, 1984.

Kral VA: The relationship between senile dementia (Alzheimer's type) and depression. *Can J Psychiatry* 28:304–306, 1983.

Kranzler HR, Cardoni A: Sodium chloride treatment of antidepressant-induced orthostatic hypotension. *J Clin Psychiatry* 49:366–368, 1988.

Krauthammer C, Klerman GL: Secondary mania. *Arch Gen Psychiatry* 35:1333–1339, 1978.

Krenzelok EP, North DS: Physostigmine's use questioned for amoxapine overdose (letter). *Am J Hosp Pharm* 38:1882–1883, 1981.

Kronfol Z, Greden J, Carroll B: Psychiatric aspects of diabetes mellitus. *Br J Psychiatry* 139:172, 1981.

Kronig MH, Roose SP, Walsh BT, et al: Blood pressure effects of phenelzine. *J Clin Psychopharmacol* 3:307, 1983.

Kulig K, Rumack BH, Sullivan JB: Amoxapine overdose: Coma and seizures without cardiotoxic effects. *JAMA* 248:1092–1094, 1982.

Kushnir SL: Lithium-antidepressant combinations in the treatment of depressed, physically ill geriatric patients. *Am J Psychiatry* 143:378–379, 1986.

Lago D, Connell CM, Knight B: Initial evaluation of PACT (People and Animals Coming Together): A companion animal program for community-dwelling older persons, in Smyer M, Gatz M (eds): *Mental Health and Aging: Programs and Evaluations*. Beverly Hills, Cal, Sage, 1983.

Laitinen L: Desipramine in treatment of Parkinson's disease. *Acta Neurol Scand* 45:109–113, 1969.

Lapierre YD, Anderson K: Dyskinesia associated with amoxapine antidepressant therapy: A case report. *Am J Psychiatry* 140:493–494, 1983.

Lazare A: Unresolved grief, in Lazare A (ed): *Outpatient Psychiatry*. Baltimore, Williams and Wilkins, 1979, pp 498–512.

Lazarus LW, Newton N, Cohle RB, et al: Frequency and presentation of depressive symptoms in patients with primary degenerative dementia. *Am J Psychiatry* 144:41–45, 1987.

Lebensohn Z, Jenkins RB: Improvement of parkinsonism in depressed patients treated with ECT. *Am J Psychiatry* 132:283–285, 1975.

Levav I, Friedlander Y, Kark JD, et al: An epidemiologic study of mortality among bereaved parents. *N Engl J Med* 318:457–461, 1988.

Liebowitz MR, Quitkin FM, Stewart JW, et al: Psychopharmacologic validation of atypical depression. *J Clin Psychiatry* 45(7, Sect 2):22–25, 1984.

Linden ME: The promise of therapy in the emotional problems of aging. Paper presented at the Fourth Congress of the International Association of Gerontology. Merano, Italy, July 1957.

Lipsey JR, Pearlson GD, Robinson RG, et al: Nortriptyline treatment of poststroke depression: A double-blind study. *Lancet* 1:297–300, 1984.

Liptzin B: Treatment of mania, in Salzman C (ed): *Clinical Geriatric Psychopharmacology*. New York, McGraw-Hill Book Co, 1984, pp 116–131.

Liston EH Jr: Diagnostic delay in presenile dementia. *J Clin Psychiatry* 39:599–603, 1978.

Litovitz TL, Trautman WG: Amoxapine overdose: Seizures and fatalities. *JAMA* 250:1069–1071, 1983.

Louie AK, Meltzer HY: Lithium potentiation of antidepressant treatment. *J Clin Psychopharmacol* 4:316–321, 1984.

Ludwig AM: The perceptual sphere in principles of clinical psychiatry. New York, Free Press, 1980.

Luohivuori KA, Hakama M: Risk of suicide among cancer patients. *Am J Epidemiol* 109:59–65, 1979.

Lydiard RB, Gelenberg AJ: Amoxapine: An antidepressant with some neuroleptic properties? *Pharmacotherapy* 1:163–175, 1981.

Maas JW: Biogenic amines and depression. *Arch Gen Psychiatry* 32:1357–1361, 1975.

MacClay WS: Death due to treatment. *Proc Roy Soc Med* 46:1–20, 1952.

Makeeva VL, Gol'davskach IL, Pozdnyakova SL: Somatic changes and side effects from the use of lithium salts in the prevention of affective disorders. *Zh Neuropatol Psikhiatr* 74:602–607, 1974.

Mann J: Altered platelet monoamine oxidase activity in affective disorders. *Psychol Med* 9:729–736, 1979.

Mann JJ, Aarons SF, Frances AJ, et al: Studies of selective and reversible monoamine oxidase inhibitors. *J Clin Psychiatry* 45(7, Sect 2):62–66, 1984.

Martin JB, Reichlin S, Brown GM: Regulation of ACTH secretion and its disorders, in Martin JB, Reichlin S, Brown GM (eds): *Clinical Neuroendocrinology*. Philadelphia, FA Davis Co, 1977, pp 179–200.

Mayeux R, Stern Y, Rosen J, et al: Depression, intellectual impairment, and Parkinson's disease. *Neurology* 31:645–650, 1981.

Mayeux R: Depression and dementia in Parkinson's disease, in Marsden CC, Fahn S (eds): *Movement Disorders*. London, Butterworth, 1982, pp 75–95.

McAllister TW, Ferrell RB, Price TRP, et al: The dexamethasone suppression test in two patients with severe depressive pseudodementia. *Am J Psychiatry* 139(4):479–481, 1982.

McCabe B, Tsuang M: Dietary consideration in MAO inhibitors regimens. *J Clin Psychiatry* 43:178–181, 1982.

McDonald WJ, Golper TA, Mass RD, et al: Adrenocorticotropin-cortisol axis abnormalities in hemodialysis patients. *J Clin Endocrinol Metab* 48:92–97, 1979.

McHugh PR, Folstein MF: Psychiatric syndromes of Huntington's chorea: A clinical and phenomenologic study, in Benson DF, Blumer D (eds): *Psychiatric Aspects of Neurologic Disease*. New York, Grune and Stratton, 1975, pp 267–286.

Merriam AE, Aronson MK, Gaston P, et al: The psychiatric symptoms of Alzheimer's disease. *J Am Geriatr Soc* 36:7–12, 1988.

Meyer D, Halfin V: Toxicity secondary to meperidine in patients on monoamine oxidase inhibitors: A case report and critical review. *J Clin Psychopharmacol* 1:319, 1981.

Michael MI, Smith RE, Hermich EM: Adrenal suppression and intranasally applied steroids. *Ann Allergy* 25:569–574, 1967.

Mielke D, Winstead D, Goethe J, et al: Multiple-monitored electroconvulsive therapy: Safety and efficacy in elderly depressed patients. *J Am Geriatr Soc* 32:180–183, 1984.

Mielke DH: Adverse reactions to thymoleptics, in Gallant DM, Simpson GM (eds): *Depression: Behavioral, Biochemical, Diagnostic and Treatment Concepts*. Holliswood, NY, Spectrum Publications, 1976.

Miller M: *Suicide After Sixty: The Final Alternative*. New York, Springer, 1979.

Miller NE: The measurement of mood in senile brain disease: Examiner ratings and self reports, in Cole JO, Barrett JE (eds): *Psychopathology in the Aged*. New York, Raven Press, 1980.

Miller TC, Crosby TW: Musical hallucinations in a deaf elderly patient. *Ann Neurol* 5:301, 1979.

Mitchell RS: Fatal toxic encephalitis occurring during iproniazid therapy and pulmonary tuberculosis. *Ann Intern Med* 42:417, 1955,

Mjones H: Paralysis agitans. *Acta Psychiatr Neurol* 54(Suppl):1–195, 1949.

Modigh K, Balldin J, Eriksson E, et al: Increased responsiveness of dopamine receptors after ECT: a review of experimental and clinical evidence, in Lerer B, Weiner RD, Belmaker RH (eds): *ECT: Basic Mechanisms*. Washington, DC, American Psychiatric Association Press, 1984.

Moffie HS, Paykel ES: Depression in medical inpatients. *Br J Psychiatry* 126:346–353, 1975.

Moriarty RW: Tricyclic antidepressant poisoning. *Drug Ther Hosp* 6(8):73–82, 1981.

Moss AJ: Prolonged QT-interval syndromes. *JAMA* 256:2985–2987, 1986.

Mulligan MA, Bennett R: Assessment of mental health and social problems during multiple friendly visits: The development and evaluation of a friendly visiting program for the isolated elderly. *Int J Aging Hum Devel* 8:43–65, 1977–1978.

Murphy DL, Garrick NA, Aulakh CS, et al: New contributions from basic science to understanding the effects of monoamine oxidase inhibiting antidepressants. *J Clin Psychiatry* 45(7, Sect 2):37–43, 1984.

Murphy JE, Ankier SI: An evaluation of trazodone in the treatment of depression. *Neuropharmacology* 19:1217–1218, 1980.

Myerson A: The effect of benzadrine on fatigue in normal and neurotic persons. *AMA Arch Neurol Psychiatry* 36:816–822, 1936.

National Center for Health Statistics: Advance Report of Final Mortality Statistics, 1983. *NCHS Monthly Vital Statistics Report* 34(6), 1985.

Neil JF, Licata SM, May SJ, et al: Dietary noncompliance during treatment with tranylcypromine. *J Clin Psychiatry* 40:33–37, 1979.

Neshkes RE, Gerner R, Jarvik LE, et al: Orthostatic effect of imipramine and doxepin in depressed geriatric outpatients. *J Clin Psychopharmacol* 5:102–106, 1985.

Newton R: The side effect profile of trazodone in comparison to an active control and placebo. *J Clin Psychopharmacol* 1(65):895–935, 1981.

Nicotra MB, Rivera M, Pool JL, et al: Tricyclic antidepressant overdose: Clinical and pharmacologic observations. *Clin Toxicol* 18:599–613, 1981.

Nies A, Robinson DS, Davis JM: Changes in monoamine oxidase with aging, in Eisdorfer C, Fann WE (eds): *Psychopharmacology and Aging*. New York, Plenum Press, 1973, pp 41–54.

Nies A: Differential response patterns to MAO inhibitors and tricyclics. *J Clin Psychiatry* 45(7, Sect 2):70–77, 1984.

Normand PS, Jenike MA: Lowered insulin requirements after ECT. *Psychosomatics* 25:418–419, 1984.

Nuller JL, Ostroumova MN: Resistance to inhibiting effect of dexamethasone in patients with endogenous depression. *Acta Psychiatr Scand* 61:169–177, 1980.

Oates JA, Seligmann AW, Clark MA, et al: The relative efficacy of guanethidine, methyldopa, and pargyline as antihypertensive agents. *N Engl J Med* 273:729–734, 1965.

Ogura C, Okuma T, Uchida Y, et al: Combined thyroid (triiodothyronine) tricyclic antidepressant treatment in depressive states. *Folia Psychiatr Neurol Jpn* 28:179–186, 1974.

Orr DA, Bramble MG: Tricyclic antidepressant poisoning and prolonged external cardiac massage during asystole. *Br Med J* 283:1107–1108, 1981.

Osgood NJ: Suicide in the elderly. *Carrier Foundation Letter* #133, April 1988.

Osgood NJ: *Suicide in the Elderly: A Practitioner's Guide to Diagnosis and Mental Health Intervention.* Rockville, Md, Aspen, 1985.

Oxenkrug GF: Dexamethasone test in alcoholics. *Lancet* 1:794, 1978.

Papp C, Benaim S: Toxic effects of iproniazid in a patient with angina. *Br Med J* 2:1070, 1958.

Parkes CM, Benjamin B, Fitzgerald RG: Broken heart: a statistical study of increased mortality among widowers. *Br Med J* 1:740–743; 1969.

Patrick HT, Levy DM: Parkinson's disease: A clinical study of 146 cases. *Arch Neurol Psychiatry* 7:711–720, 1922.

Pentel P, Sioris L: Incidence of late arrhythmias following tricyclic antidepressant overdose. *Clin Toxicol* 18:543–548, 1981.

Perry EK, Tomlinson BE, Blessed G, et al: Correlation of cholinergic abnormalities with senile plaques and mental test scores in senile dementia. *Br Med J* 2:1457–1459, 1978.

Post F: Dementia, depression, and pseudodementia, in Benson DF, Blumer D (eds): *Psychiatric Aspects of Neurologic Disease.* New York, Grune and Stratton, 1975.

Post F: Diagnosis of depression in geriatric patients and treatment modalities appropriate for the population, in Gallant EM, Simpson GM (eds): *Depression: Behavioral, Biochemical, Diagnostic and Treatment Concepts.* New York, Spectrum Publications, 1976.

Prien RF, Kupfer DJ: Continuation drug therapy for major depressive episodes: How long should it be maintained? *Am J Psychiatry* 143:18–23, 1986.

Quitkin FM, Harrison W, Liebowitz M, et al: Defining the boundaries of atypical depression. *J Clin Psychiatry* 45(7, Sect 2):19–21, 1984.

Quitkin FM, Rabkin JG, Ross D, et al: Duration of antidepressant drug treatment. *Arch Gen Psychiatry* 41:238–245, 1984a.

Raft D, Newman M, Spencer R: Suicide on L-dopa. *South Med J* 65:312, 1972.

Raskin A, Friedman AS, DiMascio A: Cognitive and performance deficits in depression. *Psychopharmacol Bull* 18:196–202, 1982.

Raskind M, Peskind E, Rivard MF, et al: DST and cortisol circadian rhythm in primary degenerative dementia. *Am J Psychiatry* 139:1468–1471, 1982.

Raskind M, Veith R, Barnes R, et al: Cardiovascular and antidepressant effects of imipramine in the treatment of secondary depression in patients with ischemic heart disease. *Am J Psychiatry* 139:1114–1117, 1982a.

Rauch PK, Jenike MA: Digoxin toxicity possibly precipitated by trazodone. *Psychosomatics* 25:334–335, 1984.

Reding M, Haycox J, Blass J: Depression in patients referred to a dementia clinic: A three-year prospective study. *Arch Neurol* 42:894–896, 1985.

Reding MJ, Orto LA, Winter SW, et al: Antidepressant therapy after stroke: A double-blind trial. *Arch Neurol* 43:763–765, 1986.

Reed E, Chandler JR: Huntington's chorea in Michigan. I. Demography and genetics. *Am J Hum Genet* 10:201–225, 1958.

Rees LH, Besser GM, Jeffcoate WJ, et al: Alcohol induced pseudo-Cushing's syndrome. *Lancet* 1:726, 1977.

Reifler BV, Larson E, Hanley R: Coexistence of cognitive impairment and depression in geriatric outpatients. *Am J Psychiatry* 139:623–626, 1982.

Reimann IW, Frolich JC: Effects of diclofenac on lithium kinetics. *Clin Pharmacol Ther* 30:348–352, 1981.

Resnick H, Cantor J: Gerifacts. *Geriatrics* 22:68, 1967.

Resnick H, Cantor J: Suicide and aging. *J Am Geriatr Soc* 22:68, 1967a.

Richelson E: Pharmacology of antidepressants in use in the United States. *J Clin Psychiatry* 43(11, Sect 2):4–11, 1982.

Robertson OH, Breznock EM, Riegle GD: *Endocrines and Aging.* New York, MSS Information Corp, 1972, pp 1–243.

Robinson DS, Davis JM, Nies A, et al: Relation of sex and aging to monoamine oxidase activity of human brain, plasma, and platelets. *Arch Gen Psychiatry* 24:536–539, 1971.

Robinson DS, Nies A, Davis JN, et al: Aging, monoamines, and monoamine oxidase levels. *Lancet* 1:290, 1972.

Robinson DS, Nies A, Revaris CL, et al: Clinical pharmacology of phenelzine. *Arch Gen Psychiatry* 35:629, 1978.

Robinson DS, Sourkes RC, Kralik P, et al: Effects of neuroleptics on platelet mono-amine oxidase activity. *Biol Psychiatry* 17:885–895, 1982.

Robinson DS: Changes in monoamine oxidase and monoamines with human development and aging. *Fed Proc* 34:103, 1975.

Robinson RG, Kubos KL, Starr LB, et al: Mood changes in stroke patients: Relationship to lesion location. *Compr Psychiatry* 24:555–566, 1983.

Robinson RG, Szetela B: Mood change following left hemisphere brain injury. *Ann Neurol* 9:447–453, 1981.

Robinson RG: Depression in aphasic patients: Frequency, severity, and clinicopathological correlations. *Brain Lang* 14:282–291, 1981.

Rogers MP, Reich P: On the health consequences of bereavement. *N Engl J Med* 318:510–511, 1988.

Ron MA, Toone BK, Garralda ME, et al: Diagnostic accuracy in presenile dementia. *Br J Psychiatry* 134:161–168, 1979.

Roose SP, Glassman AH, Giardina EGV, et al: Tricyclic antidepressants in depressed patients with cardiac conduction disease. *Arch Gen Psychiatry* 44:273–275, 1987.

Ross ED, Josman PD, Bell B, et al: Musical hallucinations in deafness. *JAMA* 231:620–622, 1975.

Roth M: The natural history of mental disorder in old age. *J Ment Sci* 101:281–301, 1955.

Rowe JW, Andres R, Tobin JD, et al: The effect of age on creatinine clearance in men: A cross-sectional and longitudinal study. *J Gerontol* 31:155–163, 1976.

Rudorfer MV, Clayton PJ: Depression, dementia, and dexamethasone suppression (letter). *Am J Psychiatry* 138:701, 1981.

Rudorfer MV, Young RC: Desipramine: Cardiovascular effects and plasma levels. *Am J Psychiatry* 137:984–986, 1980.

Sachar EJ, Asnis G, Halbreich U, et al: Recent studies in the neuroendocrinology of major depressive disorders. *Psychiatr Clin North Am* 3:313–326, 1980.

Sachar EJ, Halbreich U, Asnis GM, et al: Paradoxical cortisol responses to dextroamphetamine in endogenous depression. *Arch Gen Psychiatry* 38:1113–1117, 1981.

Sachar EJ, Hellman L, Roffwarg HP, et al: Disrupted 24-hour patterns of cortisol secretion in psychotic depression. *Arch Gen Psychiatry* 28:19–24, 1973.

Saltz R: Fostergrandparenting: A unique child-care service, in Troll LE, Israel J, Israel K (eds): *Looking Ahead: A Woman's Guide to the Problems and Joys of Growing Older.* Englewood Cliffs, NJ, Prentice-Hall, 1977.

Salzman C: A primer on geriatric psychopharmacology. *Am J Psychiatry* 139:67–76, 1982.

Schildkraut JJ: The catecholamine hypothesis of affective disorders: a review of the supporting evidence. *Am J Psychiatry* 122:509–522, 1965

Schlesser MA, Winokur G, Sherman BM: Hypothalamic-pituitary-adrenal axis activity in depressive illness: Its relationship to classification. *Arch Gen Psychiatry* 37:737–743, 1980.

Schmidt CW: Psychiatric problems of the aged. *J Am Geriatr Soc* 22:355, 1974.

Schoenfeld M, Myers RG, Cupples LA, et al: Increased rate of suicide among patients with Huntington's disease. *J Neurol Neurosurg Psychiatr* 47:1283–1287, 1984.

Scovern AW, Kilmann PR: Status of ECT: A review of the outcome literature. *Psychol Bull* 87:260, 1980.

Sendbuehler J, Goldstein S: Attempted suicide among the aged. *J Am Geriatr Soc* 25:245–248, 1977.

Sethna E: A study of refractory cases of depressive illnesses and their response to combined antidepressant treatment. *Br J Psychiatry* 124:265–272, 1974.

Shamoian CA (ed): *Treatment of Affective Disorders in the Elderly*. Washington, DC, American Psychiatric Association Press, 1985.

Sheehan DV, Claycomb JB, Kouretas N: Monoamine oxidase inhibitors: prescription and patient management. *Int J Psychiatry Med* 10:99, 1980–1981.

Sherman EL: *Counseling the Aging: An Integrative Approach*. New York, The Free Press, 1981.

Shuttleworth EC, Huber SJ, Paulson GW: Depression in patients with dementia of Alzheimer type. *J National Med Assoc* 79:733–736, 1987.

Silberman EK, Weingartner H, Post RM: Thinking disorder in depression. *Arch Gen Psychiatry* 40:775–780, 1983.

Silberman EK: Heterogeneity of amphetamine response in depressed patients. *Am J Psychiatry* 138:1302–1306, 1981.

Smith SR, Biedsoc T, Chetii MK: Cortisol metabolism and the pituitary-adrenal axis in adults with protein-calorie malnutrition. *J Clin Endocrinol Metab* 40:43–52, 1975.

Snyder SH, Yamamura HI: Antidepressants and the muscarinic acetylcholine receptor. *Arch Gen Psychiatry* 34:236–239, 1977.

Spar JE, Gerner R: Does the dexamethasone suppression test distinguish dementia from depression? *Am J Psychiatry* 139:238–240, 1982.

Spar JE, LaRue A: Major depression in the elderly: DSM III criteria and the dexamethasone suppression test as predictors of treatment response. *Am J Psychiatry* 140:844–847, 1983.

Spiker DG, Weiss JC, Dealy RS, et al: The pharmacological treatment of delusional depression. *Am J Psychiatry* 142:430–436, 1985.

Sternberg DE, Jarvik ME: Memory functions in depression. *Arch Gen Psychiatry* 33:219–224, 1976.

Steuer J: Psychotherapy for depressed elders, in Blazer DG (ed): *Depression in Late Life*. St Louis, CV Mosby, 1982.

Strang RR: Imipramine in treatment of parkinsonism: A double-blind placebo study. *Br J Med* 2:33–34, 1965.

Streeten DHP, Stevenson CT, Dalakos TC, et al: The diagnosis of hypercortisolism, biochemical criteria differentiating patients from lean and obese normal subjects and from females on oral contraceptives. *J Clin Endocrinol Metab* 29:119–121, 1969.

Stromgren LS: The influence of depression on memory. *Acta Psychiatr Scand* 56:109–128, 1977.

Sullivan G: Increased libido in three men treated with trazodone. *J Clin Psychiatry* 49:202–203, 1988.

Task Force on the Use of Laboratory Tests in Psychiatry: Tricyclic antidepressants-blood level measurements and clinical outcome. *Am J Psychiatry* 142:142–149, 1985.

Terry RD, Davies P: Dementia of the Alzheimer type. *Ann Rev Neurosci* 3:77–95, 1980.

The Medical Letter: Monoamine oxidase inhibitors for depression. July 11, 1980, p 58.

Tollefson GD: Monoamine oxidase inhibitors: A review. *J Clin Psychiatry* 44:280–288, 1983.

Tourigny-Rivard MF, Raskind M, Rivard D: The dexamethasone suppression test in an elderly population. *Biol Psychiatry* 16:1177–1184, 1981.

Tsuang MT, Woolson RF, Fleming JA: Premature deaths in schizophrenia and affective disorders. *Arch Gen Psychiatry* 37:979–983, 1980.

Tsutsui S, Yamazaki Y, Namba T, et al: Combined therapy and antidepressants in depression. *J Int Med Res* 7:138–146, 1979.

Van Praag H, Korf J, Schut D: Cerebral monoamines and depression. *Arch Gen Psychiatry* 28:827–831, 1973.

Vandenbos GR, Stapp J, Kilburg RR: Health service providers in psychology: Results of the 1978 APA Human Resources Survey. *Am Psychol* 36:1395–1418, 1981.

Veith RC, Raskind MA, Caldwell JH, et al: Cardiovascular effects of tricyclic antidepressants. *N Engl J Med* 306:954–959, 1982.

Walker JI, Davidson J, Zung WWK: Patient compliance with MAO inhibitor therapy. *J Clin Psychiatry* 45(7, Sect 2):78–80, 1984.

Wallace EZ, Rosmann P, Toshav N, et al: Pituitary-adrenocorticol function in chronic renal failure: Studies in episodic secretion of cortisol and dexamethasone suppressibility. *J Clin Endocrinol Metab* 50:46–51, 1980.

Warburton JW: Depressive symptoms in parkinsonian patients referred for thalamotomy. *J Neurol Neurosurg Psychiatr* 30:368–370, 1967.

Weiner RD: The role of electroconvulsive therapy in the treatment of depression in the elderly. *J Am Geriatr Soc* 30:710–712, 1982.

Weingartner H, Cohen RM, Murphy DL, et al: Cognitive processes in depression. *Arch Gen Psychiatry* 38:42–47, 1981.

Wellens H, Cats B, Durren D: Symptomatic sinus node abnormalities following lithium carbonate therapy. *Am J Med* 59:285–287, 1975.

Wells BG, Gelenberg AJ: Chemistry, pharmacology, pharmacokinetics, adverse effects and efficacy of the antidepressant maprotiline hydrochloride. *Pharmacotherapy* 1:121–139, 1981.

Wells CE: Pseudodementia. *Am J Psychiatry* 120:244–249, 1963.

Wells CE: Pseudodementia. *Am J Psychiatry* 136:895–900, 1979.

White K, MacDonald N, Razini J, et al: Platelet MAO activity in depression. *Compr Psychiatry* 24:453–457, 1983.

White K, Simpson G: The combined use of MAOIs and tricyclics. *J Clin Psychiatry* 45(7, Sect 2):67–69, 1984.

Wilson J, Kraus E, Bailas M, et al: Reversible sinus node abnormalities due to lithium carbonate therapy. *N Engl J Med* 294:1223–1224, 1976.

Winston F: Combined antidepressant therapy. *Br J Psychiatry* 118:301–304, 1971.

Wolf PA, Dawber TR, Thomas HE, et al: Epidemiology of stroke, in Thompson RA, Green JR (eds): *Advances in Neurology*. New York, Raven Press, 1977, pp 5–19.

Woods SW, Tesar GE, Murray GB, et al: Psychostimulant treatment of depressive disorders secondary to medical illness. *J Clin Psychiatry* 47:12–15, 1986.

Yudofsky SC: Parkinson's disease, depression, and electroconvulsive therapy: A clinical and neurobiologic synthesis. *Compr Psychiatry* 20:579–581, 1979.

Zavodnick S: Atrial flutter with amoxapine: A case report. *Am J Psychiatry* 138:1503–1504, 1981.

Zetin M: Combined use of trimipramine and phenelzine in depression. *J Nerv Ment Dis* 170:246–247, 1982.

Zisook S: Side effects of isocarboxazid. *J Clin Psychiatry* 45(7, Sect 2):53–58, 1984.

5

Alzheimer's Disease and Other Dementias

OVERVIEW

The importance of the dementia syndrome is rapidly being appreciated by the medical community. Clinicians have come to understand that dementia is not a normal and inevitable aspect of the aging process; yet it is also true that the common dementing diseases—except for the acquired immunodeficiency syndrome (AIDS) dementia and the Alzheimer-type dementia of Down's syndrome—are usually expressed in later life (Raskind, 1988).

A review of the statistics on Alzheimer's disease and other dementing illnesses makes it clear that easy solutions are not forthcoming. As noted in earlier chapters, people older than 65 years constitute the fastest-growing segment of the US population, with an eightfold increase from 1900 to 1980. Now, more than 50% of the US population reaches the age of 75 years and 25% live to be 85 years old. As this trend accelerates, the number of Americans older than 65 will more than double from 26 million in 1980 to 67 million by the middle of the next century (Heckler, 1985). Today, one in nine Americans is older than 65 years; by the year 2030, one in five will be in that group.

As the absolute number of elderly Americans increases, age-associated disorders, such as dementia, will become more prevalent. Physicians of all disciplines will come into contact with dementing patients or their families and a basic understanding of the syndrome and its management, from both family and patient perspectives, will be required.

PREVALENCE AND COST OF DEMENTIA

At present, Alzheimer's disease follows heart disease, cancer, and stroke as the fourth leading cause of death in the United States and with public health efforts decreasing the incidence of stroke, it is likely to move up into third place (Maletta, 1988). The prevalence of severe dementia in the United States has recently been estimated at about 1.3 million patients, of which 50% to 60% are of the Alzheimer's type (Terry and Katzman, 1983). Of the population over the age of 65 years, 5% to 6% have severe dementia (Myers et al, 1984); for those over the age of 80 years, it rises to 20%. An additional 2.8 million patients are estimated to have mild-to-moderate impairment on the basis of cognitive decline. The recent National Institute of Mental Health Multisite Epidemiological Catchment Area Study found six-month prevalence rates of mild dementia in persons older than 65 to be 11.5% to 18.4% in noninstitution-alized community samples (Myers et al, 1984). More than 10 billion of the 21 billion dollars spent on nursing home care in the United States in 1982 was expended on the care of patients with dementing illnesses and roughly half of all nursing home beds are presently occupied by Alzheimer's victims. As the number of people living into old age continues to rise, the number of patients will correspondingly increase; we are about to face an epidemic of dementia (Wells, 1981). It is estimated that by the year 2030 the annual cost of taking care of Alzheimer's patients alone will exceed 30 billion dollars.

DIAGNOSIS OF DEMENTIA AND ALZHEIMER'S DISEASE

Most physicians easily recognize the late stages of dementing illnesses but are often unfamiliar with earlier stages, when patient complaints may be largely subjective. The diagnosis of dementia can be made according to DSM-III-R criteria (Table 5–1). Certain progressive degenerative dementias have tradition-ally been referred to as senile and presenile dementias, the distinction being arbitrarily based on an age at onset before or after 65 years. Many of these cases are associated with the histopathologic changes of Alzheimer's disease.

Although definitive diagnosis of Alzheimer's disease is dependent on histo-pathologic data, there is growing consensus that there is a high correlation be-tween this pathology and a particular clinical picture. Since pathologically the presenile and senile onset disorders appear the same, DSM-III-R contains a sin-gle category which is called Primary Degenerative Dementia of the Alzheimer Type.

According to DSM-III-R, Alzheimer's disease (primary degenerative dementia) itself is a physical disorder, and therefore is not included as a mental disorder; it should be recorded in medical records under Axis III. Primary degenerative dementia is still subtyped, however, according to age of onset, to maintain historical continuity and compatibility with international classification systems. Thus Primary Degenerative Dementia of the Alzheimer Type, Senile Onset refers to patients with onset after the age of 65 and Primary Degenerative Dementia of the Alzheimer Type, Presenile Onset refers to patients with onset before the age of 65.

Table 5–1
Diagnostic Criteria for Dementia

A. Demonstrable evidence of impairment in short- and long-term memory. Impairment in short-term memory (inability to learn new information) may be indicated by inability to remember three objects after five minutes. Long-term memory impairment (inability to remember information that was known in the past) may be indicated by inability to remember past personal information (eg, what happened yesterday, birthplace, occupation) or facts of common knowledge (eg, past Presidents, well-known dates).
B. At least one of the following:
    (1) impairment in abstract thinking, as indicated by inability to find similarities and differences between related words, difficulty in defining words and concepts, and other similar tasks
    (2) impaired judgment, as indicated by inability to make reasonable plans to deal with interpersonal, family, and job-related problems and issues
    (3) other disturbances of higher cortical function, such as aphasia (disorder of language), apraxia (inability to carry out motor activities despite intact comprehension and motor function), agnosia (failure to recognize or identify objects despite intact sensory function), and "constructional difficulty" (eg, inability to copy three-dimensional figures, assemble blocks, or arrange sticks in specific designs)
    (4) personality change, ie, alteration or accentuation of premorbid traits
C. The disturbance in A and B significantly interferes with work or usual social activities or relationships with others.
D. Not occurring exclusively during the course of delirium.
E. Either (1) or (2):
    (1) there is evidence from the history, physical examination, or laboratory tests of a specific organic factor (or factors) judged to be etiologically related to the disturbance
    (2) in the absence of such evidence, an etiologic organic factor can be presumed if the disturbance cannot be accounted for by any nonorganic mental disorder, eg, major depression accounting for cognitive impairment

Criteria for severity of dementia:
  Mild: Although work or social activities are significantly impaired, the capacity for independent living remains, with adequate personal hygiene and relatively intact judgment.
  Moderate: Independent living is hazardous, and some degree of supervision is necessary.
  Severe: Activities of daily living are so impaired that continual supervision is required, eg, unable to maintain minimal personal hygiene; largely incoherent or mute.

Reprinted with permission from the *Diagnostic and Statistical Manual of Mental Disorders, third edition, revised.* Copyright 1987. American Psychiatric Association.

The criteria for primary degenerative dementia are listed in Table 5–2. The importance of reevaluating demented patients to document the course of their illness cannot be emphasized to improve the accuracy of diagnosis in patients suspected to have primary degenerative dementia (Shore et al, 1983).

To make the diagnosis of dementia, one must observe a patient who has both memory impairment and a loss of other intellectual abilities of sufficient

Table 5–2
Diagnostic Criteria for Primary Degenerative
Dementia of the Alzheimer Type

A. Dementia.
B. Insidious onset with a generally progressive deteriorating course.
C. Exclusion of all other specific causes of dementia by history, physical examination, and laboratory tests.

Reprinted with permission from the *Diagnostic and Statistical Manual of Mental Disorders, third edition, revised.* Copyright 1987. American Psychiatric Association.

severity to interfere with social or occupational functioning. In addition, at least one of the following must be present: impairment of abstraction; impaired judgement; personality change; or other disturbances of higher cortical function such as aphasia, apraxia, agnosia, or constructional difficulty. In addition, the patient must not be delirious; that is, if one is asked to see a patient for dementia and it turns out that the patient was functioning well at work and socially just a week previously, this would be inconsistent with dementia and the focus would shift to an evaluation for some acute cause (ie, delirium). If the criteria just mentioned are met, clinicians can make the diagnosis of dementia; this does not imply that we know what type of dementing illness it is or what has caused the cognitive decline. It is analogous to making the diagnosis of pneumonia; clinicians still need to find out the cause or type of pneumonia.

If the patient meets criteria for dementia, a clinical diagnosis of Alzheimer's disease or primary degenerative dementia can be made only if the patient's dementing illness has had an insidious onset and generally progressive deteriorating course. One must also exclude all other specific causes of dementia by history, physical examination, and laboratory tests which will be covered later in this chapter. It is best to make the diagnosis of Alzheimer's disease based on the clinical course of the illness.

As noted earlier, many clinicians are only familiar with the late stages of the disease and may fail to recognize beginning stages or attribute early changes to old age or senility (a term with no specific medical meaning). Having a good idea of the natural history of the illness not only will aid in diagnosis but also will assist the caregivers in predicting the future course.

In 1984, a work group established by the National Institute of Neurological and Communicative Disorders and Stroke (NINCDS) and the Alzheimer's Disease and Related Disorders Association (ADRDA) established diagnostic clinical criteria for Alzheimer's disease (McKhann et al, 1984). The need to refine clinical diagnostic criteria was emphasized because 20% or more of patients who had the clinical diagnosis of Alzheimer's disease were found at autopsy to have other conditions and not Alzheimer's disease. It was believed that therapeutic trials could be meaningfully compared only if uniform criteria were used for diagnosis and response to treatment. Their criteria have become accepted as the standard for clinical diagnosis and are listed in Table 5–3.

These criteria are compatible with definitions in DSM-III-R. McKhann and colleagues recommended a diagnosis of definite Alzheimer's disease only after an examination of brain tissue. The diagnosis of probable Alzheimer's disease could be made in a patient who had deficits in two or more areas of cognition, insidious onset of disease and progression, and a normal level of consciousness. The diagnosis of possible Alzheimer's disease was reserved for patients who met the criteria for probable Alzheimer's disease and who had variations in the disease course or had systemic illness that was sufficient to cause dementia but that was not believed to be responsible for the dementia (Thal, 1988).

The only way to definitely make the diagnosis is by doing a brain biopsy; histopathologic changes include senile plaques, neurofibrillary tangles, and granulovacuolar degeneration of neurons (Figure 5–1). Patients with Pick's disease may present with a different clinical picture (see next section) and show similar but different findings at autopsy (Figure 5–1).

However, the ability to diagnose Alzheimer's disease clinically has improved greatly, from a 10% to 50% error rate to at least a 90% assurance of accuracy (Katzman, 1986; Wade et al, 1987; Ron et al, 1979). Improved diagnostic accuracy may be even closer because of the discovery of specific proteins, A50 and A68, which seem to be found selectively in the brains of patients with Alzheimer's disease. These proteins were discovered using monoclonal antibodies reactive to these substances and were not found in the brains of neurologically normal individuals or patients with other neurologic disease (Wolozin et al, 1986; Wolozin and Davies, 1987). Of interest, these proteins are also found in patients with Down's syndrome, a disorder linked to Alzheimer's disease in a number of ways (see later section on genetic theory).

Demonstrating other possibilities for early diagnosis, researchers have reported global and focal cerebral blood flow deficits, by using inhaled radioactive xenon (^{133}Xe) in patients with early onset of Alzheimer's disease, which were later confirmed by results of postmortem neuropathologic examination. These deficits have been sharply discriminated from major depressive disorder, multi-infarct dementia, and diffuse frontotemporal degeneration or Pick's disease, as well as from normal aging (Prohovik et al, 1988; Risberg and Gustafson, 1983).

As more effective treatments become available, the ability to diagnose Alzheimer's disease in its earliest stages will become very important; it is unlikely that treatments will bring dead cells to life (although transplantation of fetal cholinergic cells is being considered).

DEMENTIA OF FRONTAL LOBE TYPE (PICK'S DISEASE)

A significant proportion of patients with presenile dementia caused by primary cerebral atrophy do not have Alzheimer's disease. One form of non-Alzheimer's dementia may be designated as dementia of frontal lobe type (DFT). These patients are classified in DSM-III-R under Presenile (onset before the

Table 5–3
NINCDS/ADRDA Criteria for Clinical Diagnosis
of Alzheimer's Disease*

The criteria for the clinical diagnosis of PROBABLE Alzheimer's disease include:
1. dementia established by clinical examination and documented by the Mini-Mental Test, Blessed Dementia Scale, or some similar examination, and confirmed by neuropsychological tests;
2. deficits in two or more areas of cognition;
3. progressive worsening of memory and other cognitive functions;
4. no disturbance of consciousness;
5. onset between ages 40 and 90, most often after age 65; and
6. absence of systemic disorders or other brain diseases that in and of themselves could account for the progressive deficits in memory and cognition.

The diagnosis of PROBABLE Alzheimer's disease is supported by:
1. progressive deterioration of specific cognitive functions such as language (aphasia), motor skills (apraxia), and perception (agnosia);
2. impaired activities of daily living and altered patterns of behavior;
3. family history of similar disorders, particularly if confirmed neuropathologically; and
4. laboratory results of: normal lumbar puncture as evaluated by standard techniques, normal pattern or nonspecific changes in EEG, such as increased slow-wave activity, and evidence of cerebral atrophy on CT with progression documented by serial observation.

Other clinical features consistent with the diagnosis of PROBABLE Alzheimer's disease, after exclusion of causes of dementia other than Alzheimer's disease, include:
1. plateaus in the course of progression of the illness;
2. associated symptoms of depression, insomnia, incontinence, delusions, illusions, hallucinations, catastrophic verbal, emotional, or physical outbursts, sexual disorders, and weight loss;
3. other neurologic abnormalities in some patients, especially with more advanced disease and including motor signs such as increased muscle tone, myoclonus, or gait disorder;
4. seizures in advanced disease; and
5. CT normal for age.

age of 65) or Senile (onset at the age of 65 or later) Dementia Not Otherwise Specified and the diagnosis is listed on Axis III.

This diagnosis is suggested by a characteristic neuropsychologic picture suggestive of frontal lobe disorder (Neary et al, 1988). Typically patients present, usually between the ages of 40 and 60 years (Moore and Busse, 1987), with social misconduct and personality change with an air of unconcern and disinhibition, but have physical well-being and few neurologic signs. Assessments reveal economic and concrete speech with verbal stereotypes, variable memory impairment, and marked abnormalities on tasks sensitive to frontal lobe function. Visuospatial disorder is invariably absent (Neary et al, 1988). Often behavioral abnormalities occur in the context of relatively mild memory

Table 5–3 *continued*
NINCDS/ADRDA Criteria for Clinical Diagnosis
of Alzheimer's Disease*

Features that make the diagnosis of PROBABLE Alzheimer's disease uncertain or unlikely include:
1. sudden, apoplectic onset;
2. focal neurologic findings such as hemiparesis, sensory loss, visual field deficits, and incoordination early in the course of the illness; and
3. seizures or gait disturbances at the onset or very early in the course of the illness.

Clinical diagnosis of POSSIBLE Alzheimer's disease:
1. may be made on the basis of the dementia syndrome, in the absence of other neurologic, psychiatric, or systemic disorders sufficient to cause dementia, and in the presence of variations in the onset, in the presentation, or in the clinical course;
2. may be made in the presence of a second systemic or brain disorder sufficient to produce dementia, which is not considered to be *the* cause of the dementia; and
3. should be used in research studies when a single, gradually progressive severe cognitive deficit is identified in the absence of other identifiable cause.

Criteria for diagnosis of DEFINITE Alzheimer's disease are:
1. the clinical criteria for probable Alzheimer's disease and
2. histopathologic evidence obtained from a biopsy or autopsy.

Classification of Alzheimer's disease for research purposes should specify features that may differentiate subtypes of the disorder, such as:
1. familial occurrence;
2. onset before age of 65;
3. presence of trisomy-21; and
4. coexistence of other relevant conditions such as Parkinson's disease.

---

*NINCDS = National Institute of Neurological and Communicative Disorders and Stroke, ADRDA = Alzheimer's Disease and Related Disorders Association
Reproduced with permission from McKhann G, Drachman D, Folstein M, et al: Clinical diagnosis of Alzheimer's disease. *Neurology* 34:939–944, 1984.

disturbance. Neary and associates (1988) believed that this disorder may be much more common than is often recognized and they described clinical and imaging characteristics of these patients compared with related findings in patients with Alzheimer's disease (Table 5–4).

DFT is a clinical designation that specifies the presumed major topographical emphasis of pathology, but not pathogenesis (Neary et al, 1988). The presence of circumscribed atrophy of the anterior cerebral hemispheres raises the possibility of Pick's disease (see Figure 5–1F), and the clinical profile of DFT patients is consistent with descriptions of that disease, which have emphasized the early breakdown in social behavior and personality change (Lishman, 1978; Brun and Gustafson, 1978). Kluver-Bucy symptoms (hyperphagia, hyperorality, dietary alterations, hypersexuality, placidity, agnosia) may occur early in the course of Pick's disease.

Neary and colleagues (1988) further contended that although DFT

134

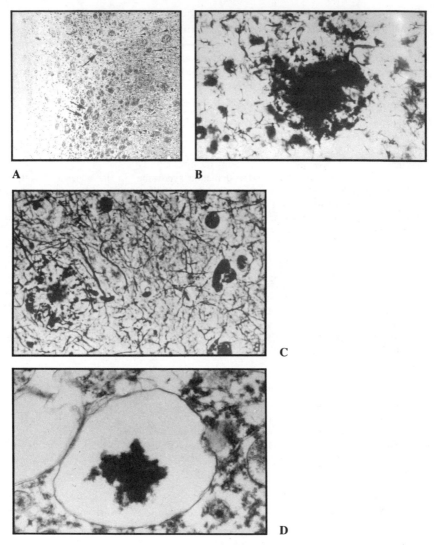

Figure 5–1   Pathologic changes in patients with Alzheimer's disease include senile plaques (low power of hippocampus [**A**]; high power of one plaque [**B**]), neurofibrillary tangles (dark patches on right side of picture [**C**]), and hippocampal granulovacular degeneration (**D**). The brain of a patient who died of Alzheimer's disease (**E**) demonstrates generalized cortical atrophy compared with that of a patient who died of Pick's disease in which atrophy is mainly in the frontal and temporal areas (**F**).

accounts for only a minority of patients with presenile dementia, the incidence appears sufficiently great to suggest that Alzheimer's disease should not be regarded as the inevitable diagnosis in patients meeting clinical criteria for primary degenerative dementia. Besides the distinction between cortical and

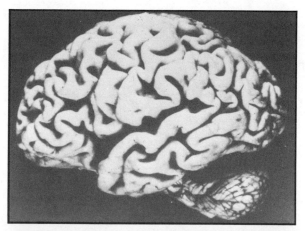

E

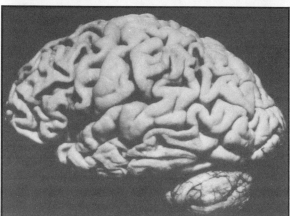

F

subcortical dementia, a further distinction appears warranted: the distinction between the relatively common posterior cortical dementia of Alzheimer's disease and the anterior dementia of DFT.

In addition to questions about diagnosis, clinicians are often consulted about the difficult behavioral problems that these patients exhibit; there is essentially no information on the efficacy of psychotropic medication in these patients. In many ways these patients are more difficult to manage than patients with Alzheimer's disease and extended care or nursing home placement is often indicated at earlier stages of the illness.

COURSE OF PRIMARY DEGENERATIVE DEMENTIA

Reisberg and colleagues (1982) divided the progression of Alzheimer's disease into seven stages (Table 5–5). Clearly, not all patients follow this pattern

Table 5–4
Characteristics of Dementia of Frontal-type and
Alzheimer's Disease

	Dementia of Frontal Lobe Type	Alzheimer's Disease
History	Early personality change and social breakdown	Early memory problems, spatial and language problems
Family history	Dementia common	Dementia less common
Physical signs	Primitive reflexes	Normal early in course of disease
EEG	Normal	Slowing
Single photon emission computed tomography imaging	Anterior abnormalities	Posterior abnormalities
Conduct and affect	Apathy, unconcern, inappropriate jocularity, disinhibition, distractibility, loss of social awareness, loss of emotional empathy, hypochondriasis, obsessionality, gluttony	Anxiety, preserved social awareness early in disease course
Language	Economical output, concrete, mutism in late stage	Often impaired, repetition, naming disorder
Spatial abilities	Preserved	Often impaired in early stage
Memory	Variable memory loss	Consistent memory problems

Reprinted in part from Neary D, Snowden JS, Northen B, et al: Dementia of frontal lobe type. *J Neurol Neurosurg Psychiatry* 51:353–361, 1988.

exactly; however, this outline serves as a rough guide for the clinician and the family concerning expected progression of the disease.

Usually during the earliest stage of the illness, patients seem mildly forgetful and frequently complain of memory deficit; they may forget names or where they have placed household items. The patient may seem concerned, but has no social or employment problems and shows no evidence of memory deficit during clinical interview. Benign senescent forgetfulness and Age Associated Memory Impairment (AAMI) are terms commonly used to describe such complaints in elderly patients whose memory difficulties are not progressive.

The next stage, mild cognitive decline, is evident by decreased performance in demanding employment or social situations. Patients complain of poor concentration and difficulty finding words and names and may report that co-workers have noticed the patient's relatively poor performance. Some patients present initially with primarily visuospatial deficits, and others may have difficulty with

Table 5–5
Stages of Alzheimer's Disease

Stage 1: No cognitive decline
Stage 2: Very mild cognitive decline
    Complaints of forgetfulness
    Forgets names
    Loses items
    No objective deficits in employment or social situations
    Patient displays appropriate concern
Stage 3: Mild cognitive decline
    May remember little of passage read from a book
    Decreased performance in demanding employment and social situations
    Co-workers become aware of patient's relatively poor performance
    Difficulty finding words and names
    May get lost when traveling to unfamiliar locations
    Anxiety is common
    Denial is likely
Stage 4: Moderate cognitive decline
    Clear-cut deficits
    Concentration deficits, eg, poor results on serial sevens test
    Decreased knowledge of recent events in their lives and of current events
    Difficulties traveling alone and in handling personal finances
    Remains oriented to time and person
    Recognizes familiar persons and faces
    Can still travel to familiar locations, eg, corner drugstore
    Withdrawal from challenging situations
    Denial becomes dominant defense
Stage 5: Moderately severe cognitive decline
    Patient can no longer survive without some assistance
    May forget address or telephone number and names of close family members, eg,
       grandchildren
    Frequently disoriented to time or place
    Remembers own names and names of spouse and children
    May clothe themselves improperly, eg, shoe on wrong foot
    Need no assistance with eating or toileting

speech early in the course of the illness (see later section on heterogeneity). Later, patients may get lost when traveling to an unfamiliar location. Anxiety and depression are common and many patients begin to deny symptoms.

In this stage, patients may be less able to handle complex occupational tasks but these deficits often can be so subtle that they are not apparent in people with less demanding social roles, such as retirees. In some jobs that are not complex, the patient may find it unnecessary to withdraw from working (Reisberg, 1988). Some professionals, in fact, are able to function in a nominal fashion even during later stages of the disease. However, teachers, salespersons, and those with similarly demanding occupations may not be able to cope with the normal requirements of their jobs. Patients are often able to function in ordinary community activities without special assistance. Physicians should

Table 5–5 *continued*
Stages of Alzheimer's Disease

Stage 6: Severe cognitive decline
  Eventually forgets spouse's name
  Largely unaware of all recent events and experiences in their lives
  Retain some sketchy knowledge of their past lives
  Unaware of surroundings, season, or year
  Sleep patterns frequently disturbed
  Personality and emotional changes frequent (often occur at earlier stages)
  Delusions, eg, spouse is an imposter, imaginary visitors, talks to own reflection in
    mirror
  Repetitive behaviors—continual cleaning, raking leaves, or lawn mowing
  Anxiety, agitation, occasional violent behavior
  Loss of initiative, abulia, apathy
Stage 7: Very severe cognitive decline
  Late dementia
  Inability to communicate, grunting
  Incontinent of urine and eventually feces
  Needs assistance with toileting and eating
  May be unable to walk
  Focal neurologic signs and symptoms common

Adapted with permission from Reisburg B, Ferris SH, DeLeon MJ, et al: The Global Deterioration Scale for Assessment of primary degenerative dementia. *Am J Psychiatry* 139:1136–1139, 1982.

counsel patients to withdraw from occupational or social tasks that have become stressful because the inability to cope can be anxiety-provoking or humiliating for the patient. Since patients in these early stages can still perform all the routine activities of daily living, the elimination of stressful situations may resolve psychological stress until or unless the patient's condition worsens.

Reisberg (1988) noted that approximately 85% of patients meeting criteria for Stage 3 of Alzheimer's disease (see Table 5–5) experience no notable deterioration of cognition or functioning after three to four years. Others have noted a smaller percentage of patients meeting criteria for mild Alzheimer's disease who do not progress (Storandt et al, 1986). Families and patients can be appraised that rapid progression is not necessarily the rule for patients who have mild dementia.

In the earlier stages of a dementing illness, tests of memory will detect deficits in the recall of recent events while recall of distant memories will remain intact (Sagar et al, 1988). That is, patients may remember where they lived, where and when they got married, and when their children were born, but may be unable to remember what they had for lunch 20 minutes ago.

As the illness progresses, patients become unable to travel alone and to handle their personal finances. Memory for recent events is drastically impaired, and patients display decreased knowledge of current events. Complex tasks are impossible, but patients remain well oriented to time and person and can travel to very familiar places like the corner drugstore. Patients instinctively withdraw from previously challenging situations. Many patients are aware of their deficits and understand what is happening to them. Patients often repeat themselves as a consequence of the illness. Some patients begin to create a protective shield of denial and emotional withdrawal, and the deficits are often more a matter of concern for the spouse than for the patient (Reisberg, 1988).

If the patient is living with a spouse or other close relative, this person can supervise the writing of checks and the handling of other financial matters. If the patient is living alone, a conservator may be useful to help the patient handle finances. Patients are still capable of independent survival and should be assisted in maintaining maximum independence. They can still transact purchases and travel, although they may get lost on occasion. Patients should be encouraged to become involved in activities in which they wish to participate; however, the patient's withdrawal from some activities is an adaptive response to decreasing cognitive abilities. The physician should discuss the diagnosis and its consequences with the family. Local support groups and the Alzheimer's Disease and Related Disorders Association (discussed in detail later) may be of help to caregivers.

During the next phase, patients can no longer survive without assistance and are unable to recall major aspects of their current lives and names of close friends or even family members. Patients cared for by a spouse or other close relative, however, may appear normal to casual acquaintances during social events or even to friends and family who are not responsible for the patient's care. This appearance of normality on the part of the patient can be frustrating for the caregiver, who is faced with very real burdens which may be unrecognized or denied by friends and family.

Delusions and personality changes are common at this stage, but may occur earlier. The spouse may be accused of being an imposter and the patient may talk to imaginary people or to his or her own reflection in the mirror. Depression, agitation, and, rarely, violent behavior may occur and patients are typically disoriented to time or place. They generally require no assistance with toileting or eating, but may have difficulty choosing the proper clothing to wear; they may put their shoes on the wrong feet or put their clothes over their pajamas, for example.

Patients can still enjoy activities that are not complex. The key to selecting activities is to exploit whatever talents and knowledge the patients retain. This is, however, not the time to try to teach them something new. Generally cognitive decline is not accompanied by commensurate physical decline and some form of physical activity can be continued.

The last stages find patients totally incapacitated and disoriented. They eventually forget their names and do not recognize their spouse. Incontinence is common. Eventually all verbal abilities are lost, motor skills deteriorate, and patients require total care. At this stage, generalized cortical and focal neurologic signs and symptoms are frequently present; if these occur earlier in the course of the illness, other causes of dementia should be considered. Death usually occurs from total debilitation or infection (eg, pneumonia or sepsis from decubital ulcerations).

HETEROGENEITY AMONG PATIENTS

Overview

During a recent National Institutes of Health symposium (Friedland, 1988), the clinical and biological heterogeneity of Alzheimer's disease was discussed. Clinicians, for many years, had noted that patients presented with an array of different traits and that not all Alzheimer's patients were alike in terms of neuropsychiatric symptomatology. The presence of considerable intersubject and intrasubject heterogeneity suggests that subtypes of the disease exist. There appear to be subtypes in regard to behavioral features, dosage of chromosome 21 (eg, presence of Down's syndrome), inheritance (eg, familial or sporadic), rate of disease progression, age of onset (eg, presenile or senile), and presence or absence of motor deficit.

Brain Metabolic and Structural Heterogeneity

Studies with positron emission tomography (PET) scans, which measure regional cerebral glucose metabolism, have demonstrated focal alterations in glucose use, with cerebral metabolic asymmetries in dementing patients that are related to the nature of the cognitive deficit (Figure 5–2). For example, patients with Alzheimer's disease who have predominantly right temporoparietal hypometabolism (eg, diminished regional cerebral metabolic rate for glucose) have dramatic visuospatial deficits, which can be demonstrated as an inability to copy a design by memory, as opposed to other patients with mainly left temporoparietal hypometabolism who are able to copy quite well. The opposite pattern (left hypometabolism more than right) is found in patients with a disproportional impairment of language relative to visuospatial function.

Serial CT scans show heterogeneous rates of lateral ventricle enlargement in patients with the disease that are related to rates of cognitive decline. Similar anatomic and physiologic abnormalities are found in persons who are 45 years or older who have Down's syndrome.

Neurochemical Heterogeneity

On a neurochemical level, much of the recent research has focused on abnormalities in the ascending cholinergic neurons in the cerebral cortex and hippocampus which have reduced function in Alzheimer's disease and whose changes correlate with clinical severity of dementia and with the extent of neuropathologic changes found in such patients (Perry et al, 1977 and 1978; Davies, 1979; Rossor et al, 1982 and 1984; Reinikainen et al, 1985, 1987,

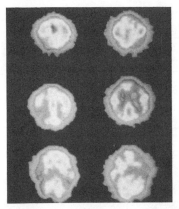 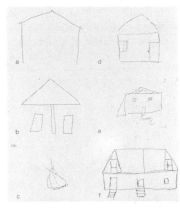

A   **B**

Figure 5–2 (**A**) Positron emission tomographic (PET) scan of a patient with predominantly left-sided hypofunction (left) and PET scan of a patient with more right-sided hypofunction (right). Both patients have the same level of functioning as assessed by memory tests. (**B**) The patient with left-sided hypofunction drew the figures on the right, exhibiting good visuospatial abilities, while the patient with right-sided hypofunction drew the figures on the left, which show a pronounced loss of visuospatial skills. This demonstrates that Alzheimer's disease is not a homogeneous disorder and that careful evaluation of each patient is necessary in order for the clinician to give the best advice to maximize function.

and 1988; Mountjoy, 1986; Neary et al, 1986; Perry, 1986). Alterations in other classic ascending neurotransmitter systems, including noradrenergic and serotonergic systems, have been less extensively documented (Rossor and Iversen, 1986; Palmer et al, 1987; Reinikainen et al, 1988) but are clearly present in many patients.

Reinikainen and colleagues (1988) studied 20 brains from patients with histologically confirmed Alzheimer's disease and compared them with 14 control patients and reported that concentrations of noradrenaline were decreased significantly in the frontal cortex, temporal cortex, hippocampus, and putamen in the dementing patients. Serotonin levels were significantly lowered in the hippocampus, hippocampal cortex, caudate nucleus, and putamen and a metabolite of serotonin, 5-HIAA, was reduced in some cortical areas, thalamus, and putamen. Overall, the damage to serotonergic neurons seemed to be more generalized and more severe than that to adrenergic neurons. These findings further confirmed the involvement of noradrenergic and serotonergic systems in patients with Alzheimer's disease. Thus, not only clinical heterogeneity among patients is common, but also neurochemical findings may vary significantly.

The possible clinical relevance of these findings as they relate to cognitive dysfunction and behavioral disturbances awaits further evaluation before it will be possible to decide whether or when these neuronal systems in patients with Alzheimer's disease should be manipulated by pharmacological agents.

Despite advances in knowledge, the clinician is still left with a trial-and-error approach when dealing with psychiatric symptoms in the dementing patient. Perhaps the time will come when physicians can perform cerebrospinal fluid assays, determine specific individual aberrations, and tailor treatment for each patient's chemical abnormalities.

Heterogeneity of Clinical Symptoms

The behavioral manifestations of Alzheimer's disease are not uniform. Some authors studied features of late-onset versus early-onset forms of the disease and noted some differences. Seltzer and Sherwin (1983) studied a total of 65 patients and found that those who had early onset of disease demonstrated a greater prevalence of language disturbance, a disproportionate prevalence of left-handedness, and a much shorter relative survival time. Folstein and Breitner (1981) found that patients with a language disorder were statistically more likely to have a family history of dementia than those who did not. Becker and associates (1988) compared 86 patients with probable Alzheimer's disease and 92 elderly control subjects and identified various patterns of impairments in the dementing patients. They identified a group of patients, all with at least mild memory impairment, who had primarily visuoconstructional deficits and another group with mainly verbal inadequacies, but found no significant differences in age at onset or rate of progression of dementia among patients with different patterns of cognitive dysfunction. These data suggest that there are different patterns of neuropsychological deficits in patients with Alzheimer's disease and that these differences may be related to the pathophysiology of the disease.

Inheritance of the disease varies among patients; although most cases are sporadic, 10% to 15% are due to autosomal dominant inheritance, usually with clinical features that are identical to the sporadic cases (Friedland, 1988).

The course of Alzheimer's disease from onset of symptoms to death is usually 5 to 10 years, but rapid progression with death within 1 or 2 years, or slow progression with plateau and survival for 12 or more years, has also been documented. The age of onset may vary, beginning in most patients after 65 years old, but the disease may occur in younger persons, as originally reported by Alzheimer in 1906. Typically, the illness progresses at a fairly constant rate; that is, if it has progressed rapidly over the past years it is likely to continue at that rate. A slowly progressive illness over the past 5 to 10 years means that the patient may survive for a number of years. These are not infallible rules, but do serve as a rough guideline (Jenike, 1987 and 1988).

The first and most salient symptom of Alzheimer's disease is usually memory loss; patients are forgetful, misplace objects, or have difficulty keeping appointments. Changes in noncognitive behaviors may include agitation or apathy, sleep disturbances, paranoid ideation, and hallucinations. As noted already, some patients first have a language deficit or visuospatial or perceptual impairment. Patients whose disease is at the same stage may have different symptoms.

Occasionally clinicians see patients who appear demented but upon closer examination, it is clear that their main problems are with communication and that if careful memory tests are performed, their memory is only slightly or not impaired. They may speak as if they have had a stroke, but give no history of stroke and neurologic examination is otherwise normal. Poeck and Luzzatti (1988) described cases of patients who had such a slowly progressive aphasic disorder with little or no dementia for a number of years. Mehler and associates (1987) also described the cases of two patients with progressive dysphasia who did eventually have profound cognitive and behavioral disturbances and asymmetric left cerebral atrophy that was also progressive. Interestingly, these patients had normal tissue levels of choline acetyltransferase activity, but reduced somatostatin-like immunoreactivity. Since cerebral somatostatin is largely present in intrinsic cortical neurons, while cholinergic innervation is largely derived from the basal forebrain, these findings suggest that this form of dysphasic dementia may be an example of a distinct class of dementia caused by intrinsic cortical degeneration, with sparing of the basal forebrain. Poeck and Luzzatti (1988) believed that this disorder is quite rare and most likely represents an atypical presentation of Alzheimer's disease; others (Mesulam, 1982; Benson et al, 1982) thought that these patients do not have Alzheimer's disease and may have some other, as yet unidentified, disorder. The vast majority of these patients do not have the behavioral abnormalities and judgement lapses that typically occur in patients with Pick's disease. Psychotropic agents are helpful to treat concomitant psychiatric symptoms and speech therapy may assist the patients' efforts to communicate.

In another study, patients with Alzheimer's disease with onset of symptoms prior to the age of 65 years had more pronounced language deficits, while those whose onset was apparent after the age of 65 years had more problems with visuospatial functions (Filley et al, 1986). Koss and Friedland (1987), however, suggested alternative interpretations of their data.

Patients with Alzheimer's disease who have extrapyramidal dysfunction or myoclonus are a distinct subgroup, with specific abnormalities of central monoamine markers of dopamine metabolism, serotonin metabolism, and the hydroxylation cofactor, biopterin.

Significance of Heterogeneity

The clinical significance of heterogeneity among dementing patients meeting criteria for primary degenerative dementia (Alzheimer's disease) remains to be determined, but it appears that the clinician cannot assume specific deficits, apart from memory loss which is essential to make the diagnosis, and must obtain detailed neuropsychologic assessment of each patient in order to know how best to be of assistance to the patient. For example, telling an elderly dementing woman who loves to knit to keep on knitting will lead to frustration and anger if this woman has pronounced visuospatial deficits that prevent her from being able to knit. Similarly, allowing a dementing patient to drive just because his eyes test adequately could lead to a dangerous situation if the patient has difficulty determining spatial relationships. Neuropsychologists are trained to identify specific areas of deficit and also to suggest ways to maximize function despite these deficits.

The concept of subtypes and heterogeneity in this disorder is based primarily on clinical observations and on data provided by the powerful tools that are now available for noninvasive quantitative assessment of important aspects of brain structure and function. It appears that the clinical picture reflects the relative degrees of involvement of different cortical regions as shown by PET studies of regional cerebral glucose metabolism. We still have no idea why certain patients have one area affected and not another. What determines the subtypes? Are these separate diseases with separate causes or do these findings reflect genetic susceptibility to some environmental toxin? We do not know why the disease develops in some patients at an early age or why the disease develops in Down's syndrome patients earlier and why they have a more benign course.

The concept of subtypes in Alzheimer's disease serves as a model with which the interactions of genetic influences with environmental factors can be examined.

Treatment studies not only must assess overall group success but also must identify subgroups of responders or nonresponders.

EVALUATION AND DIFFERENTIAL DIAGNOSIS OF THE DEMENTING PATIENT

Overview

Some authors have attempted to determine predictive factors for potentially reversible intellectual decline. Freeman and Rudd (1982) studied the records of 110 patients who had progressive cognitive decline and found 16 in whom intellectual deterioration was caused by underlying treatable disorders. These 16 patients had a shorter duration of symptoms and evidenced less cortical atrophy on CT scan than did patients who had idiopathic dementia. The average age of the two groups was not significantly different. We have noted anecdotally that fluctuating cognitive state is one clue to an organic cause; that is, one day the patient may score 16 on the MMSE (chapter 2) and the next day score 27.

Medical Workup

To make the diagnosis of Alzheimer's disease, one must exclude all other specific causes of dementia (Table 5–6 and Table 5–7). Haase (1977) listed more than 50 diseases that may cause dementia, and this list is constantly

Table 5–6
Potentially Treatable Causes of Dementia

Tumors
    Direct CNS invasion
    Remote effect, usually from lung tumor, occasionally from ovary, prostate, rectum
        or breast tumors
Nutritional
    Vitamin B_{12} deficiency (dementia may precede anemia)
    Folate deficiency, pellagra, Wernicke-Korsakoff syndrome
Infection
    Syphilis, abscess, encephalitis, AIDS
Metabolic
    Electrolytes, hepatic or renal disorder, chronic obstructive lung disease (COLD)
Inflammatory
    Lupus
Endocrine
    Thyroid (hypo- or hyperthyroid), adrenal, parathyroid
Trauma
    Subdural
Psychiatric/neurologic
    Schizophrenia, seizures, normal pressure hydrocephalus (NPH) (dementia, ataxia,
        incontinence), depression (most common, may need medication trial)

Reproduced with permission from Jenike MA: Alzheimer's disease—What the practicing clinician needs to know. *J Geriatr Psychiatr Neurol* 1:37–46, 1988.

growing. Alzheimer's disease is, however, the most common disorder producing dementia in the elderly, with postmortem studies confirming that between 50% and 60% of all patients with dementia have classic Alzheimer's changes (Jellinger, 1976; Sourander and Sjogren, 1970; Tomlinson et al, 1968 and 1970).

Other neurologic diseases produce dementia: Parkinson's disease (about 40% become demented [Cummings, 1988]), Huntington's chorea, and Creutzfeldt-Jakob disease. After Alzheimer's disease, however, multiple strokes or so-called multi-infarct dementia is the second leading cause of dementia and Hachinski and colleagues (1974) developed a group of questions that can assist the clinician and researcher in ruling out multi-infarct dementia (Table 5–8). Liston and La Rue (1983), in a comprehensive review of the literature, suggested that clinical differentiation of primary degenerative dementia from multi-infarct dementia (Table 5–9), however, is far from perfect and that only results of studies for which autopsy material has been obtained should be considered relevant. In practice, one often sees patients with clinical pictures that overlap; that is, sudden loss of function superimposed on a general picture of gradual and progressive loss of function.

Once the diagnosis of dementia has been made, the clinician must perform a thorough medical, neurologic, and psychiatric evaluation. Brain failure requires as thorough an evaluation as heart failure or renal failure. Potentially

Table 5–7
Commonly Used Medications That May Cause
Cognitive or Affective Change in the Elderly

Alcohol
Beta blockers, especially propranolol (Inderal)
Antihypertensive agents
   Beta blockers (see above)
   Methyldopa
   Reserpine
   Clonidine
   Diuretics
Neuroleptics
   Haloperidol (Haldol)
   Chlorpromazine (Thorazine)
   Thioridazine (Mellaril)
   Fluphenazine (Prolixin)
   Perphenazine (Trilafon)
   Loxapine (Loxitane)
   Molindone (Moban)
   Thiothixene (Navane)
   Trifluoperazine (Stelazine)
Benzodiazepines
   Diazepam (Valium)
   Flurazepam (Dalmane)
   Clorazepate (Tranxene)
   Chlordiazepoxide (Librium)
   Prazepam (Centrax)
   Alprazolam (Xanax)
   Halazepam (Paxipam)
   Triazolam (Halcion)
   Temazepam (Restoril)
   Oxazepam (Serax)
   Lorazepam (Ativan)
Antiseizure medications
   Barbiturates
   Carbamazepine (Tegretol)
   Phenytoin (Dilantin)
   Phenobarbital
Antihistamines
Cimetidine
Steroids
Procainamide
Disopyramide
Quinidine
Atropine and other anticholinergic agents (eg, benztropine, trihexyphenidyl, diphenhy-
   dramine, etc)

Reproduced with permission from Jenike MA: Depression and other psychiatric disorders, in Albert MS, Moss M (eds): *Geriatric Neuropsychology*. New York, Guildford Press, 1988, pp 115–144.

treatable causes of dementia are listed in Table 5–6 and 5–7 and a suggested workup to eliminate most treatable causes is listed in Table 5–10 (Jenike, 1986, 1986a, and 1988).

A thorough physical examination is important for all patients with dementia as disease in virtually any organ system can cause an acute confusional state or delirium. During a physical exam in a dementing patient, a few clues may surface: (1) Pneumonia and myocardial infarction cause acute confusion, or exacerbate a chronic condition; (2) subcortical dementias frequently produce neurologic signs, including the typical bradykinesia and gait of Parkinson's disease; (3) multi-infarct dementias frequently produce asymmetrical pyramidal and extrapyramidal signs; and (4) normal pressure hydrocephalus may be characterized by an ataxic gait in the presence of incontinence (Moore and Busse, 1987). On the other hand, the cortical degenerative diseases including Alzheimer's and Pick's disease characteristically produce unremarkable results of the physical examination until late in the course of the illness (see later section for discussion of the concepts of cortical and subcortical dementia).

The erythrocyte sedimentation rate (ESR) is a quick, inexpensive screening test for inflammatory conditions, especially collagen vascular diseases that may present with the picture of dementia.

The CT scan may help to diagnose the cause of reversible or treatable dementias such as subdural hematoma, normal pressure hydrocephalus, and brain tumor. It may also make apparent less treatable causes such as multiple strokes or Alzheimer's disease. Clinicians sometimes see patients who have been mistakenly told that they have Alzheimer's disease based on the appearance of mild or moderate atrophy on CT scan. In patients with advanced Alzheimer's disease, the CT scan typically shows marked cortical atrophy with widened sulci and shrunken gyri and ventricular dilatation. Mild-to-moderate cortical atrophy, however, is not well correlated with brain pathology or clinical condition (Lishman, 1978; Wells, 1977). That is, many healthy elderly people have moderate atrophy as determined by CT scan while some dementing patients have none. Thus, cortical atrophy itself does not establish a diagnosis of a cortical degenerative disease, as cortical atrophy correlates better with age than with presence of dementia (Moore and Busse, 1987).

To compare the merits of magnetic resonance imaging (MRI) and CT scan in assessing patients with dementia, Johnson and colleagues (1987) examined pairs of MRI and CT brain images obtained from 26 patients with Alzheimer's disease, 8 patients with vascular or mixed dementia, and 2 patients with Parkinson's disease plus dementia. They found that abnormalities in subcortical white matter and in hippocampus, enlargement of basal and sylvian cisterns, and ventriculomegaly were more evident on MRI than on CT scans, but qualitative ratings in all other brain regions were similar. Overall, severity of dementia correlated with periventricular white matter abnormalities on both MRI and CT images. An advantage of MRI was its greater image contrast between normal and abnormal brain as well as between gray and white matter structures and cerebrospinal fluid. The high sensitivity of MRI to white matter abnormalities (Bradley et al, 1984) has been a useful aid in the investigation of stroke (Dewitt et al, 1984) and demyelinating disease (Lukes et al, 1983). Whether or not MRI offers any advantage over the CT scan in the evaluation of the dementing patient without focal neurologic signs and symptoms or a history of hypertension remains to be determined (see chapter 13 for more on MRI).

PET evaluations of patients with Alzheimer's disease have shown a substantial, generalized decline in oxygen and in glucose utilization in cerebral hemisphere as the disease progressed (Katzman, 1986). One group reviewed by Katzman reported that PET scan studies in patients with Alzheimer's disease revealed decreased metabolism in parietal and frontal cortex with intact subcortical metabolism. PET scans demonstrate diminished metabolic activity in the frontal lobes in patients with progressive supranuclear palsy and show a mild diffuse decrement in metabolism of both cortical and subcortical structures in Parkinson's disease.

PET remains largely of research interest because of the expense of scans, scarcity of machines, and relative paucity of published data. Nonetheless, PET and some of the newer scans may, in the future, be of invaluable assistance in the diagnosis of dementing diseases and also in following response to treatment. One group already demonstrated, for example, that cortical hypometabolism as demonstrated by PET scan improved in response to physostigmine in occasional patients, who also improved clinically with this medication (Folstein, 1987). In Huntington's disease, decreased glucose metabolism is demonstrable in the caudate nucleus even before structural alterations are evident on CT scans and when behavioral and motor symptoms are minimal (Cummings and Benson, 1988); cerebral cortical metabolism is unaffected however (see chapter 13 for more on PET).

Differential Diagnosis

One of the most common causes of a treatable dementia is drugs, as almost any drug can cause cognitive impairment. Propranolol has been reported to mimic Alzheimer's disease. Other common offenders include methyldopa, clonidine, haloperidol, chlorpromazine, phenytoin, bromides, paraldehyde, primidone, phenacetin, phenobarbital, cimetidine, quinidine, procainamide, disopyramide, and atropine and related compounds. A trial without medication is the only way to determine if a drug is a factor. Often alcoholic patients will show greatly improved cognition over a period of months when they stop drinking.

Tumors may cause cognitive impairment either directly by interfering with the CNS or by a poorly understood remote effect. Such remote effects are associated with pulmonary neoplasms in the great majority of patients, but other reported sites include the ovary, breast, rectum, and prostate (Lishman, 1978).

Thyroid abnormalities, both hyperthyroid and hypothyroid states, are the most common endocrine dysfunctions associated with cognitive impairment. Approximately three-quarters of patients with pernicious anemia have objective memory impairment and 60% have abnormal EEGs. Most return to normal after replacement therapy. Unless replacement therapy is started early, irreversible deficits that may precede the anemia may occur. All dementing patients should be screened for megaloblastic anemia, and serum levels of vitamin B_{12} should be checked for all patients with unexplained dementia, especially when they have persistent fatigue or a history of gastric surgery. Folic acid deficiency may also present as megaloblastic anemia with dementia. Prior to starting folic acid replacement, the serum level of vitamin B_{12} should be checked because these levels tend to fall when folic acid therapy is started, and this could precipitate or aggravate neurologic disturbances in patients with undiagnosed pernicious anemia (Lishman, 1978).

Neurosyphilis, which may progress to frank dementia, if untreated, is frequently associated with concentration difficulty, faulty judgement, emotional instability, and malaise. In older persons the VDRL and fluorescent treponemal antibody absorption (FTA-ABS) tests are both done as serologic studies for syphilis. The FTA-ABS test is more specific and important because of the frequency of serum negative VDRL results for tertiary syphilis in older people. A negative VDRL result but positive FTA-ABS result calls for cerebrospinal fluid serologies to establish or rule out tertiary syphilis (O'Daniel et al, 1981).

Subdural hematomas usually follow head trauma, but may occur spontaneously in the elderly, especially in patients who have blood dyscrasias or those who are taking anticoagulants. Patients with a chronic subdural hematoma may have increasing difficulty with concentration, memory lapses, and fluctuating level of consciousness. Variability in the mental state from day to day and even from hour to hour is often the most important indicator of this condition. Sometimes headache or episodes of restlessness may occur. The EEG is abnormal in 90% of these patients. A CT scan may show a mass effect, but the subdural hematoma assumes the same density as brain tissue approximately 10 days after a bleed. After that, a brain scan is a useful diagnostic test (Lishman, 1978).

Vascular Dementias

While the earlier belief that Alzheimer's disease was related to atherosclerosis has been proven false, other forms of irreversible dementia are currently attributed to vascular disease. In general, these processes are associated with

Table 5–8
Hachinski Ischemic Score*

Feature	Value, if present	Score
Abrupt onset	2	—
Stepwise deterioration	1	—
Fluctuating course	2	—
Nocturnal confusion	1	—
Relative preservation of personality	1	—
Depression	1	—
Somatic complaints	1	—
Emotional incontinence	1	—
History of hypertension	1	—
History of strokes	2	—
Evidence of associated atherosclerosis	1	—
Focal neurological symptoms	2	—
Focal neurological signs	2	—
Total Score		—

*A total score of 5 or greater is suggestive of multi-infarct dementia.
Reproduced with permission from Hachinski VC, Iliff LD, Zilhka E, et al: Cerebral blood flow in dementia. *Arch Neurol* 32:632–637, 1975.

a history of hypertension and stroke (see Tables 5–8 and 5–9) but the syndrome can occur with atherosclerosis, diabetes, embolic disorders, or inflammatory conditions (Cummings, 1986). CT scanning may provide evidence of multifocal defects, but some infarctions may be too small to be visualized radiologically and a normal appearance on CT scan does not exclude the diagnosis of multi-infarct dementia (Cummings, 1986). Depression is common with multi-infarct dementia and seizures develop in 15% of these patients (Cummings, 1986). While the dementias associated with vascular disease are complex and somewhat controversial, there appear to be at least three main patterns of dementia caused by ischemic vascular disease (Moore and Busse, 1987). These

Table 5–9
Diagnostic Criteria for Multi-infarct Dementia

A. Dementia.
B. Stepwise deteriorating course with "patchy" distribution of deficits (ie, affecting some functions, but not others) early in the course.
C. Focal neurologic signs and symptoms (eg, exaggeration of deep tendon reflexes, extensor plantar response, pseudobulbar palsy, gait abnormalities, weakness of an extremity, etc).
D. Evidence from history, physical examination, or laboratory tests of significant cerebrovascular disease (recorded on Axis III) that is judged to be etiologically related to the disturbance.

Reprinted with permission from the *Diagnostic and Statistical Manual of Mental Disorders, third edition, revised.* Copyright 1987. American Psychiatric Association.

are multiple large cerebral infarcts, lacunar infarcts of smaller vessels, and Binswanger's disease which is also called subcortical atherosclerotic encephalopathy. While it is unclear as to the relative importance of volume of brain tissue lost versus location of the damage, it has been generally accepted that at least 90 cm^3 of brain tissue must be involved in vessel disease to produce significant dementia (Tomlinson et al, 1970).

Binswanger's disease is a confusing disorder as radiographic and pathologic descriptions are better defined than is the clinical syndrome; most patients, however, have a history of hypertension and subacute, gradual mental deterioration. The clinical spectrum appears to range from asymptomatic radiologic lesions to dementia with focal deficits, frontal signs, pseudobulbar palsy, gait difficulties, and urinary incontinence (Roman, 1987). Pathologically, patients show periventricular demyelination, most marked in the posterior frontal regions. Radiographically, Binswanger's disease is seen as areas of hypolucency on CT scan and MRI shows areas of white matter hyperintensity. Roman (1987) noted that the periventricular white matter is a watershed area irrigated by long, penetrating medullary arteries and that risk factors for this disorder are small-artery diseases such as hypertension and amyloid angiopathy, impaired autoregulation of cerebral blood flow in the elderly, and periventricular hypoperfusion due to cardiac failure, arrhythmias, and hypotension. As described in a case report, depression in a patient with typical CT findings of Binswanger's disease improved with moderate doses of MAOI (Summergrad, 1985).

Hydrocephalus

Normal pressure hydrocephalus is characterized by the development over many weeks or months of memory impairment, physical and mental slowness, unsteadiness of gait, and urinary incontinence (Hakim and Adams, 1965; Mamo et al, 1987). The mental changes usually occur first, although gait disturbance may be the presenting symptom. Urinary incontinence generally appears much later. This disorder is, unfortunately, probably not as frequently reversible as was originally hoped. It is an uncommon disorder that can resemble Alzheimer's disease. In one of the earliest extensive reviews of this disorder, Katzman (1977) found that in only one-third of the patients the disorder was idiopathic and that in two-thirds it was secondary to other processes: most commonly subarachnoid hemorrhage and trauma (Moore and Busse, 1987).

Other causes of hydrocephalus included tumors and aqueductal stenosis. These patients should be referred for a complete neurologic workup including a CT scan and Risa cisternography which may show characteristically dilated ventricles with abnormal flow of cerebrospinal fluid (Wells, 1977). Patients with this disorder are sometimes helped by permanent placement of a cerebrospinal fluid shunt to drain fluid away from the brain. It is hypothesized that the reduction in cerebral blood flow in patients with normal pressure hydrocephalus is a result of increased intraparenchymal pressure in the brain (Mamo et al, 1987). There has been much controversy about how to decide which patients to shunt and Mamo and colleagues (1987) suggested using a xenon-133 method to measure cerebral blood flow before and after a trial of cerebrospinal fluid removal. Their preliminary results suggested that shunting should be performed on patients whose cerebral blood flow increases after removal of cerebrospinal fluid. They found a significant increase in cerebral blood flow in patients with normal pressure hydrocephalus, which was confirmed by the favorable outcome of 88% of patients shunted. They used a control group of patients with presenile and senile dementia and found that they showed, in contrast, a decrease or no change in blood flow after removal of cerebrospinal fluid.

Extrapyramidal Disorders

A host of degenerative extrapyramidal syndromes are also accompanied by dementia. These include Parkinson's disease, Huntington's disease, progressive supranuclear palsy, Wilson's disease, and olivopontocerebellar atrophies. In some, the dementia is mild or is confined to the final stages of the disease. In others, dementia occurs early and is a prominent disability. CT scans may show distinctive abnormalities in Huntington's disease (caudate atrophy), Wilson's disease (putaminal alterations), and olivopontocerebellar atrophy (cerebellar atrophy). Wilson's disease has diagnostic laboratory findings (low levels of serum ceruloplasm, elevated levels of urinary copper).

Treatment is disease specific in the patients with Parkinson's disease and Wilson's disease and is directed toward controlling the chorea in Huntington's

Table 5–10
Workup of the Dementing Patient

History from patient and relative or friend
Mental status examination
Physical examination with vital signs
Neurological examination
CT scan and EEG
Thyroid functions, serum vitamin B_{12} and folic acid
Chest x-ray, ECG
Complete blood count, urinalysis, blood urea nitrogen, glucose, calcium, albumin, electrolytes, alkaline phosphatase, erythrocyte sedimentation rate, Venereal Disease Research Laboratory test for syphilis, flourescent treponemal antibody-absorption test
Others as indicated: drug levels, toxic screen, brain scan, lumbar puncture (not routinely)

Reproduced with permission from Jenike MA: Alzheimer's disease—What the practicing clinician needs to know. *J Geriatr Psychiatr Neurol* 1:37–46, 1988.

disease. The dementia may improve with levodopa therapy for Parkinson's disease or with penicillamine treatment of Wilson's disease (Cummings, 1986).

Progressive supranuclear palsy, also known as Steele-Richardson-Olszewski disorder, is a chronic progressive disorder with extrapyramidal rigidity, bradykinesia, gait impairment, bulbar palsy, dementia, and a characteristic supranuclear ophthalmoplegia often manifested as a loss of volitional downgaze. The inability to look down may be the initial presenting symptom of this disorder. This leads to frequent falls and to the telltale "dirty-tie sign," as the patient cannot look down while walking or eating (Cummings and Benson, 1983, p 86). CT and MRI scans show midbrain atrophy early and atrophy of the pontine and midbrain tegmentum and the frontal and temporal lobes later (Duvoisin et al, 1987). Psychiatric symptoms are unusual but an occasional patient has been reported to improve with treatment with amitriptyline (Kvale, 1982).

Clinical Approach to Workup

Until a diagnosis is made, a specific disorder such as Alzheimer's disease should probably not be mentioned to the patient or the family. People tend to be terrorized by the possibility that they or somebody in their family may be affected by it, and there is nothing to be gained by prematurely raising the specter of Alzheimer's disease (Moore and Busse, 1987).

CORTICAL VERSUS SUBCORTICAL DEMENTIA

The dementia accompanying Alzheimer's disease is referred to as a cortical dementia; dementia in patients with other neurologic disorders, such as Huntington's disease, Parkinson's disease, and progressive supranuclear palsy, that principally involve subcortical structures (such as the basal ganglia, brain stem, and subcortical white-matter tracts) are called subcortical dementias (Cummings and Benson, 1983, 1984, and 1988; Joynt and Shoulson, 1975). In addition, subcortical dementia can result from a variety of subcortical vascular, infectious, inflammatory, neoplastic, and traumatic conditions including spinocerebellar degeneration, idiopathic basal ganglia calcification, multiple sclerosis, and the AIDS-dementia complex (Cummings and Benson, 1988).

Some believe that these two types of dementia are clinically quite different (Table 5–11). The cortical dementias, such as Alzheimer's disease and Pick's disease, are said to be characterized by aphasia, agnosia, and apraxia; findings that are usually absent in the subcortical dementias. Language testing has proved to be among the most reliable means of distinguishing subcortical and cortical dementias. Linguistic functions are relatively spared in the subcortical

Table 5–11
Cortical versus Subcortical Dementia

	Cortical Dementia	Subcortical Dementia
Typical diseases	Alzheimer's disease, Pick's disease	Parkinson's disease, Huntington's chorea, progressive supranuclear palsy, AIDS-dementia complex
Movement disorder	None or in late stage	In early stage
Bradyphrenia	None or in late stage	In early stage
Memory disturbance	More severe, faster progression	Less severe, slowly progressive
Language disturbance	Very common in early stage	Unusual until very late stage
Apraxia	Very common in early stage	Unusual until very late stage
Depression	Uncommon	Very common
Psychosis	Uncommon	Rare with Parkinson's, common with Huntington's
PET scan	Decreased glucose metabolism cortically	Huntington's—decreased glucose metabolism in caudate, Parkinson's—decreased glucose metabolism cortically and subcortically

dementing disorders, whereas they are prominently affected from the early stages in many patients with cortical dementias (Cummings and Benson, 1988; Cummings et al, 1988). When present, language difficulties in Parkinson's patients are most likely to involve motor functions such as phrase length, speech melody, dysarthria, and agraphia (Cummings et al, 1988). Similarly, patients with multi-infarct dementia are also likely to have difficulties with the motor aspects of speech, while patients with Alzheimer's disease generally exhibit empty speech, more marked anomia, and relative sparing of motor speech functions (Powell et al, 1988).

Patients with Parkinson's disease perform normally on tests of naming unless their dementia syndrome is severe (Bayles and Tomoeda, 1983; Freedman et al, 1984; Huber et al, 1986). Mahler and colleagues (1985) failed to identify any language alterations in patients with progressive supranuclear palsy, and Caine and associates (1986) found that language changes in patients with Huntington's disease were mild and relatively less profound than alterations in memory and abstraction.

In contrast to the mild linguistic changes exhibited by patients with subcortical dementias, Alzheimer's patients exhibit marked language abnormalities (Bayles and Tomoeda, 1983; Mendez et al, 1987). In addition, the progressive intellectual and memory dysfunction of Alzheimer's disease is said to be more severe and progress more rapidly than that of the subcortical syndromes.

Patients with subcortical dementias seem to benefit from strategies that help them to encode stimulus material for later recall and clues aid the patient in recalling learned information (Butters et al, 1983; Martone et al, 1986; Wilson et al, 1987; Flowers et al, 1984; Huber et al, 1986a; Weingartner et al, 1984). In contrast, patients with Alzheimer's dementia have more difficulty encoding information for later retrieval and are aided little by encoding strategies (Butters et al, 1983; Davis and Mumford, 1984; Kopelman, 1985). Patients with subcortical dementias are often described as apathetic and depressed and suffer from bradyphrenia (cognitive slowing), whereas patients with Alzheimer's disease are said to lack insight and tend not to be depressed. Subcortical disorders are usually linked with movement disorders, such as the chorea of Huntington's disease or the tremor and rigidity of Parkinson's disease.

Pillon and associates (1986) compared patients with Alzheimer's disease (cortical dementia) and those with progressive supranuclear palsy (subcortical dementia). They matched patients for overall severity of dementia and found that the patient groups exhibited different profiles of neuropsychologic impairment; patients with progressive supranuclear palsy evidenced more marked frontal systems dysfunction than Alzheimer's patients. The former manifested more inertia, stereotypy, disinterest, and indifference to rules and had less mental control.

There appears to be some validity to the cortical-subcortical distinction, but it is not strikingly useful to the clinician. Some general principles, however, seem to hold true. Patients with Alzheimer's disease do not have neurologic signs and symptoms until very late stages of the illness, while those with a subcortical dementia have such findings early. Also, aphasia, agnosia, and apraxia are rare in the course of Parkinson's disease but are common in Alzheimer's disease. Whether depression is more common in patients with Parkinson's disease than in those with Alzheimer's disease remains to be demonstrated. Recent reports showed that there was no significant difference in the prevalence of depression with these two disorders, but that patients with both disorders were more likely to be depressed than control subjects (Huber et al, 1986; Mayeux et al, 1983). It also remains unclear whether the dementia of Parkinson's disease is likely to be less severe or to progress at a slower rate than that of Alzheimer's disease.

DONATING BLOOD

Since the antemortem diagnosis in a patient with a dementing illness is usually uncertain, a recent report of blood products from dementing patients being able to infect animals raises concern about the appropriateness of dementing patients donating blood (Manuelidis et al, 1985). The patients in this report had Creutzfeldt-Jakob disease, which has a well-documented viral cause. Because of diagnostic inadequacies, however, extreme caution is appropriate when blood is used for transfusion purposes. Blood from any donor with dementia should be rejected, even if the cause of the condition has not been proven to be infectious. In addition, the etiology of Alzheimer's disease has not been determined, and some researchers consider it likely that an infectious agent is involved.

COGNITIVE CHANGES ASSOCIATED WITH DEPRESSION

Clinically, one may find that depressed patients undergoing cognitive testing with the MMSE and other memory tests will actually perform better with time; that is, the depressed patient may remember one or none of three items after three minutes, but will remember all three if asked again after 15 minutes. Such an improvement in memory does not occur with Alzheimer's patients.

The term pseudodementia is often used to describe depression-related cognitive deficits that are reversible with adequate treatment of the affective illness. Lack of effort on the part of depressed patients is observed frequently by clinicians, who have noted patients' increased dependency, indecisiveness, and avoidance of responsibility as part of a general picture of motivational change. Depressed patients perform poorly on a number of motor performance tasks and have also been reported to show deficits in memory (Raskin et al, 1982). The data in reference to cognitive changes associated with affective illness have been reviewed in detail in chapter 4.

It was recently suggested that depression in an elderly patient is a red flag warning of an underlying early dementing illness (Reding et al, 1985). Of 225 patients referred to a dementia clinic over a three-year period, 57% of those initially thought to be depressed and nondemented developed frank dementia. Many of them had some sign, often subtle, of organic neurologic disease. Depressed elderly patients were found to be at high risk for development of dementia if any of the following were present: cerebrovascular, extrapyramidal, or spinocerebellar disease; a modified Hachinski ischemic score of 4 or greater; a Mental Status Questionnaire score of less than 8; or confusion while taking low doses of tricyclic antidepressants. Numerous patients have both depression and a structurally based intellectual impairment. Vigorous therapeutic intervention (see chapter 4) may benefit the affective state even when there is no rebound in neuropsychologic functioning. This may improve the functional status of the patient. It has been reported that depression occurs less frequently as the dementing disease progresses (Reifler et al, 1982) but others (Shuttleworth et al, 1987) found that the magnitude of depression did not differ as a function of disease severity and they recommended the use of appropriate antidepressant therapy at any stage of disease in these patients.

Ideally, the uncertain clinician will initially consider the depressed, dementing patients to have pseudodementia, for which there is hope for recovery, and begin antidepressant therapy. The dangers of assuming that cognitive deficits are secondary to neurologic disease have been outlined by several authors (Kiloh, 1961; Shamoian, 1985; Jenike, 1988a and 1988b). It is important to guard against fatalistically assuming the cognitively impaired depressed individual as irretrievably demented and withholding treatment as a result. Therapeutic interventions should be based on the presence of responsive target symptoms, and although diagnosis is important, it may not be essential for initiating effective treatment measures. As noted in chapter 4, the distinction between a psychiatric and neurologic disorder may not be necessary as long as one establishes that the course is nonprogressive or has done a complete workup to rule out other treatable causes.

THE DEXAMETHASONE SUPPRESSION TEST, DEPRESSION, AND DEMENTIA

As noted, one of the common clinical dilemmas facing the physician who treats elderly patients is the separation of the truly demented patient from the patient who has reversible cognitive impairment on the basis of depression, ie, pseudodementia. If the dexamethasone suppression test (DST) could be shown to be normal in patients with mild dementia and frequently abnormal in those with depression, the test could be used as a diagnostic aid. Much of the current literature on the DST has been reviewed in chapter 4. Results of numerous studies indicated that the DST may be useful in identifying patients with depressive illness (Carroll et al, 1981; Schlesser et al, 1980; Jenike, 1982) and in following their response to treatment (Jenike, 1983). While advanced age alone apparently does not alter the utility of the overnight DST (Tourigny-Rivard et al, 1981), its efficacy in elderly patients with Alzheimer's disease has been questioned. In particular, it has been reported that patients with dementia of the Alzheimer's type who are not depressed frequently have abnormal DST results. Spar and Gerner (1982) found that 9 of 17 Alzheimer's patients had abnormal DST results, while Raskind and colleagues (1982) reported that 7 of 15 patients had abnormal values. However, an examination of the data suggests that both groups of patients were moderately to severely demented. Spar and Gerner's patients had a mean MMSE score of 13.3 (out of a possible score of 30) and had been ill for an average of 4.3 years. The patients of Raskind and colleagues had no correct responses to the Short Portable Mental Status Questionnaire and a mean duration of illness of 7.4 years. Thus, it may be that the DST abnormalities were caused by advanced disease.

Most patients for whom the diagnostic confusion between depression and dementia is a problem are only mildly demented. Several case reports suggested that the DST may be helpful in this differential diagnosis. Rudorfer and Clayton

(1981) reported the case of a patient with pseudodementia whose abnormal DST result normalized after treatment of the underlying depressive illness. Greden and Carroll (1979) described the case of a catatonic patient with an initial diagnosis of dementia who had an abnormal DST result. As a result of this finding, a diagnosis of primary unipolar depression was entertained, and ECT was begun. The initially abnormal DST result returned to normal following two courses of ECT. Similarly, McAllister and associates (1982) reported the cases of two patients for whom the DST appeared to be useful in distinguishing depression accompanied by cognitive dysfunction from dementia.

A report of 18 well-characterized Alzheimer's patients, who were separated into two groups on the basis of degree of cognitive impairment, found that of 13 patients with mild cognitive impairment, only one had a slightly abnormal DST result (Jenike and Albert, 1984). In contrast, four of the five more advanced patients had markedly abnormal DSTs. These differences were found to be highly significant. None of the patients were depressed according to clinical interview and Hamilton Depression Rating Scale. These data indicate that the DST may be useful for identifying persons with treatable depression among those with mild cognitive dysfunction. The results further suggest that as Alzheimer's disease progresses, the DST no longer can be used as a neuroendocrine correlate of depression.

The most likely explanation for the increasing incidence of abnormal DST results among moderately to severely impaired patients is the impact on hypothalamic function of the neurochemical and neuropathologic changes associated with Alzheimer's disease (Davies, 1979). However, it remains possible that the depression in Alzheimer's patients presents in an unusual fashion. Thus, patients with abnormal DST results and low Hamilton Depression Rating Scale scores may, in fact, be depressed. Only if such patients are treated for depression can this possibility be ruled out.

It is hoped that future work will clarify these issues, since depressive pseudodementia is one of the most common causes of reversible cognitive change in the elderly.

COGNITIVE CHANGES ASSOCIATED WITH PSYCHOSIS

There are few data on the effect of psychosis on cognitive functioning in the elderly. Psychological data on the effects of psychosis on cognition have been gathered primarily from schizophrenic patients. It is frequently observed that schizophrenics and other psychotic patients have difficulty with complex cognitive tasks and abstract concepts (Goldstein, 1986; Watson et al, 1968). Many researchers believe that the apparent conceptual deficits of the schizophrenic patient may be a matter of failure to attend to the task, often because of interfering ideation, in combination with a motivational lag (Sutton, 1973).

Schizophrenic patients frequently do poorly on neuropsychologic tests that measure perceptual and motor skills, memory, visuospatial skills, and related functions. Attentional deficits have been well documented with emphasis on reaction time experiments (Zubin, 1975). Because of the presence of neuropsychologic disturbances, Chapman and Chapman (1973) referred to the "general deficit syndrome" of schizophrenia. However, decrements in function appear not to be linked to severity of the symptomatology (Goldstein, 1986).

Schizophrenics administered the Halstead-Reitan battery perform like brain-damaged patients (Heaton and Crowley, 1981; Watson et al, 1968; Levine and Feirstein, 1972; Chelune et al, 1979; Goldstein, 1986). It has been suggested that schizophrenics are indistinguishable from brain-damaged patients because they, too, are brain damaged (Goldstein, 1986). It is unclear whether these effects are the result of genetics, environmental deprivation, nutritional deficiencies, medication, or some other effects still to be identified.

Results of other studies using the Luria-Nebraska Neuropsychological Battery showed that schizophrenic patients perform significantly better than brain-injured subjects on all but four of the summary measures: Expressive Speech, Receptive Speech, Memory, and Intellectual Functioning (Purisch et al, 1978). Schizophrenia appears to produce deficits in the ability to do complex tasks in the Luria-Nebraska Battery, while brain injury produces deficits in the ability to do both simple and complex tasks (Shelly and Goldstein, 1983). The degree of discrimination between a schizophrenic and brain-damaged group may, however, depend on the severity of brain damage in the latter.

Definitive conclusions and advice from the research just reviewed will await further findings. At present, the clinician should assume that psychotic elderly patients may have some features in common with demented and brain-damaged patients. Such patients must be closely monitored in terms of medication and compliance, as well as living environment.

THEORIES OF ETIOLOGY

The cause of Alzheimer's disease remains unknown. Four main theories predominate: genetic, viral, aluminum, and immune function. Also, an association with head trauma has been suggested. Some of the relevant findings in reference to each theory will be reviewed.

Genetic

Relatives of patients diagnosed as having Alzheimer's disease commonly ask if the disorder is inherited; the answer to this question remains elusive. Population studies have shown an increased risk of dementia in first-degree relatives of probands with Alzheimer's disease (Sjogren et al, 1952; Larsson et al, 1963; Heston et al, 1981; Breitner and Folstein, 1984; Mohs et al, 1987; Breitner et al, 1988). There is also a familial form of the illness, identified in more than 50 families (Huff et al, 1988; McKusick, 1983), where it appears to be a straightforward autosomal dominant condition (Terry and Katzman, 1983; Cook et al, 1979; Goudsmit et al, 1981). There is growing evidence that the earlier the age of onset of the disease, the more likely a sibling is to have the disease. Estimates for the risk to children are not available, but the risk to brothers and sisters of individuals who initially become ill after the age of 70 is hardly different from that to the general population (Heston et al, 1981; Mortimer and Schuman, 1981; Larsson et al, 1963). Risk to relatives decreases sharply as severity of the proband's illness decreases and when compared with a control group and the general population, the relatives of Alzheimer's patients have excesses of Down's syndrome, lymphoma, and immune diatheses (Heston et al, 1981).

Huff and associates (1988) found the lifetime risk of Alzheimer's dementia to be similar among relatives of probands with early-onset or late-onset Alzheimer's disease, but relatives of probands with early-onset disease tended to have an earlier onset of dementia than did relatives of probands with late-onset disease. This result raises the possibility that age at onset of dementia in Alzheimer's disease may be genetically determined. It has been posited that expression of the gene for Alzheimer's disease is age dependent with complete penetrance, implying that Alzheimer's disease will ultimately develop in all individuals who inherit the gene if they live to the age of gene expression (Huff et al, 1988).

Studies of twins have yielded conflicting results. Incomplete concordance among identical twins has been reported (Jarvik et al, 1971 and 1980). However, another report of identical twins in whom Alzheimer's disease developed over 12 years apart casts doubt on the supposed lack of concordance in twins (Cook et al, 1981). This case implies that factors other than genetics may influence the age of onset of the disease. Perhaps if the illness develops in one twin, it will also in the other if followed long enough.

Further evidence for a genetic involvement comes from the finding that in apparently all patients with Down's syndrome, a genetic disorder, changes consistent with Alzheimer's disease develop if they reach the ages of 35 to 40. They invariably show significant numbers of plaques and tangles in cerebral cortex and hippocampus (Owens et al, 1971; Burger and Vogel, 1973; Heston, 1976).

Recent research, which capitalized on the knowledge that Alzheimer's-type dementia develops in Down's syndrome patients, demonstrated that the gene for a familial form of Alzheimer's disease is probably localized on chromosome 21 (St. George-Hyslop et al, 1987). Intensive molecular genetic studies are under way to more precisely map and characterize that gene and to address the possibility of genetic heterogeneity in Alzheimer's disease (Raskind, 1988).

In most Alzheimer's patients, however, evaluating family pedigrees has been a complex problem. In discussing the difficulties, Whitehouse (1987) noted that when patients have a late-onset disease like Alzheimer's disease—

meaning they have the gene but it does not express itself until the late 80s or 90s—they can have a relative who died at the age of 65 who was mentally intact but actually had the gene for Alzheimer's disease and just never showed it. To clarify the clinical implications of the linkage analysis with chromosome 21, Whitehouse presented the following analogy. Eye color is genetically inherited. Assume that linkage between eye color and the presence of Alzheimer's had been established; for example, in a family all people with blue eyes get Alzheimer's and all with brown eyes escape the disorder. One could use this technique to predict who would and who would not have the gene for Alzheimer's—that is, presymptomatic testing using eye color. With Huntington's disease, which is another autosomal dominant dementia, clinicians can now tell whether somebody has that gene or not with about 95% to 99% certainty. One implication of this work is that it is now known where the gene is, but it is not known what it produces. One possibility for the gene product is amyloid which has at least one of its amino acid sequences on chromosome 21 (Whitehouse, 1987). The implications for the majority of Alzheimer's patients of the finding that the gene for familial Alzheimer's disease is on chromosome 21 are yet to be determined. Certainly Alzheimer's disease is a very variable disorder that may have different causes.

These findings make the genetic theory particularly attractive, especially for the occasional familial cases, and enhances the importance of applying molecular genetic techniques to the study of Alzheimer's disease.

Viral

It is now well documented that other degenerative neurologic illnesses, such as kuru (Gajdusek and Zigos, 1957) and Creutzfeldt-Jakob disease (Roos et al, 1973) in humans, and scrapie (Hourrigan et al, 1979) and transmissable mink encephalopathy (Marsh et al, 1974) in animals, are caused by viruses or other subcellular infective agents like prions (Prusiner, 1984). It has also been demonstrated that certain strains of the scrapie agent inoculated into the CNS of certain recipient mouse strains induce the formation of neuritic plaques very much like those of Alzheimer's disease, except for an absence of paired helical filaments (Bruce and Fraser, 1975).

A number of trials have been made in an effort to transmit an infective agent from humans to primates. These have all met with no success (Terry and Katzman, 1983; Gibbs and Gajdusek, 1978), with the exception of one report where specimens from two of six patients with familial Alzheimer's disease induced a spongy encephalopathy in recipient primates (Gibbs and Gajdusek, 1978). This report was, however, retracted (Terry and Katzman, 1983) and other investigators have been unsuccessful in their attempts to reproduce or corroborate these initial findings or to isolate the virus.

In another report, an extract of brain tissue from patients with Alzheimer's disease seemed to induce the formation of paired helical filaments in cultured human fetal neurons (DeBoni and Crapper, 1978). These researchers reportedly now believe that this was a degenerative toxic phenomenon in the recipient cultures rather than a change related to the inoculum (Terry and Katzman, 1983).

The recent discovery of submicroscopic protinacious infectious particles called prions might stimulate increased interest in the infectious theory (Prusiner, 1984). It appears that prions may take as long as 20 years to induce brain damage and that they can be linked to at least one form of degenerative brain disease that has long been the focus of slow-virus investigations.

Viral theories remain of interest, but there is still no hard evidence that viruses are involved in the transmission of Alzheimer's disease.

Aluminum

Aluminum intoxication as a possible cause gained attention when it was discovered that neurofibrillary tangles developed in rabbits exposed to toxic amounts of aluminum (Klatzo et al, 1965; Cummings and Benson, 1983). These tangles were, however, somewhat different from those found in the brains of patients with Alzheimer's disease (Terry and Pena, 1965). Some investigators (Crapper et al, 1973 and 1976) found elevated levels of aluminum in brains from Alzheimer's patients, while others failed to confirm an elevation (McDermott et al, 1977 and 1979). Others (Delaney, 1979; Shore et al, 1980) found normal levels of aluminum in cerebrospinal fluid and serum, while Markesbery and colleagues (1981) reported that intraneuronal aluminum content was also normal. Also, dialysis dementia is a disease known to be associated with significantly elevated levels of aluminum in the brain; neurofibrillary tangles, however, were not found (Dunea et al, 1978; Lederman and Henry, 1978; Rozas et al, 1978).

The neurofibrillary tangles induced experimentally by aluminum administration differ from those of Alzheimer's disease in that they are straight rather than twisted and they are distributed in the brain stem and spinal cord instead of the cortex (Yates, 1979).

Others found no differences in brain aluminum content between Alzheimer's patients and age-matched control subjects; they did, however, find increased brain aluminum content associated with aging (McDermott et al, 1977 and 1979). Using sophisticated and sensitive methods to analyze the elemental content of individual cells from brains with Alzheimer's disease and normal brains, an unmistakable link between the pathology of Alzheimer's and aluminum has surfaced. Only neurons with neurofibrillary degeneration contain detectable amounts of aluminum; the element rarely appears in normal nerve cells even when adjacent to tangle-bearing nerve cells with high levels of the element. Investigators hypothesize that these high levels of aluminum are probably not causing the disease, but they do become apparent in its development and may contribute substantially to its symptoms. Thus, it appears that the weight of the cumulative evidence is against the likelihood that aluminum is the agent responsible for Alzheimer's disease (Cummings and Benson, 1983).

Immune Function

Abnormalities in immune function have been reported in Alzheimer's patients. One group (Behan and Feldman, 1970) reported that two-thirds of their patients had abnormalities in serum protein content which included decreases in albumin and increases in α_2-macroglobulin, α_1-antitrypsin, and haptoglobin fractions. Others (Jonker et al, 1982) reported normal immunoglobulin levels in the cerebrospinal fluid. Impaired cellular immune responses (Behan and Behan, 1979) as well as impaired immunoregulation (Miller et al, 1981) have been observed. Elevated levels of brain antibody have also been reported in Alzheimer's patients (Nandy, 1978), suggesting that in Alzheimer's disease the immune system loses its ability to recognize elements of the host's body and begins to attack them.

Neuritic (senile) plaques have an amyloid core which some investigators think is composed of antigen-antibody complexes catabolized by phagocytes and degraded by lysosomes (Wisniewski et al, 1970; Wisniewski and Terry, 1973; Roth et al, 1966). Altered immune function could explain the presence of amyloid in senile plaques and its occasional occurrence in cerebral vessels (Glenner, 1978). At present, it is unknown whether these immunologic abnormalities are primary and thus of etiologic significance, or secondary to some more basic process (Cummings and Benson, 1983).

Thus far, no peculiarities of histocompatibility antigens have been found among patients with Alzheimer's disease (Henschke et al, 1978; Sulkava et al, 1980; Whalley et al, 1980). Although the immune hypothesis is conceptually of interest, there is insufficient evidence to draw any definite conclusions at present.

Head Trauma

Dementia may follow repeated blows to the head (dementia pugilistica) and the pathologic findings include neurofibrillary tangles and, less frequently, neuritic plaques and congophilic angiopathy. Noting that these lesions were similar to those found in patients dying of Alzheimer's disease, Mortimer and colleagues (1985) performed a case-control study in which the frequency of head injury was assessed in 78 Alzheimer patients and 124 control subjects matched for age, sex, and race. They found a history of head injury with loss of consciousness in 26% of patients but in only 6% and 15% of hospital and community-dwelling control subjects, respectively ($P<0.01$). Their findings suggested a possible etiologic role for head injury in at least some patients with Alzheimer's disease.

PRINCIPLES OF MANAGEMENT

Overview

Once treatable causes for dementia have been ruled out, the caregiver must manage a patient with a chronic and progressive illness. The physician will be required to be familiar with the use of psychoactive drugs in the elderly (Jenike, 1985 and 1986b; Salzman, 1984) and will be asked to counsel and advise family members. Two-thirds of all persons with dementia are cared for by their families (Rabins, 1988) and the myth that Americans place family members in an institution at the first sign of a problem is not valid.

Many physicians prefer not to manage such patients and referral to another colleague or geriatric specialist is encouraged under these circumstances. Management must involve family members who may choose to keep the dementing patient at home until very late in the course of the illness and it is not uncommon for a spouse to devote almost the entire day to caring for the patient. A number of drugs are now available as potential memory enhancers; although none are dramatically effective, family members will ask about them. Drugs are available to treat depression, psychosis, and behavioral problems in dementing individuals (Jenike, 1985 and 1986b; Salzman, 1984). Also, a number of agencies can be of major assistance to physicians, patients, and families. These issues are reviewed individually.

A multidisciplinary team approach helps the patient to receive good care at home. When the primary caregiver can draw on the resources of the physician, a social worker, nursing personnel, a nutritionist, and others, he or she can better learn to cope effectively with caring for the patient (Maletta, 1986 and 1988).

The long-term management of irreversible dementia differs in several respects from that of other chronic irreversible illnesses (Council on Scientific Affairs, 1986). In devising a framework for optimizing long-term care of patients with primary dementia, several principles of the disease and its sociology must be recognized. First, the duration of the disease is long and the point at which total disability often occurs is late in the course of the illness. For most of the illness, the patient is ambulatory and able to perform some of the activities of usual daily living and the patient is able to experience and express emotions. Second, most families of demented patients are determined to care for the patient for as long as possible. Third, in most other illnesses, the focus of psychological intervention is the patient's response to the illness. In dementia, suffering occurs to a similar degree in the patient, caregiver, and other family members, so emotional support systems must be available to them all. Fourth, social milieu is a prime consideration in the management of patients with dementia because they have limited ability to adjust to change. A demented patient is much more likely to retain functional effectiveness in a familiar and stable environment.

Given these principles, management of the demented patient in the noninstitutionalized setting such as the home should be the first priority in planning long-term care. Caregivers with severe deficiencies in health, emotional state, and coping skills should be objectively assessed and encouraged to consider alternatives to home management.

Nonpharmacologic Treatments for Dementia

A number of investigators have tried to improve cognitive function in dementing patients by psychotherapy. Group therapy by means of mnemonic devices, organizational schemes, visual imagery, and a variety of cognitive structuring strategies have been successful in improving the cognitive and affective state in community volunteers (Yesavage et al, 1981; Zarit et al, 1979). Such treatment involves the enhancement of clear visual and auditory images of the item to be remembered, the formation of associations which facilitate recall, and the use of organization schemes to provide a framework on which to "place" the object to be remembered. Yesavage and associates (1981) described the classic example which integrates all these factors—the method of the Roman Forum. A Roman orator, for example, would memorize a set of places or loci in a familiar building. He would then associate with each locus a clear image of what he wanted to remember. When the time came to recall these images, the orator would imagine the first locus, and this would lead to recall of the associated image. Thus, if he wanted to remember a paragraph in a speech about war versus food, he would imagine a soldier in the first place and a sack of grain in the second.

Yesavage and colleagues (1981) noted that several similar techniques have been used by poets, orators, and actors since the earliest of times (Yates, 1966). Other authors stressed treating the social milieu around the demented patient as a way of increasing their cognitive performance (Labouvie-Vief and Gonda, 1976). Some found that the aged can improve memory through mutual sharing of ideas in a group situation without formal instruction (Labouvie-Vief and Gonda, 1976; Goulet, 1973). Deficiencies of attention and retrieval seem to be major contributors to the overall problem of amnestic syndromes in the elderly (Elias and Elias, 1976; Craik, 1976) and some investigators stressed attempted improvement in these areas (Yesavage et al, 1981). Other modalities have been employed to improve other cognitive functions such as inductive reasoning in the demented elderly, and to treat specific losses associated with brain damage (Labouvie-Vief and Gonda, 1976; Luria et al, 1969).

Yesavage and colleagues (1981) reported that it has long been known that a wide variety of drugs may either impair learning or to a slight degree facilitate learning, and that material learned under one drug regimen may not be accessible under a different drug regimen (Reus et al, 1979). This concept is referred to as state-dependent learning. In an attempt to assess the relative contribution of two different forms of psychotherapy, supportive counseling or cognitive training, to a drug regimen of Hydergine, Yesavage and colleagues gave Hydergine to 21 moderately demented subjects in a dosage of 1 mg three times daily; and supportive counseling or cognitive training for one hour every two weeks for a total of 12 weeks. The cognitive training was designed to enhance memory and other intellectual functions by the teaching of organizational schemes and mnemonic devices as already described. The patients receiving the combination of Hydergine and cognitive training performed better at the end of the study on measures of memory and learning than the group receiving Hydergine and supportive counseling. These results supported the idea that patients with Alzheimer's disease can improve memory and learning if specific efforts are made in that direction.

Occasionally environmental modifications can improve psychiatric symptoms; we have seen dementing patients whose visual hallucinations or paranoia resolved completely without medication when the level of care that they received was increased. This is not uncommon with patients who are living alone when they are really not able to handle daily life by themselves.

Hussain and Brown (1987), noting that dementing patients in institutions often perceived two-dimensional areas on the floor as three-dimensional obstacles, studied patients who tended to wander from their units. Walking into potentially dangerous areas or away from necessary monitoring can be a problem for demented patients and their caregivers. Current methods of controlling hazardous walking usually involve restraint, medication, locked doors, or physical intervention. Capitalizing on the observation that many demented individuals perceive two-dimensional patterns as barriers, they laid out masking tape in different grid patterns in an attempt to prevent walking through exit doors. The baseline condition (no tape) yielded a 98% exit-door contact for 8 demented male patients, but the addition of horizontal grids reduced exit-door contact to 42%. Often, they found complete prevention occurred at the first experimental trial; some patients, however, ignored the tape or were not able to see it. This technique may well be worth trying in wandering patients.

Karlsson and colleagues (1988) demonstrated that improving nursing care and providing emotional and intellectual stimulation for moderately demented patients not only improves concentration, absentmindedness, recent memory, and restlessness, but also produces significant changes in certain cerebrospinal metabolites (homovanillic acid [HVA] and somatostatin) when compared with a control group of patients who were maintained in a quiet, nonstimulating environment. The stimulated subjects in this study were divided into small groups (4 or 5 patients each) that were as homogeneous as possible with regard to intellectual and motor impairments. The groups met for one hour twice a week in a room equipped with a blackboard, calendar, and clock under the guidance of one or two members of the staff. They all had coffee together and looked at photographs, and efforts were made to activate all the patients and make them take part in the conversation. The patients were encouraged to discuss different topics of common interest such as former occupations, farming and fishing, the living area, and so on. In addition to the group activity there was an increase in the emotional and intellectual contact and stimulation during the daily activities.

Drugs for Memory Enhancement

Several classes of drugs have been used to treat patients with presenile and senile dementia of the Alzheimer's type (Alzheimer's disease). These include, among others, neuropeptides, cerebral metabolic enhancers, and drugs that have a direct effect on the cholinergic system (Goodnick and Gershon, 1984; Jenike, 1986b).

Less than a decade ago it was assumed that arteriosclerotic narrowing was the primary pathology responsible for Alzheimer's disease and a number of cerebral vasodilators and anticoagulants were tried in an effort to dilate stenotic vessels. With the finding that most patients had fairly normal vessels, these approaches were discontinued.

Cholinomimetic Treatments

In the past few years, new discoveries have stimulated innovative pharmacologic approaches based on the cholinergic hypothesis of memory which is supported by a number of findings: (1) Anticholinergic drugs, such as scopolamine, induce memory deficits in healthy young subjects similar to those observed in nondemented elderly subjects; (2) these deficits are reversed by physostigmine, a cholinergic agent that potentiates synaptic acetylcholine; (3) cholinergic drugs such as tetrahydroaminoacridine (THA), arecholine, and physostigmine improve aspects of learning and memory in normal subjects; (4) cholinergic neurons (in nucleus basalis of Meynert) are found to be selectively destroyed in the brains of patients with Alzheimer's disease; and (5) the activity of choline acetyltransferase, which catalyzes the synthesis of acetylcholine, is reduced in brain tissue obtained from patients with Alzheimer's disease (Bartus et al, 1982).

In normal subjects, results of experimental manipulations of the cholinergic system have supported the idea that it is involved in memory. Drachman and Leavitt (1974) used an anticholinergic agent, scopolamine, to produce measurable memory deficits in young normal subjects and demonstrated that these deficits could be reversed by intravenously administered physostigmine, a cholinomimetic agent, but not by the nonspecific activation of amphetamine.

Drachman and Sahakian (1980) later demonstrated that a single subcutaneous injection of physostigmine improved memory and other cognitive functions in normal elderly subjects. Also, Davis and associates (1978) demonstrated improvement after the administration of physostigmine in long-term memory processes in normal humans. Agnoli and colleagues (1983) demonstrated a correlation among the degree of memory loss, intellectual impairment, the quantity of senile plaques, and a decrease in choline acetyltransferase and acetylcholinesterase activity in patients affected by Alzheimer's disease. In this study, patients were subjected to a series of computerized EEG recordings and neuropsychologic evaluations after acute administration of a number of cholinergic drugs, including physostigmine, and anticholinergic drugs (scopolamine and orphenadrine). Their results showed that the acute administration of some cholinergic drugs improved memory and also attention, whereas the anticholinergic drugs induced opposite effects. In addition, cholinergic drugs exhibited a tendency to shift the EEG spectrum analysis into more normal patterns compatible with the patient's age. This study further supports the view that the cholinergic system plays an important role in memory and attention disturbances found in patients with Alzheimer's disease.

Francis and co-workers (1985) studied acetylcholine synthesis by measuring the incorporation of radiolabeled glucose into the transmitter in temporal-cortex specimens obtained at diagnostic craniotomy in 17 young patients with Alzheimer's disease (mean age, 59 years; SD, ±5 years). They found that decreased synthesis of acetylcholine was significantly correlated with cognitive impairment and they thought that these results were consistent with the view that the deficit in the presynaptic cholinergic system is a relatively early change in the development of the clinical features of the disease.

The loss of cholinergic markers is consistently found in patients with Alzheimer's disease, whereas other neurochemical markers are usually decreased to a lesser extent and not as consistently (Terry and Davies, 1980; Davies, 1979; Cross et al, 1981), especially early in the course of the illness. In addition, quantitative measurements of cholinergic cell loss correlate with an increase in the number of senile plaques and a reduction in memory function (Perry et al, 1978).

Cholinergic precursors Based on these abnormalities of the cholinergic system in Alzheimer's disease and its association with memory deficits in normal subjects, various pharmacologic approaches to the treatment of Alzheimer's disease have been undertaken. This situation was analogous to that a number of years ago when it was found that dopaminergic cells, pathways, and enzymes were decreased in particular areas of brains of patients with Parkinson's disease. Giving a dopaminergic precursor, such as L-dopa, did improve disease symptoms in many patients.

Researchers attempted to increase extracellular concentration of choline by directly administering choline itself or its precursor, lecithin, in hopes of increasing brain acetylcholine levels. The results of such precursor therapy have been largely disappointing (Albert, 1983; Jenike et al, 1986). Dementing patients and their families frequently ask about cholinergic precursors, such as choline and lecithin, and some patients take lecithin that they have purchased from so-called health food stores. Unfortunately, as noted, these cholinergic precursors have not been useful.

Physostigmine Following failures with cholinergic precursors, attempts were made to inhibit synaptic acetylcholine breakdown in the brains of Alzheimer's patients with an anticholinesterase inhibitor, such as physostigmine which is now available for research purposes in an oral form. Previously, a major limitation to the use of physostigmine was its intravenous or subcutaneous route of administration. Physostigmine does improve cognitive test scores in some patients, but its overall clinical effect is less dramatic, and its effect on the progression of Alzheimer's disease remains to be determined (Thal et al, 1983; Mohs et al, 1985; Davis et al, 1983; Smith and Swash, 1979; Jenike et al, 1989). While results of some initial studies were encouraging (Smith and Swash, 1979; Davis et al, 1979; Christie et al, 1981; Davis and Mohs, 1982; Muramoto et al, 1979; Peters and Levin, 1979; Denber, 1982; Mohs and Davis, 1982), others demonstrated little or no improvement (Wettstein, 1983; Ashford et al, 1981; Caltagirone et al, 1982).

Preliminary investigations with the oral form of physostigmine found that some patients showed significant improvement in performance (Thal and Fuld, 1983; Mohs et al, 1985; Davis et al, 1983; Smith and Swash, 1979; Jenike et al, 1989). Overall, it appears that about a third of the patients treated with oral physostigmine showed clinically significant improvement, a third were marginally improved, and a third demonstrated inconsistent or no improvement. Physostigmine has been reported to improve constructional abilities (Muramoto et al, 1979) and decrease the number of intrusion errors on recall tasks (Smith and Swash, 1979). In those studies in which some efficacy was noted, a dose-finding phase was included to find an optimal dose for each individual patient. Studies using fixed-dose schedules have generally yielded negative results (Caltagirone et al, 1982; Delwaide et al, 1980).

Mayeux and associates (1987), noting that myoclonus occurs in about 15% of patients with Alzheimer's disease, reported that in two patients taking chronic oral physostigmine myoclonus developed and then reversed upon stoppage of physostigmine. They hypothesized that physostigmine reduced the sensitivity of the remaining muscarinic receptors in these two patients, altering the interaction between cholinergic and either serotonergic or dopaminergic neurotransmitter systems. There are few data on the effects of cholinergic alterations on other brain systems.

Tetrahydroaminoacridine (THA) THA, a centrally acting anticholinesterase, has been reported to lead to dramatic improvement in some Alzheimer's patients (Summers et al, 1986). This report has been sharply criticized on many fronts because of inadequate study design, presence of confounding factors, and the fact that investigators charged patients and family members substantial sums ($12,000 for the first year of treatment) for participation in the study (Marx, 1987). Although many are skeptical of these preliminary results, firm conclusions cannot be made at this time. A large multicenter trial of THA is presently in progress to evaluate efficacy of this agent.

Intracranial infusions of bethanechol A report of continuous intra-cranial infusion of the muscarinic agonist, bethanechol chloride, received national attention (Harbaugh et al, 1984). The initial study was done in only four patients with Alzheimer's disease that was documented by biopsy. At first, the subjective response to this treatment was encouraging, with reports of improved cognition and social functioning during drug infusion. Unfortunately, results of follow-up studies with 12 patients who received bethanechol for three months and an inert saline solution for another three months have been disappointing, and the researchers now believe that there was too little improvement in patients to justify the risks of treatment, which involves surgically implanting a pump that supplies the drug to the brain.

The improvement noted initially may have been biased by psychological cues given unintentionally by investigators. They are now looking for a more effective drug to use with the implanted pump.

Hydergine

Ergoloid mesylates, consisting of three hydrogenated alkaloids of ergot, has been used for over 30 years to treat patients with senile dementia or other age-related problems and is the eleventh most widely prescribed drug in the world (Hollister and Yesavage, 1984). With a 30-year history of use, it has been shown to be extremely safe, even with long-term administration (Spiegel et al, 1983). This drug was classified as a cerebral vasodilator in the past but is now labeled a metabolic enhancer. Hollister and Yesavage (1984), in a review of available data, noted that despite years of experience with this drug the optimal dose is unknown. Usual prescribed doses of the drug range from 1.5 mg/day to as much as 12 mg/day.

At least 12 placebo-controlled studies have compared Hydergine either with placebo alone or with placebo and papaverine (Bazo, 1973; Rosen, 1975; Rehman, 1973; McConnachie, 1973; Thibault, 1974; Banen, 1972; Rao and Norris, 1972; Jennings, 1972; Triboletti and Ferri, 1969; Ditch et al, 1971; Gerin, 1969; Roubicek et al, 1972; Thiehaus et al, 1987). Thirteen of 36 behavioral variables, assessed in three or more studies, showed a statistically significant improvement with Hydergine in at least 50% of the studies (Reisberg et al, 1981). Variables that improved significantly were mental alertness, orientation, confusion, recent memory, depression, emotional lability, anxiety, fear, motivation, initiative, agitation, vertigo, and locomotion; overall impression and global therapeutic change also showed significant improvement. The most consistently improved variable, however, was mood. Hollister and Yesavage (1984) also reported that in their clinical experience an occasional patient shows a dramatic response to the drug.

A review of the literature suggests that a treatment trial of several months is more likely to yield improvement than treatment of a shorter duration and Hollister and Yesavage (1984) concluded that a six-month course of drug may be most beneficial. While daily doses of 3 mg to 4.5 mg have most often been employed in American studies of Hydergine, doses of 6 mg are commonly used in Europe, and doses as large as 12 mg/day have been given without serious side effects (Hollister and Yesavage, 1984).

In a recently completed double-blind study (Jenike et al, 1989a) Alzheimer's patients received either a 3-mg or a 12-mg dosage per day for one year in a double-blind protocol. There had been some discussion in the literature that ergoloid mesylates has some antidepressant effects and that many of the variables that improved with this agent were actually secondary to improved mood. The study just described would refute this contention as there was no relationship between scores on Hamilton Depression Scale (HAM-D) and improvement on any other test. There was also no difference in mood scores between low-dose and high-dose groups.

In summary, individual effects with Hydergine are generally small and the variable that showed the most significant change was mood in many studies (Rosen, 1975; Thibault, 1974; Banen, 1972; Jennings, 1972; Ditch et al, 1971; Reisberg et al, 1981). Even though study results are weak, experienced clinicians occasionally report an individual patient with a good response to a three-month to six-month trial of this agent. If there is no improvement after six months, Hydergine should be discontinued.

Other Drugs

Piracetam, another metabolic enhancer, may influence cerebral energy reserves and increase the ratio of adenosine triphosphate (ATP) to adenosine diphosphate (ADP) in the brain. There is preliminary evidence that piracetam and related drugs may be useful in improving functioning in patients with mild-to-moderate senile dementia, but not in severely demented patients. More research is needed to see if clinically significant results are obtained (Reisberg et al, 1981; Crook and Cohen, 1981).

Psychostimulants, such as methylphenidate hydrochloride, may improve mood in depressed demented patients (see chapter 4), but do not enhance cognition. Procaine hydrochloride, which inhibits MAO activity, has similar actions. There is some research in progress looking at the effectiveness of vasopressin and its analogs on memory in Alzheimer's patients. Vasopressin and other brain peptides, such as ACTH and melanocyte-stimulating hormone (MSH), have been shown to affect the learning process, particularly in animals (Reisberg et al, 1981).

Other agents including neuropeptides, other metabolic enhancers, and gangliosides are presently being investigated; there is, however, no dramatically effective drug available at this time.

Even though the body of basic information about Alzheimer's disease has increased dramatically in the last few years, pharmacologic treatment remains in its infancy. Research has thus far produced no consistently effective agents that the primary care physician can use to treat Alzheimer's patients. It is likely, however, that breakthroughs will occur in the next decade. All patients with mild or moderate Alzheimer's disease should be referred to research centers for experimental protocols when this is feasible.

Chelation Therapy

Chelation therapy is offered by an estimated 1,000 practitioners and clinics in the United States that frequently announce that they can treat angina, reverse atherosclerosis, reverse blindness, open blocked arteries, dissolve kidney stones, dissolve small cataracts, reduce arthritis symptoms, decrease the effects of aging, and improve memory. Many families of Alzheimer's patients inquire into these treatments and understandably will invest huge sums of money in the hope that some benefit will be forthcoming (Harvard Medical School Health Letter, 1984).

Before chelation therapy is begun, most centers proceed with an expensive battery of tests which may exceed $1,000 in cost. These tests rarely serve to disqualify a willing candidate. The treatment consists of 30 to 40 sessions in which the chemical ethylenediaminetetraacetic acid (EDTA) is given intravenously over three or four hours. Sessions are generally spread out over 8 to 10 weeks with intervening periods of "rest." Since EDTA binds to a variety of dissolved minerals or metals present in the body to form a complex which is renally excreted, it is very useful if one is suffering from heavy-metal poisoning, such as lead poisoning.

Advocates of chelation therapy have come up with a number of vague and highly improbable theories which have never been subjected to rigorous testing (Jenike, 1988). All of the evidence in favor of chelation therapy is in the form of anecdotes or uncontrolled trials. A course of chelation therapy costs from $3,000 to $6,000 and is not covered by insurance providers.

After reviewing the available information on chelation therapy for heart disease and other ailments, the editors of a distinguished newsletter (Harvard Medical School Health Letter, 1984) reached the following conclusions: (1) There is no credible evidence that chelation therapy works as claimed; (2) there is good theoretical reason to think that it does not work, except as an elaborate placebo; and (3) as a placebo, the treatment is very expensive and, far from being unprofitable, chelation can afford quite a high income to those who promote it.

We have seen a number of patients who have been urged to undergo chelation therapy for Alzheimer's disease. Proponents of the therapy state that chelation somehow acts as a vasodilator and increases blood flow to the brain. This rationale seems particularly illogical in light of the fact that most Alzheimer's patients have normal cerebral vessels and that the pathology of

Alzheimer's disease is no longer thought to be secondary to brain vascular insufficiency.

Until controlled scientific studies have demonstrated some benefit, it seems unreasonable to recommend chelation therapy, particularly in light of the significant cost and doubtful benefit to the individual patient.

Euthanasia and the Caregiver

Severely demented patients, such as those in the later stages of Alzheimer's disease, may live for years after the brain functions responsible for normal activities of daily living, cognitive performance, and interpersonal interaction are lost. In the later stages of dementia these patients are often in wheelchairs or are bedridden, and many are dependent on constant nursing attention and medical interventions to sustain life. The ethical issues involved in treating these patients are staggering and controversial. With the numbers of patients growing rapidly, clinicians are faced with decisions that range from extreme life maintenance, to passive euthanasia, and even to active euthanasia.

Waxman and colleagues (1988) noted that many of these issues are faced daily in institutional settings. For example, should tube feeding be initiated routinely for all severely demented patients? Should a patient's previously expressed wishes be regarded? How aggressively should antibiotic therapy be pursued? Who should make decisions regarding treatment options, and how should the decisions be made?

Those working with severely demented persons face considerable stress. As caregivers, they naturally desire to empathize with and nurture their patients to the best of their abilities. At the same time, however, they experience little positive feedback for their efforts. Working with these patients allows identification with parents and grandparents and also causes one to come to face with one's own deterioration and death. Family members' anxieties add to the stress. Natural anxiety and guilt may arouse feelings of anger and resentment. Some staff are able to resolve these feelings in a positive fashion and remain empathic, while many others, however, experience severe psychological burden that can be evidenced through symptoms of burnout, such as low self-esteem, feelings of helplessness, high job turnover, and even patient abuse (Waxman et al, 1984; Crawford et al, 1983; Stannard, 1973). Still others may react defensively by distancing themselves from the patients—both emotionally and physically. This adaptive response by some staff members leads to neglect of the patient's physical, social, and emotional needs and reduces the quality of the ward milieu.

Surprisingly little research has investigated the attitudes of those caregivers who are called on to make these difficult decisions. Waxman's group (1988) performed a survey study of 1,798 Swedish health care workers in 31 acute and chronic institutional settings and found, not surprisingly, considerable disagreement between staff concerning euthanasia. For example, attitudes of aides and licensed practical nurses were significantly more favorable toward active euthanasia (39% of aides and 29% of licensed practical nurses were neutral or approved) than were registered nurses and physicians (20% and 19%, respectively). This disagreement was most apparent among those staff in institutions with many demented patients. Favorable attitudes were also more frequent among aides experiencing job dissatisfaction and burnout, younger staff, and those without a relative in long-term care. Overall, the majority of health care personnel in this survey disapproved of active euthanasia as an option for severely demented patients; more than 30% of the staff in this study, however, were neutral or favorable of this policy.

Reflecting on possible reasons for the discrepant attitudes, Waxman and colleagues (1988) noted more opposed to active euthanasia among staff with supervisory roles (registered nurses and physicians) and elucidated some possible reasons why they might be more likely to be against this policy. These were persons (a) with more years of health care education, (b) with greater choice over their careers in geriatric medicine, (c) who were more removed from actual daily patient care, and (d) who would also have increased responsibility for the actual implementation of active euthanasia if the policy existed.

Clearly, staff attitudes toward treating severely demented patients need to be considered in any effort to enhance patient care. The extremely difficult burden of the caregivers needs to be more fully appreciated and acknowledged, especially by those in supervisory positions in long-term care settings.

Currently, staff are placed in the most difficult position of having to make life and death decisions without a well-developed, socially sanctioned structure for doing so. To meet the physical, social, and emotional needs of severely demented patients, the burdens of being an empathic caregiver must be considered. Even though solutions to these difficult problems are not available at present, the sheer burden of the numbers of afflicted patients coupled with dwindling resources will force us to make a number of difficult decisions as a society in the next few decades.

PSYCHIATRIC SYMPTOMS ASSOCIATED WITH COMMON NEUROLOGIC ILLNESSES

Many patients with neurologic illnesses have associated psychiatric symptoms as well as cognitive difficulties. Even though the underlying neurologic illness may not be treatable, the resolution of concomitant psychiatric symptoms will often improve the quality of both the patient's and the caregiver's life. As many clinicians will only read individual chapters of this book, this section will be covered here as well as in chapter 4.

Alzheimer's Disease

As noted, depression may occur concomitantly with Alzheimer's disease (Jenike, 1988b). A few clues may help to differentiate the two. Onset of Alzheimer's dementia is typically insidious, whereas the beginning of endogenous depression with pseudodementia is more often acute and recent. A careful history may reveal that cognitive impairment was not evident until the onset of depressive symptoms.

Cummings and associates (1987) found that 5 of 30 Alzheimer's patients manifested depressive symptoms but none had experienced a major depressive episode. Similarly, Knesevich and co-workers (1983) found no evidence of depression in a group of Alzheimer's patients when they were first seen or when they were reexamined one year later.

If there is any doubt whether a patient is depressed, he or she should be treated. Many patients are both demented and depressed and the only way to clearly separate the two is by response to treatment. Depression, even in a patient with an underlying dementing process, can usually be resolved. Cognition may not improve, but patients will become less negative and more interested in hobbies, social activities, and sex.

Psychosis may be present (Caine and Shoulson, 1983; Cummings et al, 1987) with delusions of persecution, infidelity, and theft occurring at some time in the course of the illness in 50% of patients (Cummings et al, 1987).

Personality changes in the patient with Alzheimer's disease occur but are usually not as troubling as those observed in patients with subcortical dementias (Cummings and Benson, 1988). Alzheimer's patients tend to maintain a facade of acceptable social behaviors despite intellectual deterioration and occasional emotional indifference.

Stroke

As discussed in chapter 4, depression also occurs commonly in stroke patients and these depressions can and should be treated aggressively. Each year 440,000 people have thromboembolic strokes in the United States (Wolf et al, 1977). Between 30% and 60% become clinically depressed and the period of high risk lasts for two years after stroke (Robinson, 1981; Lipsey et al, 1984). Statistically, patients with damage to the left frontal lobe are most likely to have severe depression (Robinson et al, 1983). Robinson and colleagues concluded from animal studies that brain levels of catecholamines are depleted in cerebrovascular accidents, and suggested that antidepressant medications might be used to treat these conditions (Robinson et al, 1983; Robinson and Szetela, 1981).

Information from close friends, family members, or caregivers will be helpful in diagnosing depression. In general, cognitive impairment in stroke patients does not prevent them from giving accurate responses concerning depressive symptoms, although this is not invariably so. Patients with right-sided brain damage (for right-handed and most left-handed individuals) may have aprosody and either have impaired ability to receive the emotional meaning of words and situations or may be unable to communicate emotional distress or depression.

Recent evidence indicates that half the depressions occurring in the acute period after stroke fulfill DSM-III-R diagnostic criteria for major depression (Robinson et al, 1983) and that untreated, these disorders last more than six months (Robinson et al, 1984). Patients with major depression after stroke and patients with functional major depression have very similar depressive symptoms (Lipsey et al, 1986).

There are case reports that psychostimulants, which may exert their effects by blocking the reuptake of depleted catecholamines, may be useful in stroke-induced depressions (Kaufmann et al, 1984; Robinson, 1981; Woods et al, 1986). They may exert their antidepressant effects by blocking the reuptake of depleted catecholamines.

A recent study by Lipsey and co-workers (1984) showed that the tricyclic nortriptyline significantly improved depression after stroke when compared in a double-blind manner to placebo. Successfully treated patients had nortriptyline levels in the therapeutic range (50–150 ng/mL). Because the number of patients in this study was small (34) they were unable to determine the relationship between lesion location and response to medication. Another controlled trial demonstrated the safety and efficacy of trazodone in treating depressed stroke patients. The demonstration of the success of antidepressants in the treatment of depression after stroke represents an important advance in the treatment of these patients.

Stroke patients have many difficulties dealing with issues of rehabilitation and loss of function and should not be forced to suffer concomitant depression when clinicians have the tools at hand to effectively treat such symptoms.

Parkinson's Disease

Parkinson's disease is complicated by depression in one-quarter to one-half of patients (Mayeux, 1982). Depressive symptoms have been reported in as many as 34% of patients prior to the onset of motor manifestations (Patrick and Levy, 1922). Most studies in which severity of symptoms was recorded found them to be of mild-to-moderate intensity (Celesia and Wanamaker, 1972; Mayeux et al, 1981; Warburton, 1967). Suicidal thoughts are common, but actual attempts are rare (Mjones, 1949). Some patients may experience depression as a reaction to the knowledge of the disease or its disability, but affective symptoms develop in others prior to obvious indications of the disease. Most investigators concur that neither the presence nor the intensity of depression can be consistently related to any factor such as age, sex, degree of disability, or type of treatment (Mayeux 1982; Horn, 1974; Mayeux et al, 1981).

L-Dopa, the drug most commonly used to treat Parkinson's disease, may also provoke depression, sometimes with suicidal tendencies (Raft et al, 1972). It may also induce other mental symptoms, such as paranoid ideation and psychotic episodes (Adams and Victor, 1981). Patients with a history of depression prior to onset of motor symptoms may be particularly prone to L-dopa–induced depression (Mayeux, 1982).

A number of reports of favorable responses to tricyclic antidepressants in depressed parkinsonian patients (Anderson et al, 1980; Laitinen, 1969; Strang, 1965) exist. Imipramine and its major metabolite desipramine have been effective in placebo-controlled trials (Laitinen, 1969; Strang, 1965) in reducing depression and fatigue. A few reports of improvement in mood (as well as in bradykinesia and rigidity) have been reported following ECT (Asnis, 1977; Lebensohn and Jenkins, 1975; Yudofsky, 1979). ECT is a reasonable option in depressed parkinsonian patients for whom medication trials fail.

Psychosis is uncommon in untreated idiopathic Parkinson's disease (Cummings and Benson, 1988).

Cummings (1988) in a review of 27 studies representing 4,336 patients with Parkinson's disease found that the prevalence of overt dementia was 39.9%. The studies reporting the highest incidence of intellectual impairment (69.9%) used psychologic assessment techniques, whereas studies identifying the lowest prevalence of dementia (30.2%) depended on nonstandardized clinical examinations. Neuropsychologic investigations revealed that patients with Parkinson's disease manifested impairment in memory, visuospatial skills, and set aptitude. Language function was largely spared. Intellectual deterioration in Parkinson's disease correlated with age, akinesia, duration, and treatment status. Neuropathologic and neurochemical observations demonstrated that Parkinson's disease is a heterogeneous disorder: the classic subcortical pathology with dopamine deficiency may be complicated by atrophy of nucleus basalis and superimposed cortical cholinergic deficits, with few patients having the histopathologic hallmarks of Alzheimer's disease. Mild intellectual deterioration also occurs with the classic pathology, and the more severe dementia syndromes have cholinergic alterations of Alzheimer's disease. Cummings concluded that Parkinson's disease includes several syndromes of intellectual impairment with variable pathologic and neurochemical correlates.

When the clinician is faced with a patient who has Parkinson's disease, it is likely that cognitive and/or psychiatric symptoms will complicate the clinical picture.

Huntington's Disease

Personality changes may occur early in the course of Huntington's chorea and may be of two general types (McHugh and Folstein, 1975). In one, the patient becomes generally apathetic and tends to neglect himself or herself, his or her job, and his or her former interests. In the other, the patient becomes increasingly irritable and oversensitive with a tendency toward angry outbursts and violence.

Psychiatric symptoms occur commonly in patients with Huntington's chorea. Episodes of depression can last from weeks to months and may persist for several years. When patients with Huntington's chorea who had disease-related affective symptomatology were examined with the Schedule for Affective Disorders and Schizophrenia (SADS) (Endicott and Spitzer, 1978), 20% received a diagnosis of dysthymic syndrome and 17% were diagnosed with a major depressive syndrome. Caine and Shoulson (1983) found that approximately 50% of patients with Huntington's disease exhibited significant affective disturbances (major depressive episodes or dysthymic disorders). If the mood disorders precede the motor disturbance or dementia, it may be impossible to differentiate them from functional disorders without the family history of Huntington's chorea.

The depression occasionally can reverse into mania in which the patient is elated, expansive and grandiose, and may overeat and talk incessantly. Schizophrenia-like symptoms may also precede motor symptoms and may consist of feelings of unreality, delusions of influence and control, and hallucinations and illusions. Patients typically are convinced of the reality of these hallucinations and delusions and may act on them.

Depression in patients with Huntington's disease appears to be responsive to antidepressant agents and ECT (McHugh and Folstein, 1975; Brothers and Meadows, 1955). It occasionally will resolve spontaneously. The manic state can last for weeks and also resolve spontaneously.

Suicide is the cause of death in as many as 7% of nonhospitalized patients with Huntington's disease (Reed and Chandler, 1958). Suicide rates in at-risk individuals are significantly greater than those for the general population (Schoenfeld et al, 1984).

Psychosis is common in Huntington's disease (Caine and Shoulson, 1983; Cummings et al, 1987).

DRUGS TO CONTROL PSYCHIATRIC SYMPTOMS

As many as 92% of institutionalized elderly patients receive psychotropic drugs (Salzman, 1982; Small, 1988). Some dementing patients have concomitant behavioral abnormalities, depression, psychosis, and/or anxiety which can be treated (Hyman and Jenike, 1987). Most patients with Alzheimer's disease, however, do not have depression and it is not inevitable in the course of the disease. Depression should be sought and, when present, treated vigorously (see chapter 4). Low doses of secondary amine tricyclics with relatively low anticholinergic activity, such as desipramine and nortriptyline, or newer agents, such as trazodone, maprotiline, or fluoxetine, should be the drugs of first choice. If a depressed patient is not sleeping well, trazodone or nortriptyline or maprotiline, given at bedtime, may improve insomnia during the early stages of treatment. In hypersomnic patients, daytime doses of desipramine, protriptyline, or fluoxetine may help to activate the patient (Jenike, 1988a and 1988b). As noted in chapter 4, sometimes these so-called activating agents actually sedate the patient and should then be given around bedtime.

Patients who fail to improve with heterocyclic antidepressants may respond to MAOIs (Jenike, 1984 and 1985a). MAO levels increase with age in human plasma, platelets, and brain (Robinson et al, 1972; Robinson, 1975; Horita, 1978), and demented patients have even higher MAO levels than age-matched control subjects, making the use of MAOIs to treat depression in dementing patients even more attractive (Gottfries et al, 1983; Jenike, 1985a). Also, the central cholinergic deficits make dementing patients prone to further cognitive decline when anticholinergic drugs are used. MAOIs lack central or peripheral anticholinergic effects (see chapter 9). If the main side effects, orthostatic hypotension and insomnia, are tolerable, these drugs can be used safely in elderly patients when certain precautions (see chapter 4) are observed (Jenike, 1984).

The following two cases illustrate the beneficial results of aggressive pharmacologic treatment of patients with concomitant major depression and Alzheimer's disease. Both patients failed to respond to standard agents but improved greatly when an MAOI was begun.

Case 1. Mrs A, a 73-year-old woman, had progressive memory deficit, typical of Alzheimer's disease, for the past four years. Results of a workup to rule out treatable causes for her cognitive decline were completely normal with the exception of the CT scan which showed moderate cortical atrophy. The Dementia Rating Scale (Mattis, 1976) score was 125 out of a possible 144 which placed her in the category of mild dementia (Jenike and Albert, 1984). Results of other neuropsychologic tests were completely consistent with the diagnosis of Alzheimer's disease. Mrs A had no history of depression, but her father had had numerous depressive episodes. Her family psychiatric history was otherwise negative.

At interview, Mrs A admitted to dysphoric feelings and appeared on the verge of tears. She had lost interest in work, hobbies, and social activities and felt lethargic throughout the day. Her appetite had decreased and she had recently lost about 10 lbs. She had to force herself to eat. She had no psychotic symptoms, but intermittently felt hopeless and had become very obsessive.

She had been depressed for over a year and numerous medication trials had failed. On amitriptyline and nortriptyline she failed to improve with low doses and developed an anticholinergic delirium at higher doses. Maprotiline, desipramine, and methylphenidate were of no help and alprazolam worsened her symptoms. The patient did not remember the medication dosages and her old records could not be located. They were, however, administered by an experienced geriatric psychiatrist.

She was begun on a regimen of tranylcypromine, 10 mg twice a day. Her daughter called the next week to report a dramatic improvement in her mother's mood and activity level. Over the next two weeks her appetite improved and she gained 5 lbs. Two weeks later she was beginning to feel slightly more depressed and tranylcypromine was gradually increased to 20 mg twice daily, with rapid improvement. Her daughter stated that the change in her mother's mood allowed her to lead a much happier and independent life despite her progressive memory loss. Six months later, Mrs A continued to be active and socially involved.

Case 2. Mr B, a 68-year-old retired laborer, was evaluated for a one-year history of worsening memory. He had also become increasingly withdrawn and was losing interest in his past hobbies—traveling and reading. His daughter frequently found him sitting alone in the dark. He had stopped driving, had lost his appetite with a resultant 14-lb weight loss, and seemed frequently confused with inability to concentrate. He felt very hopeless and depressed. His mother had, on one occasion, received ECT for severe depression with good result and his older brother had been chronically depressed with at least one episode of psychotic depression requiring hospitalization. Mr B denied a history of depressive episodes and his daughter confirmed that he had always been a very active and optimistic person.

Results of Mr B's neuropsychologic tests were consistent with Alzheimer's disease. His Dementia Rating Scale score was 135 out of a possible 144 and all other neuropsychologic tests were consistent with the diagnosis of Alzheimer's disease. It was clear that he also had a superimposed disabling depression. Treatable causes for cognitive decline were ruled out.

Mr B was begun on desipramine, 25 mg at bedtime, and the dose was increased slowly to 200 mg daily. He had no side effects, but also got no better over the next six weeks despite having blood levels in the therapeutic range. Desipramine eventually was discontinued and nortriptyline was begun, again starting with low dosage. Once again he failed to respond despite a blood level measurement in the therapeutic range.

Since Mr B had not improved on two antidepressants, and the family feared ECT, a MAOI was begun. After a 10-day drug-free period, tranylcypromine was started at 10 mg twice a day and slowly increased to 20 mg twice daily. After two weeks, Mr B was much improved and within six weeks described himself as being "back to my former self" despite his persistent cognitive deficits. At eight-month follow-up, he remained affectively stable despite considerable cognitive decline.

Sometimes moderate doses of a psychostimulant, such as methylphenidate (10 to 40 mg/day), may help to motivate and energize a lethargic or abulic (lack of initiative) demented patient (see chapter 4). If there is no response within a few days, it should be discontinued.

Severe behavioral disturbances and psychosis can usually be managed effectively by low doses (ie, 0.5 mg once or twice daily initially) of a high potency neuroleptic, such as haloperidol or fluphenazine (see chapter 6). Patients with preexisting movement disorders, such as Parkinson's disease, may be better treated with low doses of thioridazine (ie, 10 mg once or twice daily initially). The low-potency neuroleptics like thioridazine are more likely to cause excessive sedation, anticholinergic effects (tachycardia, urinary retention, dry mouth, confusion, etc), and orthostatic hypotension, but are less likely to worsen extrapyramidal symptoms than the high-potency drugs (see chapter 6). These drugs may allow many demented patients, who would otherwise have to be managed in chronic care facilities or in state psychiatric institutions, to live at home.

Other options to control severe agitation, violence, or psychosis (see chapter 6 for more complete discussion) include beta-blockers, serotonergic agents such as a combination of tryptophan and trazodone (Greenwald et al, 1986; O'Neil et al, 1986; Simpson and Foster, 1986) or buspirone (Colenda, 1988), a novel anxiolytic with partial (5-HT$_{1A}$) serotonergic agonist properties. Disruptive sexual behaviors in dementing patients, such as public masturbation and attempts to molest female patients, are reported to respond to medroxy-progesterone acetate (MPA). Within two weeks after the start of MPA therapy, grossly inappropriate sexual behaviors reportedly stopped in four demented male patients (Cooper, 1987). The changes in behavior were accompanied by reductions in serum testosterone levels and luteinizing hormone (LH). In this report, MPA was used for one year without side effects and only one patient returned to the disturbing behavior when the drug was discontinued.

MANAGEMENT OF THE FAMILY

Initial Reactions and Plans

Family members may well react to the fact that their relative has Alzheimer's disease as the worst news they have ever received. Others will have suspected the diagnosis and may be relieved to have an understanding clinician available and helpful over the course of the illness. Family members who have a preexisting psychiatric illness may decompensate and the clinician may have to contact the treating psychotherapist to coordinate care. Family members may be stunned initially and ask few questions. Further tests should be explained and a follow-up appointment scheduled. Common questions include: How long will my spouse live? Will he or she deteriorate rapidly? A child may ask what his or her chances are of developing the disease—is it hereditary? Is there a treatment?

Within the first few weeks after making the diagnosis, family members should see a social worker aware of community resources such as visiting nurse availability, meals-on-wheels, financial resources, and nursing home procedures. For the patient in the very early stages of Alzheimer's disease, this may seem premature, but family members will be reassured that help will be available when needed. Most families read about and become acutely aware of the devastating course of the illness. Even with a compassionate and empathic physician, many families feel alone with this illness and embarrassment may make them withdraw from previous social contacts.

Alzheimer's Disease and Related Disorders
Association (ADRDA)

Families have established volunteer organizations that welcome members concerned about all dementing illnesses, of which Alzheimer's disease is the most common. The number of such support groups is growing rapidly and families consistently rave about their helpfulness. These groups offer friendship and information about the diseases and about resources and local doctors, and they give members the opportunity to exchange ideas and experiences. These local volunteer organizations have established a national organization, ADRDA, whose goals are family support, education, advocacy, and encouraging research. This association has had an extraordinary growth since its founding in 1980 and it now has more than 600,000 people on its mailing list and over 170 chapters nationwide (Rabins, 1988). The address of ADRDA is: 70 East Lake Street, Chicago, IL 60601 and the telephone number is 1-800-621-0379. The national organization will give family members the addresses of local groups and will put them on the mailing list for the ADRDA newsletter. Local chapters of ADRDA can be found in most cities and are generally listed in local telephone books or can be located by calling the social services department of a local hospital.

Results of several studies (Barnes et al, 1981; Priddy et al, 1985) demonstrated improved family morale in people attending support groups. Improvement is probably the result of the emotional support received and an increase in knowledge about the diseases and the community resources available to help the caregivers. Support groups are useful for many family members but are not necessary for all caregivers.

Legal Consultation

Legal consultation is mandatory as financial ruin may result if finances are not handled appropriately. In the middle stages of the illness, patients can no longer adequately handle finances and major financial decisions should be turned over to the caregiver. It is probably best to inquire at the local ADRDA chapter about reputable and knowledgeable local lawyers. Many lawyers have special training in this area, while others mismanage financial resources and charge unreasonable fees. Even though patients are unable to make financial decisions alone, attention should be paid to their wishes with respect to issues such as living arrangement and wills, that may affect them or their assets.

A number of legal issues often arise in the care of elderly dementing patients and some of these are briefly covered. There may be minor variations in these procedures from state to state so local attorneys should be consulted about specifics.

Durable Power of Attorney

It is often helpful to consider assignment of "durable power of attorney" which authorizes an agent to act in an individual's behalf with regard to property and financial matters. The individual does not, however, relinquish control as power of attorney is granted only for the financial matters expressly set forth in the relevant document; the individual who grants power of attorney is merely agreeing to have another person exercise power that is similar to his or her own. It is called a durable power of attorney because it may continue even when the person is incapacitated. It may be written to go into effect upon its signing, or may be designed to go into effect only when disability occurs. Thus, when disability does occur, bills can continue to be paid and revenues can continue to be collected while other more permanent arrangements are being made, such as the appointment of a conservator or guardian.

Durable power of attorney documents may also facilitate the appointment of a conservator or guardian by nominating an individual to serve in that capacity if disability develops. It is not necessary to specify the disability in the document. At the time disability occurs, a certificate from a physician describing the disability will be reviewed by the court to determine whether a conservator or a guardian is necessary. If the court decides to appoint a conservator or guardian, it will usually appoint the person named in the durable power of attorney document unless it finds that that person is unfit.

Living Wills

Living wills are not legally binding but may be used as guidance by a probate court. A court or legal guardian will generally refer to it in making decisions concerning resuscitation and surgery in persons with a loss of mental competence.

Conservatorship

Conservatorship is another legal planning tool that relates to control of financial matters. In this instance, the probate court appoints a person to care for the subject's property and finances because of that person's inability to do so by reason of advanced age, mental weakness, or physical incapacity. This information must be attested to by a physician and signed no more than 10 days before the probate court hearing. A subject may nominate a particular person to be conservator by assenting to that person's petition if the doctor's certificate states that the subject has sufficient mental ability to comprehend the nature of his or her act in assenting to the petition. After appointment, the conservator will be required to file an inventory of all of the subject's assets and to report annually all income and expenses. The conservator is legally accountable to the subject and to the subject's family. The subject, however, loses actual control over his or her property and finances.

Guardianship

Guardianship is a legal tool that establishes control over a person's body as well as financial affairs. In a guardianship, the probate court appoints a person to care for the subject's person, property, and finances because of the person's inability to care for himself or herself by reason of mental illness. The appointed person has a responsibility for directing the medical treatment of the subject, as well as housing, personal needs, finances, and property. To establish the guardianship, a medical certificate from a physician must state that the individual in question is incapable of caring for himself, as well as his estate, because of mental illness. As with conservatorships, the medical certificate of the physician must be made not more than 10 days before the probate court hearing. In this sense, guardianship cannot be arranged in advance of need. However, through a durable power of attorney, an individual may nominate someone they would like to act as guardian in the event that such a need develops. All of the subject's affairs are managed by the guardian while the subject loses all control. Therefore, guardianship is generally considered a last resort because the process essentially eliminates an individual's legal rights.

Medicaid Eligibility

It is important to understand that Level II and III skilled nursing care facilities are not eligible for Medicare insurance reimbursement. However, these expenses will generally be paid by Medicaid if the subject's "countable" assets are less than $2,000. "Countable" assets are all of the subject's assets except his or her residence, life insurance with a cash value of $1,500 or less, burial asset of less than $2,500, burial trust, furniture, jewelry, and automobile, which are termed "noncountable" assets. A gift or transfer of countable assets within two years prior to application for Medicaid may make the subject ineligible for Medicaid for two years following the gift or transfer; thus, transfer of funds from an afflicted individual to other family members is allowed, but long waiting periods after such a transfer may be required to get government financial assistance.

It is important to note that possessions such as residence, furniture, jewelry, automobile, etc, which are considered noncountable assets while the subject is alive become part of the subject's probate estate after his or her death, if they are in a subject's name alone during his or her life. If the assets are held in a trust, joint tenancy, life estate, etc, they pass outside the probate estate and, therefore, are not subject to the claim of the Department of Welfare. If such arrangements have not been made, the Department of Welfare has the right to claim from the subject's estate an amount equal to the benefits paid to or for the benefit of the subject during his or her life whether or not transferred by will. Procedures for transferring wealth outside of probate should be arranged for at the time Medicaid eligibility is being planned.

Advice for the Family

Each family member should be encouraged to read one of the available lay books on Alzheimer's disease. The *36-Hour Day* is required reading for anyone (including physicians) who is dealing with an individual with a progressive dementing illness (Mace and Rabins, 1981). *Alzheimer's Disease: A Guide for Families* (Powell and Courtice, 1984) also offers helpful advice for family members. Another similar book useful both to family and other caregivers is

Care of Alzheimer's Patients: A Manual for Nursing Home Staff (Gwyther, 1985). *Confronting Alzheimer's Disease* (Kalicki, 1987) also offers practical suggestions for family members.

Families need to be encouraged to maintain a structured, predictable environment for the patient. Any change can be devastating and stressful to a demented patient and may produce a so-called catastrophic reaction, ie, a massive emotional overresponse to seemingly minor stress. A schedule in which activities such as arising, eating, medication-taking, and exercise occur at the same time each day maximizes the patient's familiarity with his personal environment. At times an orientation center in the home displaying pertinent information such as the date, time, schedule of household events, and pictures of relevant people is very helpful (Jenike, 1988).

Guilt, unrealistic expectations, and assumption of excessive responsibility are common responses of families (Rabins et al, 1982; Rabins, 1984). In discussing these and similar issues, the physician should focus both on physical realities and on the family's emotional responses to the patient. A frequently encountered difficulty is the reversal of parent/child roles. There is no one way to handle such problems and physicians may try to avoid such discussions for fear that they may not know how to handle the conflicts. In the overwhelming majority of cases, just allowing family members to discuss these and other issues will be therapeutic in and of itself.

Certain behaviors are particularly troublesome to family members; those cited most frequently include: physical violence and hitting, catastrophic reactions, suspiciousness and accusatory behavior, waking at night, and incontinence (Rabins et al, 1982). The following suggestions are helpful in dealing with these behaviors.

Catastrophic reactions or massive overreactions precipitated by task failure or seemingly minor stress can be minimized by teaching caregivers to avoid or remove the precipitating task or stress, to remain quiet and calm, and to gently change the focus of attention. Neuroleptic drugs are sometimes helpful, but only as an adjunct to these techniques. Hitting and violent resistance to care are extreme catastrophic reactions and often can be eliminated or lessened in severity and frequency in these ways. Caregivers should be advised that all activities must be adapted to the abilities of the dementing patient and that instructions should be worded in a simple, concrete, one-step manner. Mistakes should not be directly corrected; rather, praise for accomplishments should be the rule. Caregivers should avoid taking over and performing tasks that might still be within the patient's functional abilities; this might encourage dependence and feelings of low self-esteem. Conversely, patients should not be required to engage in activities that are beyond their capacities which can produce anxiety, frustration, anger, and sometimes even violence (Reisberg, 1988).

Caregivers frequently complain of chronic fatigue and when the patient awakens at night and wanders, this further deprives the caregiver of much-needed rest. Some environmental interventions are helpful. Locks can be placed on doors to keep the patient from wandering out of the house at night, and patients can be kept physically active during the day and not allowed to nap. Sedative-hypnotics, such as short-acting benzodiazepines or chloral hydrate, may be helpful (Jenike, 1983a; see chapters 7 and 8). Occasionally, low doses of neuroleptics may be needed (see chapter 6).

Suspiciousness and accusatory behaviors probably result from the brain-injured person's efforts to explain misplaced possessions or misinterpreted events. If the family understands this, frustration, hurt, and anger may be reduced. Simple interventions, such as keeping an orderly house or making a sign pointing to where objects are kept, may help. Again, neuroleptics may be used as a last resort. Patience, flexibility, and tolerance in the face of frequently monotonous or inappropriate behavior should be encouraged. Most essential is the understanding of the use of humor over time. Additionally, the caregiver should be brought to acknowledge, understand, and anticipate his or her own ongoing grief (Maletta, 1988). It is important for others, especially other family members, friends, and health care professionals, to validate frequently the caregiver's efforts. Despite denials, caregivers do care that they are not being thanked by the patient, for whom they expend incredible amounts of time and energy. The caregiver has to do his or her best to remain optimistic and adopt a positive approach despite the deteriorating situation. It is essential that the caregiver maintain his or her own health in order to successfully cope physically with attending to the patient. Sometimes the caregiver can be helped with psychotherapy and/or pharmacotherapy, on either a short-term or even long-term basis (Maletta, 1988).

Incontinence is typically a late manifestation of Alzheimer's disease and, when present early, warrants a careful search for other causes, such as urinary tract infection.

Patients with Alzheimer's disease may decompensate cognitively and behaviorally when they experience even a minor superimposed illness. Coexistent medical problems, such as asthma, diabetes, and congestive heart failure, should be optimally controlled. Even a minor upper respiratory tract or urinary tract infection can worsen behavior. Patients are susceptible to medication-induced delirium (see chapter 9) and close supervision of drug regimens is also imperative.

Sometimes something untoward may arise, such as surgery for a bowel obstruction, or repair of a fracture following a fall. Because Alzheimer's patients have no "stress reserve," there may be a notable decline in the patient's cognitive abilities following the trauma. The patient may be unable to bounce back, either permanently or for a time. This will, of course, upset the caregiver and family, who may blame the physician. Thus, the physician should advise the family in advance that these types of declines often occur, and that at such a time additional stress on the patient should be minimized (Maletta, 1988). Just going into a new environment in the hospital may precipitate an increase in confusion and disorientation; some patients, for example, will urinate in the corner of the hospital room when this has never happened at home.

Inappropriate sexual behavior is very uncommon and in the rare instances when it occurs, self-stimulation is the usual form. Alzheimer's patients are not child molesters.

Most patients stop driving by themselves, but when they wish to continue when no longer safe on the roads, techniques such as hiding the keys, disconnecting distributor wires, or giving the patient a nonfunctional set of keys have usually been successful in discouraging patients from driving without the need for confrontation. Sometimes a letter from the doctor which can be posted in a conspicuous place is helpful. Firearms should not be kept in the home for obvious reasons. In addition, smoking and cooking become potentially dangerous activities. Environmental modifications, such as removing stove knobs, having a stove cutoff switch placed in an inconspicuous place, locking rooms or closets, or locking up matches, are important for safety.

Because there is not a definitive treatment for Alzheimer's disease, the identification and correction of any medical or psychological factors that contribute to disability become of paramount importance. A relationship between impaired hearing and the progression of Alzheimer's disease has been suggested, and results of a recent longitudinal study have tentatively confirmed this relationship (Uhlmann et al, 1986). Until more data are available, clinicians should pay special attention to deficits in hearing and vision in dementing patients and correct them when possible.

Family members report that lack of time for themselves and dealing with sleep disturbances in patients are the least tolerable aspects of home care (Mace and Rabins, 1981; Rabins, 1984). Studies have shown that family support was the major variable in keeping the cognitively impaired elderly at home. Families do best when relatives and friends visit frequently and when provisions are made for the primary caregiver to have regularly scheduled breaks in his or her responsibilities. Visiting nurses or day-care centers can be invaluable. In helping the caregivers to cope, the physician should make them aware of the informal and formal support facilities that are available (Maletta, 1988). For instance, respite can be provided either by bringing a day worker into the home or by taking the patient to a day-care center one or more days during the week.

Patients generally thrive better at home where they feel more like individuals, receiving individual care and attention, as opposed to being part of an institution's patient population. This seems so no matter how devoted that institution's care may be; the longer that patients can hold on to their individuality and sense of self-worth, the better off they are (Maletta, 1988).

As noted earlier, the goal of the overwhelming majority of family members is to keep the patient at home as long as possible and it is unusual for them to try to get a patient into a nursing home when home care is still feasible. Good home care is composed of a number of factors and a breakdown in any one of these can jeopardize effective home care (Maletta, 1988). A primary caregiver must be physically and emotionally able to cope with the patient in terms of day-to-day routines as well as respond adequately when crises arise. They must be able to follow instructions and to accept help from outside sources when needed. A strong support system built on the active involvement of family members and friends as well as community facilities is of great assistance. For the patient, day-care centers, ideally provided in a group in which there are other cognitively impaired patients, provide increased socialization, physical activity, and even medical care. The patient's forgetfulness, repetitiveness, and general cognitive inadequacies may annoy or irritate other elderly persons with physical and emotional problems of their own.

Patients with severe behavioral problems, such as violent outbursts, hostility, or severe depression, cannot be managed in most day-care centers. The physician, by alleviating these troubling behaviors, either pharmacologically or by environmental manipulation, can greatly facilitate the family's efforts to keep the patient in day-care. Home health care is another means of caregiver support; a nurse or other qualified attendant at home ensures care for the patient as well as relief for the caregiver and family. This may not, however, be a viable option for most families because of economic constraints.

During the latest stages of Alzheimer's disease, nursing home placement is usually required. When considering institutionalization, the physician should raise the subject and discuss issues including the quality of care the patient will receive in an institutional setting and the importance of the family's continued involvement if and when the decision to institutionalize is made. The nursing home location should therefore be as close to the family as possible. Patients in nursing homes who do not have visitors die much sooner than those who continue to receive attention from their families (Reisberg, 1988). Decisions about placement in a nursing home should be raised sooner rather than later, since waiting lists exist for many nursing homes and the process of gaining admission can extend for several months or even years. The caregiver may resist the decision to institutionalize the patient because of overwhelming feelings of guilt, shame, or failure. Frustration, anger, anxiety, or a fear of loss of personal value may also interfere with a rational decision. Precipitating factors for nursing home placement include continuously disruptive behavior or total failure of the patient's ability to carry out routine activities of daily living such as toileting, bathing, grooming, dressing, mobility, and the ability to feed oneself. Some caregivers can appropriately handle more severe difficulties than others and the clinician's assessment of the total picture is invaluable. When nursing home placement is inevitable, consultation with fellow caregivers, often located through ADRDA, who have been through this devastating experience is often of major importance in facilitating the process. Caregivers are delighted to find that, after a period of adjustment, the majority of patients do fine and that frequent visits fulfill the need to keep the relationship going.

SUMMARY

Alzheimer's disease is reaching epidemic proportions as the percentage of older Americans continues to rise. It is estimated that 20% of those over the age of 80 have this illness and that half of all nursing home beds are filled by Alzheimer's patients. Because of these startling figures, all physicians will come into contact with these patients, both in their practices as well as in their personal lives.

The diagnosis is best made by looking at the overall course of the illness (slowly progressive decline) and by ruling out other causes of dementia. Many other illnesses, some treatable, can produce dementia. Every patient deserves a complete workup which has been outlined. Brain failure requires as thorough an evaluation as heart failure or renal failure.

The cause of Alzheimer's disease remains unknown. Four main theories have been discussed: genetic, viral, aluminum, and immune system. The role of head trauma in some patients was reviewed.

Once treatable causes for dementia have been eliminated, the primary care physician must manage a patient with a chronic and progressive illness. Physicians who prefer not to handle such patients should refer them to a colleague or geriatric specialist. Management necessitates that the physician assist family members, who may keep the patient at home until very late in the course of the illness, and be familiar with the use of psychotropic drugs. Many Alzheimer's patients will have concomitant depression, psychosis, anxiety, or behavior abnormalities which are generally responsive to medication. Extensive research on specific drugs for memory enhancement is now under way and the finding that the cholinergic system is altered early in brains of Alzheimer's patients has suggested a number of innovative approaches. Although small improvements in test scores can be achieved with some drugs, overall clinical improvement is unlikely. A six-month trial of Hydergine may be of some benefit. Chelation therapy has no proven benefit and is very expensive. Patients should be referred to research centers when possible.

Management of the family is discussed in terms of optimizing the patient's care at home. It is recommended that those involved in the care of a demented patient join the ADRDA.

REFERENCES

Adams RD, Victor M (eds): *Principles of Neurology*. New York, McGraw-Hill, 1981.

Agnoli A, Martucci N, Manna L, et al: Effect of cholinergic and anticholinergic drugs on short-term memory in Alzheimer's dementia: A neuropsychological and computerized electroencephalographic study. *Clin Neuropharmacol* 6:311–323, 1983.

Albert MA: Treating memory disorders in the elderly. *Drug Ther* 10:257–265, 1983.

Andersen J, Aabro E, Gulmann N, et al: Antidepressive treatment of Parkinson's disease. *Acta Neurol Scand* 62:210–219, 1980.

Ashford W, Soldinger S, Schaeffer J, et al: Physostigmine and its effect on six patients with dementia. *Am J Psychiatry* 138:829–830, 1981.

Asnis G: Parkinson's disease, depression and ECT: A review and case study. *Am J Psychiatry* 134:191–195, 1977.

Banen DM: An ergot preparation (Hydergine) for relief of symptoms of cerebrovascular insufficiency. *J Am Geriatr Soc* 20:22–24, 1972.

Barnes RF, Raskind MA, Scott M, et al: Problems of families caring for Alzheimer patients: Use of a support group. *J Am Geriatr Soc* 29:80–85, 1981.

Bartus RT, Dean RL, Beer R, et al: The cholinergic hypothesis of geriatric memory dysfunction. *Science* 217:408–416, 1982.

Bayles KA, Tomoeda CK: Confrontation naming impairment in dementia. *Brain Lang* 19:98–114, 1983.

Bazo AJ: An ergot alkaloid preparation (Hydergine) versus papaverine in treating common complaints of the aged: Double-blind study. *J Am Geriatr Soc* 21:63–71, 1973.

Becker JT, Huff J, Nebes RD, et al: Neuropsychological function in Alzheimer's disease. *Arch Neurol* 45:263–268, 1988.

Behan PO, Behan WMH: Possible immunological factors in Alzheimer's disease, in Glen AIM, Whatley LJ (eds): *Alzheimer's Disease. Early Recognition of Potentially Reversible Deficits*. London, Churchill Livingstone, 1979, pp 33–35.

Behan PO, Feldman RG: Serum proteins, amyloid, and Alzheimer's disease. *J Am Geriatr Soc* 18:792–797, 1970.

Benson DF, Cummings JL, Tsai SY: Angular gyrus syndrome simulating Alzheimer's disease. *Arch Neurol* 39:616–620, 1982.

Bradley WG, Waluch V, Brandt-Zawadzki M, et al: Patchy periventricular white matter lesions in the elderly: A common observation during NMR imaging. *Noninvas Med Imaging* 1:35–41, 1984.

Breitner J, Folstein M: Familial Alzheimer dementia: a prevalent disorder with specific clinical features. *Psychol Med* 14:63–80, 1984.

Breitner JCS, Silverman JM, Mohs RC, et al: Familial aggregation in Alzheimer's disease: comparison of risk among relatives of early- and late-onset cases, and among male and female relatives in successive generations. *Neurology* 38:207–212, 1988.

Brothers CRD, Meadows AW: An investigation of Huntington's chorea in Victoria. *Ment Sci* 101:548–563, 1955.

Bruce ME, Fraser H: Amyloid plaques in the brains of mice infected with scrapie: Morphological variation and staining properties. *Neuropathol Appl Neurobiol* 1:189–202, 1975.

Brun A, Gustafson L: Limbic lobe involvement in presenile dementia. *Arch Psychiatr Nervankr* 226:79–93, 1978.

Burger PC, Vogel FS: The development of the pathologic changes of Alzheimer's disease and senile dementia in patients with Down's syndrome. *Am J Pathol* 73:457–476, 1973.

Butters N, Albert MS, Sax DS, et al: The effect of verbal mediation on the pictorial memory of brain-damaged patients. *Neuropsychologia* 21:307–323, 1983.

Caine ED, Bamford KA, Schiffer RB, et al: A controlled neuropsychological comparison of Huntington's disease and multiple sclerosis. *Arch Neurol* 43:249–254, 1986.

Caine ED, Shoulson I: Psychiatric syndromes in Huntington's disease. *Am J Psychiatry* 140:728–733, 1983.

Caltagirone C, Gainotti G, Masullo C: Oral administration of chronic physostigmine does not improve cognitive or mnesic performances in Alzheimer's presenile dementia. *Intern J Neurosci* 16:247–249, 1982.

Carroll BJ, Feinberg M, Greden JF, et al: A specific laboratory test for the diagnosis of melancholia. *Arch Gen Psychiatry* 38:15–22, 1981.

Celesia GG, Wanamaker WM: Psychiatric disturbances in Parkinson's disease. *Dis Nerv Sys* 33:577–583, 1972.

Chapman LJ, Chapman JP (eds): *Disordered Thought in Schizophrenia.* New York, Appleton-Century-Crofts, 1973.

Chelune GJ, Heaton RK, Lehman RA, et al: Level versus pattern of neuropsychological performance among schizophrenic and diffusely brain damaged patients. *J Consult Clin Psychol* 47:155–163, 1979.

Christie JE, Shering A, Ferguson J, et al: Physostigmine and arecholine: effects of intravenous infusions in Alzheimer presenile dementia. *Br J Psychiatry* 138:46–50, 1981.

Colenda CC: Buspirone in treatment of agitated demented patient. *Lancet* 1:1169, 1988.

Cook RH, Schneck SA, Clark DB: Twins with Alzheimer's disease. *Arch Neurol* 38:300–301, 1981.

Cook RH, Ward BE, Austin JH: Studies in aging of the brain. IV. Familial Alzheimer's disease: Relation to transmissible dementia aneuploidy and microtubular defects. *Neurology (NY)* 29:1402–1412, 1979.

Cooper AJ: Medroxyprogesterone acetate (MPA) treatment of sexual acting out in men suffering from dementia. *J Clin Psychiatry* 48:368–370, 1987.

Council on Scientific Affairs: Dementia. *JAMA* 256:2234–2238, 1986.

Craik FIM: Age differences in human memory, in Birren JE, Schaie KE (eds): *Handbook of the Psychology of Aging.* New York, Van Nostrand, 1976, p 384.

Crapper DR, Krishnan SS, Dalton AJ: Brain aluminum distribution in Alzheimer's disease and experimental neurofibrillary degeneration. *Science* 180:511–513, 1973.

Crapper DR, Krishnan SS, Quittkat S: Aluminum, neurofibrillary degeneration and Alzheimer's disease. *Brain* 99:67–80, 1976.

Crawford SA, Waxman HM, Carner EA: Research in long term care: Discovering the need for staff recognition and reward. *Am Health Care Assoc J* 9:59–66, 1983.

Crook T, Cohen G (eds): *Physicians' Handbook on Psychotherapeutic Drug Use in the Elderly.* New Canaan, Conn, Mark Powley Associates, 1981.

Cummings JL, Benson DF: *Dementia: A Clinical Approach.* Boston, Butterworth, 1983.

Cummings JL, Benson DR: Psychological dysfunction accompanying subcortical dementias. *Ann Rev Med* 39:53–61, 1988.

Cummings JL, Benson DR: Subcortical dementia: Review of an emerging concept. *Arch Neurol* 41:874–879, 1984.

Cummings JL, Darkins A, Mendez M, et al: Alzheimer's disease and Parkinson's disease: Comparison of speech and language alterations. *Neurology* 38:680–684, 1988.

Cummings JL, Miller BL, Hill M, et al: Neuropsychiatric aspects of multi-infarct dementia and dementia of the Alzheimer type. *Arch Neurol* 44:389–393, 1987.

Cummings JL: Better diagnosis of dementia. *The Psychiatric Times* Sep 1986.

Cummings JL: Intellectual impairment in Parkinson's disease: Clinical, pathologic, and biochemical correlates. *J Geriatr Psychiatry Neurol* 1:24–36, 1988.

Davies P: Neurotransmitter-related enzymes in senile dementia of the Alzheimer type. *Brain Res* 171:319–327, 1979.

Davis KL, Mohs RC, Rosen WG, et al: Memory enhancement with oral physostigmine in Alzheimer's disease. *N Engl J Med* 308:721, 1983.

Davis KL, Mohs RC, Tinklenberg JR, et al: Physostigmine: Improvement of long-term memory processes in normal humans. *Science* 201:272–274, 1978.

Davis KL, Mohs RC, Tinklenberg JR: Enhancement of memory by physostigmine. *N Engl J Med* 10:946, 1979.

Davis KL, Mohs RC: Enhancement of memory processes in Alzheimer's disease with multiple-dose intravenous physostigmine. *Am J Psychiatry* 139:1421–1424, 1982.

Davis PE, Mumford SJ: Cued recall and the nature of the memory disorder in dementia. *Br J Psychiatry* 144:383–386, 1984.

DeBoni U, Crapper DR: Paired helical filaments of the Alzheimer's type in cultured neurones. *Nature* 271:566–568, 1978.

Delaney JF: Spinal fluid aluminum levels in patients with Alzheimer's disease. *Ann Neurol* 5:581, 1979.

Delwaide PJ, Devoitille JM, Ylieff M: Acute effect of drugs upon memory of patients with senile dementia. *Acta Psychiatr Belg* 80:748–754, 1980.

Denber HCB: Physostigmine in the treatment of memory disorders: A case report. *Psychiatr J Univ Ottawa* 7:8–12, 1982.

Dewitt LD, Buonanno FS, Kistler JP, et al: Nuclear magnetic resonance imaging in evaluation of clinical stroke syndromes. *Ann Neurol* 16:535–545, 1984.

Diagnostic and Statistical Manual of Mental Disorders, ed 3, revised. (DSM-III-R). Washington, DC, American Psychiatric Association Press, 1987.

Ditch M, Kelly FJ, Resnick O: An ergot preparation (Hydergine) in the treatment of cerebrovascular disorders in the geriatric patient: double-blind study. *J Am Geriatr Soc* 19:208–217, 1971.

Drachman DA, Leavitt J: Human memory and the cholinergic system. *Arch Neurol* 30:113–121, 1974.

Drachman DA, Sahakian BJ: Memory and cognitive function in the elderly: A preliminary trial of physostigmine. *Arch Neurol* 37:674–675, 1980.

Dunea G, Mahurkar SD, Mamdani B, et al: Role of aluminum in dialysis dementia. *Ann Intern Med* 88:502–504, 1978.

Duvoisin RC, Golbe LI, Lepore FE: Progressive supranuclear palsy. *Can J Neurol Sci* 14:547–554, 1987.

Elias M, Elias P: Motivation and activity, in Birren JE, Schaie KE (eds): *Handbook of the Psychology of Aging*. New York, Van Nostrand, 1976, p 357.

Endicott J, Spitzer RL: A diagnostic interview: The schedule for affective disorders and schizophrenia. *Arch Gen Psychiatry* 35:837–844, 1978.

Filley CM, Kelly J, Heaton RK: Neuropsychologic features on early- and late-onset Alzheimer's disease. *Arch Neurol* 43:574–576, 1986.

Flowers KA, Pearce I, Pearce JMS: Recognition memory in Parkinson's disease. *J Neurol Neurosurg Psychiatry* 47:1174–1181, 1984.

Folstein MF, Breitner JCS: Language disorder predicts familial Alzheimer's disease. *Johns Hopkins Med J* 149:145–147, 1981.

Folstein MF: *Clin Psychiatry News* May 1987, p 17.

Francis PT, Palmer AM, Sims NR, et al: Neurochemical studies of early-onset Alzheimer's disease: Possible influence of treatment. *N Engl J Med* 313:7–11, 1985.

Freedman M, Rivoira P, Butters N, et al: Retrograde amnesia in Parkinson's disease. *Can J Neurol Sci* 11:297–301, 1984.

Freeman FR, Rudd SM: Clinical features that predict potentially reversible progressive intellectual deterioration. *J Am Geriatr Soc* 30:449–451, 1982.

Friedland RP, moderator: Alzheimer disease: clinical and biological heterogeneity. *Ann Intern Med* 109:298–311, 1988.

Gajdusek DC, Zigos V: Degenerative disease of the central nervous system in New Guinea: The epidemic occurrence of "kuru" in the native population. *N Engl J Med* 257:974–978, 1957.

Gerin J: Symptomatic treatment of cerebrovascular insufficiency with Hydergine. *Curr Ther Res* 11:539–546, 1969.

Gibbs CJ Jr, Gajdusek DC: Subacute spongiform virus encephalopathies: The transmissible virus dementias, in Katzman R, Terry RD, Bick KL (eds): *Alzheimer's Disease: Senile Dementia and Related Disorders*. New York, Raven Press, 1978, pp 559–577.

Glenner GG: Current knowledge of amyloid deposits as applied to senile plaques and congophilic angiopathy, in Katzman R, Terry RD, Bick KL (eds): *Alzheimer's Disease: Senile Dementia and Related Disorders*. New York, Raven Press, 1978, pp 493–501.

Goldstein G: The neuropsychology of schizophrenia, in Grant I, Adams KM (eds): *Neuropsychological Assessment of Neuropsychiatric Disorders*. New York, Oxford, 1986, pp 167–171.

Goodnick P, Gershon S: Chemotherapy of cognitive disorders in geriatric subjects. *J Clin Psychiatry* 45:196–209, 1984.

Gottfries CG, Adolfsson R, Aquilonius SM, et al: Biochemical changes in dementia disorders of Alzheimer's type (AD/SDAT). *Neurobiol Aging* 4:261–271, 1983.

Goudsmit JAAP, White BJ, Weitkamp LR, et al: Familial Alzheimer's disease in two kindreds of the same geographic and ethnic origin. *J Neurol Sci* 49:79–89, 1981.

Goulet LR: The interfaces of acquisition, in Nesselroade JR, Reese H (eds): *Life-Span Developmental Psychology*. New York, Academic Press, 1973.

Greden JF, Carroll BJ: The dexamethasone suppression test as a diagnostic aid in catatonia. *Am J Psychiatry* 136:1199, 1979.

Greenwald BS, Marin DB, Silverman SM: Serotonergic treatment of screaming and banging in dementia. *Lancet* 2:1464–1465, 1986.

Gwyther LP: *Care of Alzheimer's Patients: A Manual for Nursing Home Staff*. Chicago, American Health Care Associates and Alzheimer's Disease and Related Disorders Association, 1985.

Haase GR: Diseases presenting as dementia, in Wells CE (ed): *Dementia*, ed 2. Philadelphia, FA Davis Co, 1977, pp 27–67.

Hachinski VC, Iliff LD, Zilhka E, et al: Cerebral blood flow in dementia. *Arch Neurol* 32:632–637, 1975.

Hachinski VC, Lassen NA, Marshall J: Multi-infarct dementia. A cause of mental deterioration in the elderly. *Lancet* 2:207–210, 1974.

Hakim S, Adams RD: The special clinical problem of symptomatic hydrocephalus with normal cerebrospinal fluid pressure. *J Neurol Sci* 2:307, 1965.

Harbaugh RE, Roberts DW, Coombs DW, et al: Preliminary report: Intracranial cholinergic drug infusion in patients with Alzheimer's disease. *Neurosurgery* 15:514–517, 1984.

Harvard Medical School Health Letter, July 1984.

Heaton, Crowley TJ: Effects of psychiatric disorders and their somatic treatments on neuropsychological test results, in Filskov SB, Boll TJ (eds): *Handbook of Clinical Neuropsychology*. New York, Wiley-Interscience, 1981, pp 481–535.

Heckler MM: The fight against Alzheimer's disease. *Am Psychologist* 40:1240–1244, 1985.

Henschke PJ, Bell DA, Cape RDT: Alzheimer's disease and HLA. *Tissue Antigens* 12:132–135, 1978.

Heston LL, Mastri AR, Anderson VE, et al: Dementia of the Alzheimer type: Clinical genetics, natural history and associated conditions. *Arch Gen Psychiatry* 38:1085–1090, 1981.

Heston LL: Alzheimer's disease, trisomy 21, and myeloproliferative disorders: Associations suggesting a genetic diathesis. *Science* 196:322–323, 1976.

Hollister LE, Yesavage J: Ergoloid mesylates for senile dementia: Unanswered questions. *Ann Intern Med* 100:894–898, 1984.

Horita A: Neuropharmacology and aging, in Roberts J, Adelman RC, Cristafalo VJ (eds): *Pharmacological Intervention in the Aging Process*. New York, Plenum Press, 1978.

Horn: The psychological factors in parkinsonism. *J Neurol Neurosurg Psychiatry* 37:27–31, 1974.

Hourrigan J, Klingsporn A, Clark WW, et al: Epidemiology of scrapie in the United

States, in Prusiner SJ, Hadlow WJ (eds): *Slow Transmissible Diseases of the Nervous System*. New York, Academic Press, 1979.

Huber SJ, Shuttleworth EC, Paulson GW, et al: Cortical vs subcortical dementia. *Arch Neurol* 43:392–394, 1986a.

Huber SJ, Shuttleworth EC, Paulson GW, et al: Dementia in Parkinson's disease. *Arch Neurol* 43:987–990, 1986.

Huff FJ, Auerbach J, Chakravarti A, et al: Risk of dementia in relatives of patients with Alzheimer's disease. *Neurology* 38:786–790, 1988.

Hussain RA, Brown DC: Use of two-dimensional grid patterns to limit hazardous ambulation in demented patients. *J Gerontol* 42:558–560, 1987.

Hyman SE, Jenike MA: Approach to the patient with depression, in Goroll AH, May L, Mulley A (eds): *Primary Care Medicine*. Philadelphia, JB Lippincott, 1987, pp 907–915.

Jarvik LF, Altshuler KZ, Kato T, et al: Organic brain syndrome and chromosome loss in aged twins. *Dis Nerv Syst* 32:159–169, 1971.

Jarvik LF, Ruth V, Matsuyama SS: Organic brain syndrome and aging: A six year follow-up of surviving twins. *Arch Gen Psychiatry* 37:280–286, 1980.

Jellinger J: Neuropathological agents and dementia. *Acta Neurol Belg* 76:83–102, 1976.

Jenike MA, Albert MS, Baer L, et al: Ergot mesylates for Alzheimer's disease: A year-long double-blind trial of 3 mg vs. 12 mg daily. Submitted for publication.

Jenike MA, Albert MS, Heller H, et al: Combination lecithin and Hydergine in the treatment of Alzheimer's disease. *J Clin Psychiatry* 47:249–251, 1986.

Jenike MA, Albert MS, Heller H, et al: Oral physostigmine treatment for patients with presenile and senile dementia of the Alzheimer's type: A double-blind placebo-controlled trial. In press, 1989.

Jenike MA, Albert MS: The dexamethasone suppression test in patients with presenile and senile dementia of the Alzheimer's type. *J Am Geriatr Soc* 32:441–444, 1984.

Jenike MA: Alzheimer's disease—What the practicing clinician needs to know. *J Geriatr Psychiatr Neurol* 1:37–46, 1988.

Jenike MA: Alzheimer's disease. *Sci Am Med* 9:1–4, 1986a.

Jenike MA: Alzheimer's disease: Clinical management. *Psychosomatics* 27:407–416, 1986.

Jenike MA: Assessment and treatment of affective illness in the elderly. *J Geriatr Psychiatry Neurol* 1:89–107, 1988a.

Jenike MA: Depression and other psychiatric disorders, in Albert MS, Moss M (eds): *Geriatric Neuropsychology*. New York, Guildford Press, 1988b, pp 115–144.

Jenike MA: Dexamethasone suppression test as a clinical aid in elderly depressed patients. *J Am Geriatr Soc* 31:45–48, 1982a.

Jenike MA: Dexamethasone suppression: A biological marker of depression. *Drug Ther* 12:203–212, 1982.

Jenike MA: Drugs for cognitive and psychiatric symptoms. *Drug Ther* 10:97–108, 1986b.

Jenike MA: *Handbook of Geriatric Psychopharmacology*. Littleton, Mass, PSG Publishing Co, 1985.

Jenike MA: Management of Alzheimer's disease, in Goroll AH, May L, Mulley A (eds): *Primary Care Medicine*. Philadelphia, JB Lippincott, 1987, pp 755–759.

Jenike MA: MAO inhibitors as treatment for depressed patients with primary degenerative dementia (Alzheimer's disease). *Am J Psychiatry* 142:763–764, 1985a.

Jenike MA: Monoamine oxidase inhibitors in elderly depressed patients. *J Am Geriatr Soc* 32:571–575, 1984.

Jenike MA: The dexamethasone suppression test in the elderly: An update. *Clin Gerontologist* 2:3–11, 1983.

Jenike MA: Treating anxiety in elderly patients. *Geriatrics* 38:115–119, 1983a.

Jennings WG: An ergot alkaloid preparation (Hydergine) versus placebo for treatment of symptoms of cerebrovascular insufficiency: double-blind study. *J Am Geriatr Soc* 20:407–412, 1972.

Johnson KA, Davis KR, Buonanno FS, et al: Comparison of magnetic resonance and roentgen ray computed tomography in dementia. *Arch Neurol* 44:1075–1080, 1987.

Jonker C, Eikelenboom P, Tavenier P: Immunological indices in the cerebrospinal fluid of patients with presenile dementia of the Alzheimer's type. *Br J Psychiatry* 140:44–49, 1982.

Joynt RF, Shoulson I: Dementia, in Heilman KM, Valenstein E (eds): *Clinical Neuropsychology*. Oxford, England, Oxford University Press, 1975, pp 475–502.

Kalicki AC (ed): *Confronting Alzheimer's Disease*. Owings Mills, Md, National Health Publishing, 1987.

Karlsson I, Brane G, Melin A, et al: Effects of environmental stimulation on biochemical and psychological variables in dementia. *Acta Psychiatr Scand* 77:207–213, 1988.

Katzman R: Normal pressure hydrocephalus, in Wells CE (ed): *Dementia*, ed 2. Philadelphia, FA Davis, 1977, pp 69–92.

Katzman R: Alzheimer's disease. *N Engl J Med* 314:964–967, 1986.

Kaufmann MW, Cassem NH, Murray GB, et al: Use of psychostimulants in medically ill patients with neurological disease and major depression. *Can J Psychiatry* 29:46–49, 1984.

Kiloh LG: Pseudodementia. *Acta Psychiatr Scand* 37:336–361, 1961.

Klatzo I, Wisniewski H, Streicher E: Experimental production of neurofibrillary degeneration. 1. Light microscopic observations. *J Neuropathol Exp Neurol* 24:187–199, 1965.

Knesevich JW, Martin RL, Berg L, et al: Preliminary report on affective symptoms in the early stages of senile dementia of the Alzheimer type. *Am J Psychiatry* 140:233–235, 1983.

Kopelman MD: Rates of forgetting in Alzheimer-type dementia and Korsakoff's syndrome. *Neuropsychologia* 23:623–628, 1985.

Koss E, Friedland RP: Neuropsychological features of early and late-onset Alzheimer's disease. *Arch Neurol* 44:797, 1987.

Kvale JN: Amitriptyline in the management of progressive supranuclear palsy. *Arch Neurol* 39:387–388, 1982.

Labouvie-Vief G, Gonda JN: Cognitive strategy training and intellectual performance in the elderly. *J Gerontol* 31:327, 1976.

Laitinen L: Desipramine in treatment of Parkinson's disease. *Acta Neurol Scand* 45:109–113, 1969.

Larsson T, Sjogren T, Jacobson G: Senile dementia. *Acta Psychiatr Scand* 39(suppl 167):3–259, 1963.

Lebensohn Z, Jenkins RB: Improvement of parkinsonism in depressed patients treated with ECT. *Am J Psychiatry* 132:283–285, 1975.

Lederman RJ, Henry CE: Progressive dialysis encephalopathy. *Ann Neurol* 4:199–204, 1978.

Levine J, Feirstein A: Differences in test performance between brain-damaged, schizophrenic and medical patients. *J Consult Clin Psychol* 39:508–511, 1972.

Lipsey JR, Pearlson GD, Robinson RG, et al: Nortriptyline treatment of poststroke depression: A double-blind study. *Lancet* 1:297–300, 1984.

Lipsey JR, Spencer WC, Rabins PV, et al: Phenomenological comparison of poststroke depression and functional depression. *Am J Psychiatry* 143:527–529, 1986.

Lishman WA: *Organic Psychiatry*. London, Blackwell Scientific Publications, 1978.

Liston EH Jr: Diagnostic delay in presenile dementia. *J Clin Psychiatry* 39:599–603, 1978.

Liston EH, La Rue A: Clinical differentiation of primary degenerative and multi-infarct dementia: A critical review of the evidence: Part I: clinical studies, Part II: pathological studies. *Biol Psychiatry* 18:1451–1483, 1983.

Lukes SA, Crooks LE, Aminoff MJ, et al: Nuclear magnetic resonance imaging in multiple sclerosis. *Ann Neurol* 13:592–601, 1983.

Luria A, Naydin V, Tsvetkova L, et al: Restoration of higher cortical function following focal brain damage, in Bruyn G, Vinken PJ (eds): *Handbook of Clinical Neurology*. Amsterdam, North-Holland, 1969, p 368.

Mace NI, Rabins PV: *The 36-Hour Day*. Baltimore, The Johns Hopkins University Press, 1981.

Mahler ER, Smith E, Lees AJ: Cognitive deficits in Steel-Richardson-Olszewski syndrome (progressive supranuclear palsy). *J Neurol Neurosurg Psychiatry* 48:1234–1239, 1985.

Maletta GJ, Hepburn K: Helping families cope with Alzheimer's: The physician's role. *Geriatrics* 41:81–90, 1986.

Maletta GJ: *Alzheimer's Disease: Management*. DuPont Monograph Series, Reisberg B (ed). Wilmington, Del, DuPont Pharmaceutical Company, 1988.

Mamo HL, Meric PC, Ponsin JC, et al: Cerebral blood flow in normal pressure hydrocephalus. *Stroke* 18:1074–1080, 1987.

Manuelidis EE, Kim JH, Mericangas JR, et al: Transmission to animals of Creutzfeldt-Jakob disease from human blood. *Lancet* 2:896–897, 1985.

Markesbery WR, Ehmann WD, Hossain TIM, et al: Brain trace element levels in Alzheimer's disease by instrumental neutron activation analysis. *J Neuropathol Exp Neurol* 40:359, 1981.

Marsh RF, Semancik JS, Medappa KC, et al: Scrapie and transmissible mink encephalopathy: Search for infectious nucleic acid. *J Virol* 13:993–996, 1974.

Martone M, Butters N, Trauner D: Some analyses of forgetting of pictorial material in amnesic and demented patients. *J Clin Exp Neuropsychol* 8:161–178, 1986.

Marx JL: Alzheimer's drug trial put on hold. *Science* 238:1041–1042, 1987.

Mattis S: Dementia Rating Scale, in Bellack R, Karasu B (eds): *Geriatric Psychiatry*. New York, Grune and Stratton Inc, 1976.

Mayeux R, Albert M, Jenike M: Physostigmine-induced myoclonus in Alzheimer's disease. *Neurology* 37:345–346, 1987.

Mayeux R, Stern Y, Rosen J, et al: Depression, intellectual impairment, and Parkinson's disease. *Neurology* 31:645–650, 1981.

Mayeux R, Stern Y, Rosen J, et al: Is "subcortical dementia" a recognizable clinical entity? *Ann Neurol* 10:278–284, 1983.

Mayeux R: Depression and dementia in Parkinson's disease, in Marsden CC, Fahn S (eds): *Movement Disorders*. London, Butterworth, 1982, pp 75–95.

McAllister TW, Ferrell RB, Price TRP, et al: The dexamethasone suppression test in two patients with severe depressive pseudodementia. *Am J Psychiatry* 139:479, 1982.

McConnachie RW: A clinical trial comparing "Hydergine" with placebo in the treatment of cerebrovascular insufficiency in elderly patients. *Curr Med Res Opin* 1:463–468, 1973.

McDermott JR, Smith AI, Lqbal K, et al: Aluminum and Alzheimer's disease. *Lancet* 2:710–711, 1977.

McDermott JR, Smith AI, Lqbal K, et al: Brain aluminum in aging and Alzheimer's disease. *Neurology* 29:809–814, 1979.

McHugh PR, Folstein MF: Psychiatric syndromes of Huntington's chorea: A clinical and phenomenologic study, in Benson DF, Blumer D (eds): *Psychiatric Aspects of Neurologic Disease*. New York, Grune and Stratton, 1975, pp 267–286.

McKhann G, Drachman D, Folstein M, et al: Clinical diagnosis of Alzheimer's disease. *Neurology* 34:939–944, 1984.

McKusick VA: *Mendelian Inheritance in Man*, ed 6. Baltimore, The John Hopkins University Press, 1983, pp 30–31.

Mehler MF, Horoupian DS, Davies P, et al: Reduced somatostatin-like immunoreactivity in cerebral cortex in nonfamilial dysphasic dementia. *Neurology* 37:1448–1453, 1987.

Mendez M, Cummings JL, Darkins AW, et al: Alzheimer's disease: comparison of speech and language alterations. *Neurology* 37(suppl 1):227, 1987.

Mesulam MM: Slowly progressive aphasia without generalized dementia. *Ann Neurol* 11:592–598, 1982.

Miller AE, Neighbor A, Katzman R, et al: Immunological studies in senile dementia of the Alzheimer's type: Evidence for enhanced suppressor cell activity. *Ann Neurol* 10:506–510, 1981.

Mjones H: Paralysis agitans. *Acta Psychiatr Neurol* 54(suppl):1–195, 1949.

Mohs RC, Breitner JCS, Silverman JM, et al: Alzheimer's disease: morbid risk among first-degree relatives approximates 50% by 90 years of age. *Arch Gen Psychiatry* 44:405–408, 1987.

Mohs RC, Davis BM, Johns CA, et al: Oral physostigmine treatment of patients with Alzheimer's disease. *Am J Psychiatry* 142:28–33, 1985.

Mohs RC, Davis KL: A signal detectability analysis of the effect of physostigmine on memory in patients with Alzheimer's disease. *Neurobiol Aging* 3:105–110, 1982.

Moore JT, Busse E: Diagnosis and management of senile dementia patients. McNeil Pharmaceutical Company Monograph Series, 1987.

Mortimer JA, French LR, Hutton JT, et al: Head injury as a risk factor for Alzheimer's disease. *Neurology* 35:264–267, 1985.

Mortimer JA, Schuman LM (eds): *The Epidemiology of Dementia*. New York, Oxford University Press, 1981.

Mountjoy CQ: Correlations between neuropathological and neurochemical changes. *Br Med Bull* 42:81–85, 1986.

Muramoto O, Sugishita M, Sugita H, et al: Effect of physostigmine on constructional and memory tasks in Alzheimer's disease. *Arch Neurol* 36:501, 1979.

Myers JK, Weissman MM, Tischler G, et al: Six-month prevalence of psychiatric disorders in three communities. *Arch Gen Psychiatry* 41:959, 1984.

Nandy K: Brain-reactive antibodies in aging and senile dementia, in Katzman R, Terry RD, Bick KL (eds): *Alzheimer's Disease: Senile Dementia and Related Disorders*. New York, Raven Press, 1978, pp 503–512.

Neary D, Snowden JS, Mann DMA, et al: Alzheimer's disease: a correlative study. *J Neurol Neurosurg Psychiatry* 49:157–162, 1986.

Neary D, Snowden JS, Northen B, et al: Dementia of frontal lobe type. *J Neurol Neurosurg Psychiatry* 51:353–361, 1988.

O'Daniel R, Lippmann S, Piyush P: Depressive pseudodementia. *Psychiatr Ann* 11:10–15, 1981.

O'Neil M, Page N, Adkins WN, et al: Tryptophan-trazodone treatment of aggressive behaviour. *Lancet* 2:859–860, 1986.

Owens D, Dawson JC, Lowsin S: Alzheimer's disease in Down's syndrome. *Am J Ment Defic* 75:606–612, 1971.

Palmer AM, Wilcock GK, Esiri MM et al: Monoaminergic innervation of the frontal and temporal lobes in Alzheimer's disease. *Brain Res* 401:231–238, 1987.

Patrick HT, Levy DM: Parkinson's disease: A clinical study of 146 cases. *Arch Neurol Psychiatry* 7:711–720, 1922.

Perry EK, Gibson PH, Blessed G, et al: Neuro-transmitter enzyme abnormalities in senile dementia. *J Neurol Sci* 34:247–265, 1977.

Perry EK, Tomlinson BE, Blessed G, et al: Correlation of cholinergic abnormalities with senile plaques and mental test scores in senile dementia. *Br Med J* 2:1457–1459, 1978.

Perry EK: The cholinergic hypothesis—ten years on. *Br Med Bull* 42:63–69, 1986.

Peters BH, Levin HS: Effects of physostigmine and lecithin on memory in Alzheimer disease. *Ann Neurol* 6:219–221, 1979.

Pillon B, Bubois B, Lhermitte F, et al: Heterogeneity of cognitive impairment in progressive supranuclear palsy, Parkinson's disease, and Alzheimer's disease. *Neurology* 36:1179–1185, 1986.

Poeck K, Luzzatti C: Slowly progressive aphasia in three patients. *Brain* 111:151–168, 1988.

Powell AL, Cummings JL, Hill MA, et al: Speech and language alterations in multi-infarct dementia. *Neurology* 38:717–719, 1988.

Powell LS, Courtice K: *Alzheimer's Disease: A Guide for Families*. Reading, Mass, Addison-Wesley Publishing Company, 1983.

Priddy JM, Gallagher DE, Lovett SB: Caregiver support groups: Structured vs. unstructured interventions. Presented at the 38th Annual Scientific Meeting of the Gerontological Society, New Orleans, 1985.

Prohovik I, Mayeux R, Sackheim HA, et al: Cerebral perfusion as a diagnostic marker of early Alzheimer's disease. *Neurology* 38:931–937, 1988.

Prusiner SD: Prions. *Sci Am* 251:50–59, 1984.

Purisch AD, Golden CJ, Hammeke TA: Discrimination of schizophrenic and brain-injured patients by a standardized version of Luria's neuropsychological tests. *J Consult Clin Psychol* 46:1266–1273, 1978.

Rabins PV, Mace NL, Lucas MJ: The impact of dementia on the family. *JAMA* 248:333–335, 1982.

Rabins PV: Management of dementia in the family context. *Psychosomatics* 25:369–375, 1984.

Rabins PV: Psychosocial aspects of dementia. *J Clin Psychiatry* 49(Suppl):29–31, 1988.

Raft D, Newman M, Spencer R: Suicide on L-dopa. *South Med J* 65:312, 1972.

Rao DB, Norris JR: A double-blind investigation of Hydergine in the treatment of cerebrovascular insufficiency in the elderly. *Johns Hopkins Med J* 130:317–324, 1972.

Raskin A, Friedman AS, DiMascio A: Cognitive and performance deficits in depression. *Psychopharmacol Bull* 18:196–202, 1982.

Raskind M, Peskind E, Rivard MF, et al: Dexamethasone suppression test and cortisol circadian rhythm in primary degenerative dementia. *Am J Psychiatry* 139:1468, 1982.

Raskind MA: Introduction: faces of dementia: Current concepts. *J Clin Psychiatry* 49(Suppl):3–4, 1988.

Reding M, Haycox J, Blass J: Depression in patients referred to a dementia clinic: A three-year prospective study. *Arch Neurol* 42:894–896, 1985.

Reed E, Chandler JR: Huntington's chorea in Michigan. I. Demography and genetics. *Am J Hum Genet* 10:201–225, 1958.

Rehman SA: Two trials comparing "Hydergine" with placebo in the treatment of patients suffering from cerebrovascular insufficiency. *Curr Med Res Opin* 1:456–462, 1973.

Reifler BV, Larson E, Hanley R: Coexistence of cognitive impairment and depression in geriatric outpatients. *Am J Psychiatry* 139:623–626, 1982.

Reinikainen K, Soininen H, Kosma V-M, et al: Neurotransmitters in senile dementia of the Alzheimer type and in vascular dementia, in Rose FC (ed): *Modern Approaches* to the Dementias, Part I: Etiology and Pathophysiology. Basel, Karger, 1985, pp 184–197.

Reinikainen KJ, Paljarvi L, Huuskonen M, et al: A post-mortem study of noradrenergic, serotonergic and GAGAergic neurons in Alzheimer's disease. *J Neurol Sci* 84:101–116, 1988.

Reinikainen KJ, Riekkinen PJ, Paljarvi L, et al: Cholinergic deficit in Alzheimer's disease: a study based on CSF and autopsy data. *Neurochem Res.* In press, 1987.

Reisberg B, Ferris SH, DeLeon MJ, et al: The Global Deterioration Scale for assessment of primary degenerative dementia. *Am J Psychiatry* 139:1136–1139, 1982.

Reisberg B, Ferris SH, Gershon S: An overview of pharmacologic treatment of cognitive decline in the aged. *Am J Psychiatry* 138:593–600, 1981.

Reisberg B: *Alzheimer's Disease: Management.* DuPont Monograph Series, Reisberg B (ed). Wilmington, Del, DuPont Pharmaceutical Company, 1988.

Reus V, Weingartner H, Post R: Clinical implications of state-dependent learning. *Am J Psychiatry* 136:927, 1979.

Risberg J, Gustafson L: Xe cerebral blood flow in dementia and in neuropsychiatry research, in Magistretti P (ed): *Functional Radionuclide Imaging of the Brain.* New York, Raven Press, 1983.

Robinson DS, David JM, Nies A, et al: Ageing, monoamines, and monoamine oxidase levels. *Lancet* 1:290–291, 1972.

Robinson DS: Changes in monoamine oxidase and monoamines with human development and aging. *Fed Proc* 34:103–107, 1975.

Robinson RG, Starr LB, Kubos KL, et al: Mood changes in stroke patients: Relationship to lesion location. *Compr Psychiatry* 24:555–566, 1983.

Robinson RG, Starr LB, Price TR: A two year longitudinal study of mood disorders following stroke: Prevalence and duration at six months follow-up. *Br J Psychiatry* 144:256–262, 1984.

Robinson RG, Szetela B: Mood change following left hemisphere brain injury. *Ann Neurol* 9:447–453, 1981.

Robinson RG: Depression in aphasic patients: Frequency, severity, and clinicopathological correlations. *Brain Lang* 14:282–291, 1981.

Roman GC: Senile dementia of the Binswanger type: A vascular form of dementia in the elderly. *JAMA* 258:1782–1788, 1987.

Ron MA, Toone BK, Garralda ME, et al: Diagnostic accuracy in presenile dementia. *Br J Psychiatry* 134:161–168, 1979.

Roos R, Gajdusek DC, Gibbs CJ: The clinical characteristics of transmissible Creutzfeldt-Jakob disease. *Brain* 96:1–20, 1973.

Rosen HJ: Mental decline in the elderly: Pharmacotherapy (ergot alkaloids versus papaverine). *J Am Geriatr Soc* 23:169–174, 1975.

Rossor MN, Iversen LL: Non-cholinergic neurotransmitter abnormalities in Alzheimer's disease. *Br Med Bull* 42:70–74, 1986.

Rossor MN, Garrett NJ, Johnson AL, et al: A post-mortem study of the cholinergic and GABA systems in senile dementia. *Brain* 105:313–330, 1982.

Rossor MN, Iversen LL, Reynolds GP, et al: Neurochemical characteristics of early and late onset types of Alzheimer's disease. *Br Med J* 288:961–964, 1984.

Roth M, Tomlinson BE, Blessed G: Correlation between scores for dementia and counts of "senile plaques" in grey matter of elderly subjects. *Nature* 209:109, 1966.

Roubicek J, Geiger C, Abt K: An ergot alkaloid preparation (Hydergine) in geriatric therapy. *J Am Geriatr Soc* 20:222–229, 1972.

Rozas VV, Port FK, Rutt WM: Progressive dialysis encephalopathy from dialysate aluminum. *Arch Intern Med* 138:1375–1377, 1978.

Rudorfer MV, Clayton PJ: Depression, dementia, and dexamethasone suppression (letter). *Am J Psychiatry* 138:701, 1981.

Sagar HJ, Cohen NJ, Sullivan EV, et al: Remote memory function in Alzheimer's disease and Parkinson's disease. *Brain* 111:185–206, 1988.

Salzman C (ed): *Clinical Geriatric Psychopharmacology*. New York, McGraw-Hill Book Co, 1984.

Salzman C: A primer on geriatric psychopharmacology. *Am J Psychiatry* 139:67–74, 1982.

Schlesser MA, Winokur G, Sherman BM: Hypothalamic-pituitary-adrenal axis activity in depressive illness: Its relationship to classification. *Arch Gen Psychiatry* 37:737, 1980.

Schoenfeld M, Myers RG, Cupples LA, et al: Increased rate of suicide among patients with Huntington's disease. *J Neurol Neurosurg Psychiatry* 47:1283–1287, 1984.

Seltzer B, Sherwin I: A comparison of clinical features in early- and late-onset primary degenerative dementia. *Arch Neurol* 40:143–146, 1983.

Shamoian CA (ed): *Treatment of Affective Disorders in the Elderly*. Washington DC, American Psychiatric Association Press, 1985.

Shelly C, Goldstein G: Discrimination of chronic schizophrenia and brain damage with the Luria-Nebraska battery: A partially successful replication. *Clin Neuropsychol* 5:82–85, 1983.

Shore D, Millson M, Holtz JL, et al: Serum aluminum in primary degenerative dementia. *Biol Psychiatry* 15:971–977, 1980.

Shore D, Overman CA, Wyatt RJ: Improving accuracy in the diagnosis of Alzheimer's disease. *J Clin Psychiatry* 44:207–212, 1983.

Shuttleworth EC, Huber SJ, Paulson GW: Depression in patients with dementia of Alzheimer type. *J Nat Med Assoc* 79:733–736, 1987.

Simpson DM, Foster D: Improvement in organically disturbed behaviour with trazodone treatment. *Gen Clin Psychiatry* 47:192–193, 1986.

Sjogren T, Sjogren H, Lundgren G: Morbus Alzheimer and morbus Pick. *Acta Pychiatr Neurol Scand* (Suppl) 82:9–51, 1952.

Small GW: Psychopharmacological treatment of elderly demented patients. *J Clin Psychiatry* 49:5 (Suppl):8–13, 1988.

Smith C, Swash M: Physostigmine in Alzheimer's disease. *Lancet* 1:42, 1979.

Sourander P, Sjogren H: The concept of Alzheimer's disease and its clinical implications, in Wolstenholme GEW, O'Connor M (eds): *Alzheimer's Disease and Related Conditions: A Ciba Foundation Symposium*. London, Churchill, 1970, pp 11–36.

Spar JE, Gerner R: Does the dexamethasone suppression test distinguish dementia from depression? *Am J Psychiatry* 139:238, 1982.

Spiegel R, Huber F, Koberle S: A controlled long-term study of ergoloid mesylates (Hydergine) in healthy volunteers. *J Am Geriatr Soc* 31:549–555, 1983.

St. George-Hyslop PH, Tanzi RE, Polinsky JL, et al: The genetic defect causing familial Alzheimer's disease maps on chromosome 21. *Science* 235:885–889, 1987.

Stannard CI: Old folks and dirty work: The social consideration for patient abuse in a nursing home. *Social Problems* 20:319–324, 1973.

Storandt M, Botwinick J, Danzinger WL: Longitudinal changes: Patients with mild SDAT and matched healthy controls, in Poon LW (ed): *Clinical Memory Assessment of Older Adults*. Washington DC, American Psychological Association, 1986, pp 277–284.

Strang RR: Imipramine in treatment of parkinsonism: A double-blind placebo study. *Br J Med* 2:33–34, 1965.

Sulkava R, Kiskimies S, Wikstrom J, et al: HLA antigens in Alzheimer's disease. *Tissue Antigens* 16:191–194, 1980.

Summergrad P: Depression in Binswanger's encephalopathy responsive to tranylcypromine: case report. *J Clin Psychiatry* 46:69–70, 1985.

Summers WK, Majovski LV, Marsh GM, et al: Oral tetrahydroaminoacridine in long-term treatment of senile dementia, Alzheimer type. *N Engl J Med* 315:1241–1245, 1986.

Sutton S: Fact and artifact in the psychology of schizophrenia, in Hammer M, Salzinger K, Sutton S (eds): *Psychopathology: Contributions from the Biological, Behavioral and Social Sciences.* New York, Wiley, 1973, pp 197–213.

Terry RD, Davies P: Dementia of the Alzheimer type. *Ann Rev Neurosci* 3:77–95, 1980.

Terry RD, Katzman R: Senile dementia of the Alzheimer type. *Ann Neurol* 14:497–506, 1983.

Terry RD, Pena C: Experimental production of neurofibrillary degeneration. II. Electron microscopy, phosphatase histochemistry and electron probe analysis. *J Neuropathol Exp Neurol* 24:200–210, 1965.

Thal L, Masur D, Fuld P, et al: Memory improvement with oral physostigmine and lecithin in Alzheimer's disease, in Katzman R (ed): *Banbury Report 15: Biological Aspects of Alzheimer's Disease.* New York, Cold Spring Harbor Laboratory, 1983, pp 461–469.

Thal LJ, Fuld PA: Memory enhancement with oral physostigmine in Alzheimer's disease. *N Engl J Med* 6:720, 1983.

Thal LJ: Dementia update: diagnosis and neuropsychiatric aspects. *J Clin Psychiatry* 49:5(Suppl):5–7, 1988.

Thibault A: A double-blind evaluation of "Hydergine" and placebo in the treatment of patients with organic brain syndrome and cerebral arteriosclerosis in a nursing home. *Curr Med Res Opin* 2:482–487, 1974.

Thiehaus OJ, Wheeler BG, Simon S, et al: A controlled double-blind study of high-dose dihydroergotoxine mesylate (Hydergine) in mild dementia. *J Am Geriatr Soc* 35:219–223, 1987.

Tomlinson BE, Blessed G, Roth M: Observations on the brains of demented old people. *J Neurol Sci* 11:205–242, 1970.

Tomlinson BE, Blessed G, Roth M: Observations on the brains of nondemented old people. *J Neurol Sci* 7:331–356, 1968.

Tourigny-Rivard MF, Raskind M, Rivard D: The dexamethasone suppression test in an elderly population. *Biol Psychiatry* 16:1177, 1981.

Triboletti F, Ferri H: Hydergine for treatment of symptoms of cerebrovascular insufficiency. *Curr Ther Res* 11:609–620, 1969.

Uhlmann RF, Larson EB, Koepsell TD: Hearing impairment and cognitive decline in senile dementia of the Alzheimer's type. *J Am Geriatr Soc* 34:207–210, 1986.

Wade JPH, Mirsen TR, Hachinski VC, et al: The clinical diagnosis of Alzheimer's disease. *Arch Neurol* 44:24–29, 1987.

Warburton JW: Depressive symptoms in parkinsonian patients referred for thalamotomy. *J Neurol Neurosurg Psychiatry* 30:368–370, 1967.

Watson CG, Thomas RW, Andersen D, et al: Differentiation of organics from schizophrenics at two chronicity levels by use of the Reitan-Halstead organic test battery. *J Consult Clin Psychol* 32:679–684, 1968.

Waxman HM, Astrom S, Norberg A, et al: Conflicting attitudes toward euthanasia for severely demented patients of health care professionals in Sweden. *J Am Geriatr Soc* 36:397–401, 1988.

Waxman HM, Carner EA, Berkenstock G: Job turnover and job satisfaction among nursing home aides. *The Gerontologist* 24:503–509, 1984.

Weingartner H, Burns S, Diebel R, et al: Cognitive impairments in Parkinson's disease:

distinguishing between effort-demanding and automatic cognitive processes. *Psychiatr Res* 11:223–235, 1984.

Wells CE: A deluge of dementia. *Psychosomatics* 22:836–840, 1981.

Wells CE: Diagnostic evaluation and treatment in dementia, in Wells CE (ed): *Dementia*, ed 2. Philadelphia, FA Davis Co, 1977, pp 247–273.

Wettstein A: No effect from double-blind trial of physostigmine and lecithin in Alzheimer disease. *Ann Neurol* 13:210–212, 1983.

Whalley LJ, Urbaniak SJ, Darg C, et al: Histocompatibility antigens and antibodies to viral and other antigens in Alzheimer's presenile dementia. *Acta Psychiatr Scand* 61:1–7, 1980.

Whitehouse PJ: Reviewing the "breakthroughs" in Alzheimer's research. *Geriatrics* 42:107–111, 1987.

Wilson RS, Como PG, Garron D, et al: Memory failure in Huntington's disease. *J Clin Exp Neuropsychol* 9:147–154, 1987.

Wisniewski HM, Terry RD, Hirano A: Neurofibrillary pathology. *J Neuropathol Exp Neurol* 29:163–176, 1970.

Wisniewski HM, Terry RD: Reexamination of the pathogenesis of the senile plaque, in Zimmerman HM (ed): *Progress in Neuropathology*. New York, Grune and Stratton Inc, 1973.

Wolf PA, Dawber TR, Thomas HE, et al: Epidemiology of stroke, in Thompson RA, Green JR (eds): *Advances in Neurology*. New York, Raven Press, 1977, pp 5–19.

Wolozin BL, Davies P: Alzheimer-related neuronal protein A68: Specificity and distribution. *Ann Neurol* 22:521–526, 1987.

Wolozin BL, Pruchnicki A, Dickson DW, et al: A neuronal antigen in the brains of Alzheimer patients. *Science* 232:648–651, 1986.

Woods SW, Tesar GE, Murray GB, et al: Psychostimulant treatment of depressive disorders secondary to medical illness. *J Clin Psychiatry* 47:12–15, 1986.

Yates CM: Aluminum and Alzheimer's disease, in Glen AIM, Whalley LJ (eds): *Alzheimer's Disease. Early Recognition of Potentially Reversible Deficits*. London, Churchill Livingstone, 1979, pp 53–56.

Yates FA: *The Art of Memory*. London, Routledge and Kegan Paul, 1966.

Yesavage JA, Westphal J, Rush L: Senile dementia: combined pharmacologic and psychologic treatment. *J Am Geriatr Soc* 29:164–171, 1981.

Yudofsky SC: Parkinson's disease, depression, and electroconvulsive therapy: A clinical and neurobiologic synthesis. *Compr Psychiatry* 20:579–581, 1979.

Zarit S, Cole K, Gallagher D, et al: Memory concerns of the aging: cognitive and affective interventions. Proceedings of the XIth International Congress on Gerontology, Tokyo, 1979.

Zubin J: Problem of attention in schizophrenia, in Kietzman M, Sutton S, Zubin J (eds): *Experimental Approaches to Psychopathology*. New York, Academic Press, 1975, pp 139–166.

6

Psychosis, Violence, and Behavioral Problems in Later Life

OVERVIEW

Elderly patients who are psychotic, are violent, or exhibit inappropriately aggressive behavior are particularly disruptive and present a therapeutic challenge to the clinician. Although in the elderly these problems do not occur as often as depression and anxiety, when they do arise, prompt attention is usually demanded by family members or nursing home staff.

Medications used to control such symptoms, on the one hand, are very effective, but on the other, may produce side effects of a serious nature. Patients who require major tranquilizers or neuroleptics usually fall into a few general categories; the majority of such patients have moderate-to-severe dementia while a smaller percentage may have a lifelong psychotic process. Schizophrenics live into old age and, with recent thrusts toward deinstitutionalization, they are finding their way into nursing homes or are living in the community. Disturbances of behavior and thinking are also present in delirious or acutely confused patients (see chapter 9) as well as in some elderly patients whose affective illnesses (see chapter 4) have reached psychotic proportions.

DIAGNOSTIC CATEGORIES

Organic Mental Syndromes and Disorders

In DSM-III-R (1987) a distinction is made between organic mental syndromes and organic mental disorders. Organic mental syndrome is used to refer to a constellation of psychological or behavioral signs and symptoms without reference to cause; organic mental disorder designates a particular organic mental syndrome in which the cause is known or presumed. The DSM-III-R categorization of patients who have dementia, delirium, and drug and alcohol disorders are covered in detail in chapters 5, 9, and 10, respectively, and is not duplicated here.

Schizophrenia

Schizophrenic patients invariably have characteristic disturbances in several of the following areas: content and form of thought, perception, affect, sense of self, volition, relationship to the external world, and psychomotor behavior (DSM-III-R, 1987).

Thought content involves delusions that are often multiple, fragmented, or bizarre. Simple persecutory delusions involving the belief that others are spying on, spreading false rumors about, or planning to harm the person are common. Ideas of reference, in which events, objects, or other people are given particular and unusual significance, usually of a negative or perjorative nature, are also common. For example, the person may be convinced that a television commentator is mocking him.

Elderly schizophrenic patients may feel that their thoughts are transmitted from their heads and that everyone can hear them (thought broadcasting) or that other's thoughts are entering their heads (thought insertion). Occasionally they may feel that their thoughts are being removed by someone else (thought withdrawal) or that some external force is controlling them (delusions of being controlled).

Another common feature of the schizophrenic patient is the presence of errors of logic (form). Such formal thought disorders are most often manifested as loosening of associations in which ideas shift from one subject to another which seem to the observer completely unrelated or only obliquely connected.

Chronic elderly schizophrenics may demonstrate poverty of content of speech where little information is conveyed in a vague, abstract, or overly concrete manner. Emotionality and affect may be greatly blunted. Various hallucinations are frequently reported, auditory hallucinations being the most common. Most frequently the patient hears many voices as coming from outside his or her head which are often commenting in a derogatory manner about the patient. Command hallucinations, where the voices issue mandates to the patient, sometimes create dangerous situations for the patient or others. Occasionally, auditory hallucinations are of sounds rather than voices. Tactile hallucinations may occur. Visual, gustatory, and olfactory hallucinations can infrequently occur and always raise the possibility of an organic mental disorder (DSM-III-R, 1987).

Difficulty in and extreme sensitivity to interpersonal relationships are the rule with resultant social withdrawal and emotional detachment. Odd mannerisms and ways of movement are often observed.

When the physician is consulted about a psychotic elderly patient who may be schizophrenic, it is important to speak to family members and to review the old records. Since the onset of schizophrenia is usually during adolescence or early adulthood, there is usually a long history of bizarre or ineffective behavior. Occasionally the disorder may begin in middle or late adult life; in these cases, differential diagnosis is more complicated.

DSM-III-R (1987) notes that the disorder generally can be divided into three phases. The prodromal phase precedes the active phase and consists of clear deterioration from a previous level of functioning and is characterized by social withdrawal, impairment in role functioning, peculiar behavior, neglect of personal hygiene and grooming, blunted or inappropriate affect, disturbances in communication, lack of initiative, and loss of energy. There are almost no data describing the prodromal phase in late-onset schizophrenia, but it is clear that elderly patients who meet this description could also have a number of disorders such as early-stage dementia, early-stage Huntington's chorea, drug side effects, etc. A careful psychiatric history, mental status exam, and physical and neurologic exam may lead to the diagnosis. Sometimes the patient will have to be observed for a few weeks to a few months to make the diagnosis.

The active phase follows the prodromal phase and is typified by delusions, hallucinations, loosening of associations, incoherence, and/or catatonic behavior (Table 6–1). Usually a residual phase follows the active phase of the illness; the patient may be totally unable to function with affective blunting. Delusions, hallucinations, or other psychotic symptoms may persist, but may no longer be accompanied by strong affect. Full remissions have been reported to occur but are extremely unlikely.

The schizophrenic disorders are separated into various types based on particular symptom clusters. These include catatonic type, disorganized type, paranoid type, undifferentiated type, and residual type (Table 6–2).

DSM-III-R requires a continuous six-month period for diagnosis; prior to this, patients meeting these criteria but with the symptoms less than six continuous months would be classified under schizophreniform disorder.

Life expectancy is shorter for people with schizophrenia because of an increased suicide rate and death from other causes. Violent and inappropriate acts occur and these may be the primary reason for consultation.

The diagnosis of schizophrenia is made when all organic factors have been eliminated. Extensive medical workups are generally not required for patients who present with a clear-cut lifelong psychotic process, but for elderly patients who have recently become psychotic, medical evaluation is of supreme importance.

Although treatment of violent or severely agitated patients may often have to be started prior to a firm diagnosis, resolution of symptoms with medication should not lead the physician to cut the medical evaluation short.

PATIENT SYMPTOMS

Severe Agitation

Some of the most disruptive patients encountered in clinical practice are those with dementia who scream loudly, bang their heads, or try to assault other

Table 6–1
Diagnostic Criteria for Schizophrenia

A. Presence of characteristic psychotic symptoms in the active phase: either (1), (2), or (3) for at least one week (unless the symptoms are successfully treated):
  (1) two of the following:
    (a) delusions
    (b) prominent hallucinations (throughout the day for several days or several times a week for several weeks, each hallucinatory experience not being limited to a few brief moments)
    (c) incoherence or marked loosening of associations
    (d) catatonic behavior
    (e) flat or grossly inappropriate affect
  (2) bizarre delusions (ie, involving a phenomenon that the person's culture would regard as totally implausible, eg, thought broadcasting, being controlled by a dead person)
  (3) prominent hallucinations [as defined in (1)(b) above] of a voice with content having no apparent relation to depression or elation, or a voice keeping up a running commentary on the person's behavior or thoughts, or two or more voices conversing with each other
B. During the course of the disturbance, functioning in such areas as work, social relations, and self-care is markedly below the highest level achieved before onset of the disturbance (or, when the onset is in childhood or adolescence, failure to achieve expected level of social development).
C. Schizoaffective disorder and mood disorder with psychotic features have been ruled out, ie, if a major depressive or manic syndrome has ever been present during an active phase of the disturbance, the total duration of all episodes of a mood syndrome has been brief relative to the total duration of the active and residual phases of the disturbance.
D. Continuous signs of the disturbance for at least six months. The six-month period must include an active phase (of at least one week, or less if symptoms have been successfully treated) during which there were psychotic symptoms characteristic of schizophrenia (symptoms in A), with or without a prodromal or residual phase, as defined below.
  Prodromal phase: A clear deterioration in functioning before the active phase of the disturbance that is not due to a disturbance in mood or to a psychoactive substance use disorder and that involves at least two of the symptoms listed below.
  Residual phase: Following the active phase of the disturbance, persistence of at least two of the symptoms noted below, these not being due to a disturbance in mood or to a psychoactive substance use disorder.

patients or caregivers often in response to internal stimuli or minimal external stimuli. These patients are very difficult to treat and often do not respond to conventional drug treatments. Treatment options, which include neuroleptics, lithium, beta-blockers, buspirone, and other serotonergic agents, are discussed in later sections of this chapter.

Psychosis

Several authors examined the nature and progression of personality changes associated with mild Alzheimer's disease in otherwise healthy subjects (Rubin

Table 6–1 *continued*
Diagnostic Criteria for Schizophrenia

Prodromal or Residual Symptoms:
  (1) marked social isolation or withdrawal
  (2) marked impairment in role functioning as wage-earner, student, or homemaker
  (3) markedly peculiar behavior (eg, collecting garbage, talking to self in public, hoarding food)
  (4) marked impairment in personal hygiene and grooming
  (5) blunted or inappropriate affect
  (6) digressive, vague, overelaborate, or circumstantial speech, or poverty of speech, or poverty of content of speech
  (7) odd beliefs or magical thinking, influencing behavior and inconsistent with cultural norms, eg, superstitiousness, belief in clairvoyance, telepathy, "sixth sense," "others can feel my feelings," overvalued ideas, ideas of reference
  (8) unusual perceptual experiences, eg, recurrent illusions, sensing the presence of a force or person not actually present
  (9) marked lack of initiative, interests, or energy
  Examples: Six months of prodromal symptoms with one week of symptoms from A; no prodromal symptoms with six months of symptoms from A; no prodromal symptoms with one week of symptoms from A and six months of residual symptoms.
E. It cannot be established that an organic factor initiated and maintained the disturbance.
F. If there is a history of autistic disorder, the additional diagnosis of schizophrenia is made only if prominent delusions or hallucinations are also present.
Classification of course. The course of the disturbance is coded in the fifth digit:
  1-Subchronic. The time from the beginning of the disturbance, when the person first began to show signs of the disturbance (including prodromal, active, and residual phases) more or less continuously, is less than two years, but at least six months.
  2-Chronic. Same as above, but more than two years.
  3-Subchronic with Acute Exacerbation. Reemergence of prominent psychotic symptoms in a person with a subchronic course who has been in the residual phase of the disturbance.
  4-Chronic with Acute Exacerbation. Reemergence of prominent psychotic symptoms in a person with a chronic course who has been in the residual phase of the disturbance.
  5-In Remission. When a person with a history of schizophrenia is free of all signs of the disturbance (whether or not on medication), "in Remission" should be coded. Differentiating schizophrenia in remission from no mental disorder requires consideration of overall level of functioning, length of time since the last episode of disturbance, total duration of the disturbance, and whether prophylactic treatment is being given.
  0-Unspecified.

et al, 1987 and 1987a) and found that in these patients passive, agitated, and self-centered behaviors develop. In addition, psychotic symptoms are reportedly common in Alzheimer's disease, occurring in at least 25% of subjects with mild dementia and in about 50% who progress to severe dementia

Table 6–2
Diagnostic Criteria for Schizophrenia Types

Diagnostic Criteria for 295.2x Catatonic Type
A type of schizophrenia in which the clinical picture is dominated by any of the following:
    (1) catatonic stupor (marked decrease in reactivity to the environment and/or reduction in spontaneous movements and activity) or mutism
    (2) catatonic negativism (an apparently motiveless resistance to all instructions or attempts to be moved)
    (3) catatonic rigidity (maintenance of a rigid posture against efforts to be moved)
    (4) catatonic excitement (excited motor activity, apparently purposeless and not influenced by external stimuli)
    (5) catatonic posturing (voluntary assumption of inappropriate or bizarre postures)
Diagnostic Criteria for 295.1x Disorganized Type
A type of schizophrenia in which the following criteria are met:
A. Incoherence, marked loosening of associations, or grossly disorganized behavior.
B. Flat or grossly inappropriate affect.
C. Does not meet the criteria for Catatonic Type.
Diagnostic Criteria for 295.3x Paranoid Type
A type of schizophrenia in which there are:
A. Preoccupation with one or more systematized delusions or with frequent auditory hallucinations related to a single theme.
B. *None* of the following: incoherence, marked loosening of associations, flat or grossly inappropriate affect, catatonic behavior, grossly disorganized behavior.
Specify stable type if criteria A and B have been met during all past and present active phases of the illness.
Diagnostic Criteria for 295.9x Undifferentiated Type
A type of schizophrenia in which there are:
A. Prominent delusions, hallucinations, incoherence, or grossly disorganized behavior.
B. Does not meet the criteria for paranoid, catatonic, or disorganized type.
Diagnostic Criteria for 295.6x Residual Type
A type of schizophrenia in which there are:
A. Absence of prominent delusions, hallucinations, incoherence, or grossly disorganized behavior.
B. Continuing evidence of the disturbance, as indicated by two or more of the residual symptoms listed in criterion D of schizophrenia.

Reprinted with permission from the *Diagnostic and Statistical Manual of Mental Disorders, third edition, revised*. Copyright 1987. American Psychiatric Association.

(Rubin and Drevets, 1987). There is some speculation that the early presence of psychotic symptoms may delineate a subgroup of patients in whom there is more rapid progression of cognitive impairment (Rubin and Drevets, 1987; Mayeux et al, 1987).

Among community-dwelling elderly persons, the prevalence of generalized persecutory ideation is reportedly as high as 4% (Christenson and Blazer, 1984).

Psychotic patients can present with various symptoms. Rubin and associates (1988) evaluated the nature of psychotic symptoms in 110 patients who met the criteria for primary degenerative dementia (Alzheimer's disease) and who were free of other potentially complicating medical, neurologic, and psychiatric disorders. Of 12 patients who subsequently died, all met autopsy criteria for Alzheimer's disease, suggesting that the authors were accurate in their antemortem diagnoses. Using this relatively homogeneous population, they characterized psychotic symptoms associated with dementia into three groups: paranoid delusions, misidentification syndromes, and hallucinations.

Paranoid Delusions

Paranoid delusions occurred in 31% of the subjects of Rubin and colleagues (1988) and could be separated into "stealing" and "suspiciousness" groups. The subjects with stealing delusions (26% of patients) were convinced that possessions were being taken away. This type of delusion manifested as a feeling either that someone was entering the home or that a certain person stole a specific item. Sometimes these fears led patients to hide things or even barricade themselves in their houses fearing robbery; occasionally violent accusations occurred. Marked suspiciousness unrelated to stealing was evident in at least 9% of the subjects; most commonly, they believed that people were plotting against them.

Christenson and Blazer (1984), attempting to identify the prevalence of paranoia and risk factors for its development, performed a survey of 997 community-dwelling elderly persons and found that the prevalence of generalized persecutory ideation was 4%. Their study canvassed a stratified, random, one-in-ten sample of the residents of an entire county, who were 65 years or older. They asked the individuals if they were willing to be interviewed, and an 85% positive response rate yielded 997 responders. Interviewers were sent to the subjects' homes to complete questionnaires. Subjects living in any type of institution were not included in the sample.

The questionnaire focused on individual assessment in five separate areas of functioning: social resources, economic resources, sensory and cognitive abilities, mental health, and activities of daily living. The group with persecutory ideation was significantly less likely to be married, but was not more likely to be living alone than were others.

Significant impairment in several areas of functioning appeared to be important factors for subjects with persecutory ideation. Almost 54% of those with persecutory ideation were rated as having their social resources impaired, compared with 13% of those without persecutory ideation. Economic resources were rated as being impaired in 73% of the symptomatic subjects, whereas only 38% of the nonsymptomatic subjects were economically impaired.

Another major point of their findings was that sensory and cognitive impairment appeared to be significant risk factors for developing persecutory ideation. Nearly 78% of subjects with persecutory ideation had impaired vision compared with 51% without such ideation; hearing was impaired in 58% of the symptomatic subjects compared with 37% of nonsymptomatic subjects. In addition, 58% of subjects with persecutory ideation had some degree of cognitive impairment, while only 20% of nonparanoid subjects had cognitive impairment.

These studies demonstrated that paranoid ideation is a significant problem, even in those living within a community setting. Identification of sensory and cognitive impairment as risk factors in developing paranoid ideation has important clinical implications; reduction of these impairments may result in a decreased likelihood of impaired individuals developing persecutory ideation. When one is treating symptomatic individuals, correction of any sensory or cognitive impairment should be part of the treatment plan whenever possible. Also, Christenson and Blazer (1984) found that many individuals in later life who exhibit persecutory ideation were reluctant to seek psychiatric services or perceived significant barriers to the receipt of such services.

Misidentification Syndromes
Misidentification syndromes occurred in 23% of the patients of Rubin and associates (1988) and they subdivided them into three types: confusion concerning the presence or identity of people in the house, confusion concerning the recognition of self, and confusion concerning the television.

The belief that imagined people, either relatives or strangers, were in the house occurred in at least 8% of subjects. On occasion, a subject would set the table for these imagined people or become afraid and agitated. Another 4% did not recognize a close relative and did not believe their spouses or children were who they claimed to be. Eight subjects (7%) were unable to recognize their faces in a mirror and would attempt to converse with their mirror reflection and might try to open the door to which the mirror was attached to invite the person in. As many as 8% of subjects were unable to recognize that people on television were not real. One subject did not want the people on television watching her undress and left the room to change. Another was frightened by television violence and felt that "they" were shooting at him; while another, watching a ballgame, was convinced the players were in the room with her.

Hallucinations
Hallucinations occurred frequently in these subjects (Rubin et al, 1988) and were often fragmented and fleeting. A total of 25% of the subjects experienced hallucinations; 10% had auditory; 15%, visual; and 2%, olfactory experiences which involved the smell of either onions or burning rubber. They excluded subjects from this category who saw imaginary people in the house and classified that as a misidentification syndrome.

Auditory experiences varied from subjects having full conversations with voices lasting for hours to subjects hearing "noises" that could not be more fully described. One subject described command hallucinations that instructed her to put her clothes on backward. Visual hallucinations usually involved seeing people or animals; some were frightening to the patient. Several subjects described faces in trees and one was convinced that she saw flowers exploding and injuring her sister.

Casey and Wandzilak (1988) described visual hallucinations (of dust particles) in two elderly patients (aged 80 and 85) which were associated with senile macular degeneration and loss of vision. In contrast to the Charles Bonnet syndrome (described later), these patients developed delusional explanations for their hallucinations. These cases illustrate the possible role of impaired vision attributable to macular degeneration in the development of psychopathology in the elderly. Only one of their patients suffered from cognitive decline and both were resistant to trials of antipsychotic medication, although only low doses were used. Neither patient had insight into the psychosis or motivation for psychiatric treatment.

Overall, in the study of Rubin and associates (1988), 55% of demented subjects had psychotic symptoms; 62% had symptoms in only one of the categories just described while 27% had symptoms in two.

Folie à Deux
Folie à deux has been reported in both nondemented and demented elderly people (Brooks, 1987; Layman and Cohen, 1957; McNeil et al, 1972; Fishbain, 1987). Fishbain (1987) reported the cases of two elderly dementing sisters (aged 78 and 76) who lived alone and shared the same delusion—that one of the sisters had a 3 1/2-year-old son who was a musical genius currently living in Florida who played the organ with F. Lee Bailey. In addition, they were both quite suspicious and paranoid.

Both sisters were treated with neuroleptics and, at one-year follow-up, were functioning well in nursing home facilities and were not paranoid but still maintained the same delusion about the son. Apparently, since the symptom was not distressing to either patient or to the caregivers, more aggressive attempts at treatment were not considered.

Psychotic Symptoms Related to Severity of Cognitive Decline

Teri and colleagues (1988) studied 127 well-characterized patients with a primary diagnosis of dementia of the Alzheimer's type (mean age, 77 years) by means of a standardized dementia rating scale and also a checklist of behavioral problems. They found that the overall number of behavioral problems significantly increased with worsening cognitive impairment and that the types of problems reported varied with cognitive severity. For example, four or more behavioral problems were reported for 55% of the severely impaired patients (MMSE score, ≤10), for 28% of the moderately impaired patients (MMSE score, between 10 and 24), and for only 8% of the mildly impaired group (MMSE score, >24). Restlessness affected approximately one-half of all patients, regardless of the level of cognitive impairment. Behavioral problems were not significantly associated with patient's age, gender, duration, or age at onset of dementia. They believed that problems found associated with level of cognitive impairment such as wandering, agitation, incontinence, and poor personal hygiene are characteristic of the disease and therefore predictable. Thus families, patients, and clinicians should probably be provided knowledge about what to expect and assisted accordingly. Problems found not associated with level of impairment such as hallucinations, irrational suspicions, falls, and restlessness are likely to be idiosyncratic and should be dealt with on an individual basis.

Inappropriate Sexual Behaviors

These may include compulsive public masturbation, genital exposure, attempts to fondle the sexual organs of members of both sexes, and attempts at coitus in inappropriate circumstances. These problems are rare in dementing patients.

These behaviors, if they take place in a nursing home or chronic-care hospital, can be extremely disruptive and cause great distress to residents, relatives, and staff. Cooper (1987) hypothesized that such behaviors in dementing patients reflect a weakening of the cerebrocortical inhibitory mechanisms that underlie self-control. Libido may also have been altered with a resultant "release" of antisocial sexual behavior. Except in a very few instances, these behaviors are not dangerous physically, but, nevertheless, are undesirable, and in a public setting may be intolerable.

There is a dearth of information on the management of sexual behaviors in dementing patients and neuroleptics and benzodiazepines have been employed (Winograd and Jarvik, 1986), as have physical restraints and incarceration in an isolated room.

Noting previous success with medroxyprogesterone acetate (MPA) in suppression of libido and unacceptable sexual behaviors in younger patients with personality disorders, in chronic schizophrenics who manifest sexual delusions and compulsive masturbation, in mental retardees, and in a small number of sexually disinhibited, cognitively intact elderly men (Hoffet, 1968; Davies, 1974), Cooper (1987) reported that four demented male patients who manifested disruptive sexual behavior, including public masturbation and attempts to molest female patients, who could not be managed by other means received a therapeutic trial of MPA. Within two weeks after the start of MPA therapy, grossly inappropriate sexual behaviors stopped in all four demented patients (Cooper, 1987). Changes in behavior were accompanied by reductions in serum testosterone and leutinizing hormone (LH). In this report, MPA was used for one year without side effects and only one patient returned to the disturbing behavior when the drug was discontinued. None of the four men had been physically assaultive, but their behavior was a nuisance. Each man had received major and minor tranquilizers in an unsuccessful attempt to control their sexual behaviors. Because of cognitive impairment, none of the study patients were able to give informed consent; written consent was obtained from next of kin following a detailed discussion of the likely beneficial and side effects of the drug. MPA was injected at a dose of 300 mg/week for the entire year; higher doses could have been used but were not necessary because of the success of this dosage in rapidly decreasing the sexual behaviors which were in complete abeyance after 10 to 14 days. No side effects were detected on physical examination, and laboratory values remained within normal limits.

MPA, originally developed as an oral contraceptive, is the best known and most available antilibidinal progestogen in the United States. Its main hormonal effect is to block testosterone synthesis in the testes; it does, however, also reduce circulating levels of gonadotrophins presumably by a direct action at the hypothalamic-pituitary level (Goodman and Gilman, 1980). Unwanted effects of MPA include increased sleepiness; mild diabetes; increased appetite and weight gain; fatigue; loss of body hair; hot and cold flashes; mild depression; and diminution of the frequency, quality, and volume of ejaculation. In practice, however, serious consequences have not been observed after as much as three years of continuous use in a dose range of 75 to 600 mg/week administered intramuscularly.

In discussing possible ethical concerns, Cooper (1987) noted that many civil libertarians oppose the use of MPA on any grounds and he recommended that fully informed written consent from a near relative or, failing that, from the court be obtained. In fact, MPA, which has specific antilibidinal effects, is inherently safer than neuroleptics, which are more often used and likely to stir less controversy (Halleck, 1981; Rosenfield, 1983).

Visual Hallucinations in Sane Elderly Patients (Charles Bonnet Syndrome)

Occasionally elderly patients who have decreased visual acuity complain of formed visual hallucinations despite the presence of normal mental function. These patients are generally not dementing and have no other stigma of mental illness. Even though this syndrome was described over 200 years ago (Bonnet, 1769), it is not well recognized in clinical practice and patients are often misdiagnosed (Rosenbaum et al, 1987).

Rosenbaum and colleagues (1987) recently described the cases of two patients with this syndrome. The first was an 82-year-old woman with no previous psychiatric disease who presented with a 14-month history of formed visual hallucinations in all visual fields of vivid figures. She usually saw people, for example, "four women dressed alike in the living room with books in hand." The images typically occurred at night and they disappeared when she closed her eyes or when it was totally dark. She was aware that the hallucinations were not real and, therefore, she was not frightened, but merely curious about their persistence. Although she could clearly see the characters'

214

lips moving, she never heard them speak. Occasionally, particularly at the onset, she would approach the figures and attempt to touch them, but the images would disappear and she would find herself waving her hand through the air. Her medical and psychiatric history was unremarkable except for bilateral cataracts, for which she had been followed for several years by an ophthalmologist. Findings on CT scan, EEG, and neurologic exam were normal (except eyes) and she was taking no medication and never abused alcohol. Visual acuity was 20/70 in the right eye and 20/50 in the left eye. Following extraction of the right cataract, visual acuity improved to 20/20 and the visual hallucinations disappeared.

The second case was a 66-year-old man who also had no psychiatric history who presented with the complaint of visual hallucinations which began approximately six months earlier, coinciding with the gradual onset of loss of visual acuity. As his sight worsened, he experienced the hallucinations more frequently, as often as three to four times each week. With further deterioration of vision, however, the hallucinations disappeared. The hallucinations were well-formed, detailed images of people engaging in ordinary activities such as walking around the room or sitting on the sofa. Generally, he observed total strangers, although he saw his sister on one occasion and his wife another time. The figures appeared in old-fashioned costumes, the colors of which were very mute and washed-out. He saw people speaking without hearing their voices, and once watched one of the figures slam a door but heard no sound. The hallucinations were devoid of emotional content and the imagined people neither interacted with the patient nor aroused fear in him. Although he initially believed them to be real, he soon realized that they were not and accepted them as hallucinations. His medical history was remarkable for a four-year history of a sporadic form of spinocerebellar degeneration manifested by the gradual onset of an unsteady gait and pigmentary macular degeneration in both eyes. Neurologic examination revealed visual acuity to be 20/400 in the right eye and 20/800 in the left eye with normal visual fields. CT scan showed very mild cerebellar atrophy and an EEG was normal. There was no evidence of dementia or other psychiatric illness.

One patient that we observed was an elderly woman who saw, but never heard, a number of leprechauns. With her Irish brogue, she described them as small, about a foot tall, and "quite smelly little fellers." She never heard them talk but they did interact with her. During an interview she was able to reach out and touch one of them. She said they did not really bother her, but that she would just as soon get rid of them because they were so dirty and smelly. Considering a temporal lobe seizure focus, despite a normal EEG, she was started on a trial of carbamazepine but did not improve. Low-dose neuroleptics did not improve her symptoms. Because she had progressive macular degeneration, vision improvement was not an option. She was able to lead a fairly normal life even though the hallucinations persisted.

Although the association between formed visual hallucinations and decreased visual acuity in an elderly individual with preserved insight was initially described in 1769 by Charles Bonnet, this syndrome has received little attention in the English literature. As a consequence of this, hallucinating elderly patients with this syndrome are often dismissed as being demented or psychotic, and potentially treatable conditions are ignored. Both cases of Rosenbaum and colleagues (1987) illustrated the salient features of this syndrome, which always occurs in elderly persons in the setting of diminished visual acuity. The hallucinations, usually people, animals, or other forms, are well organized, clearly defined, and often animated. However, despite the vividness of the scenes, patients are rarely frightened and rapidly recognize the unreality of the illusions. Progressive visual failure as a result of any ocular disease may be implicated (White, 1980) and, in fact, the phenomenon has been described in blind patients (Kolmel, 1985; McNamara et al, 1982).

A number of hypotheses have been generated in an attempt to explain this disorder. With removal of normal visual impulses, a "release" mechanism has been proposed where, in the face of sensory deprivation, indigenous cerebral activity produces hallucinations. Clearly, this disorder would be much more common if only a loss of sensory input were the mechanism. An irritative focus has been theorized and there is one report of an anticonvulsant alleviating hallucinations in a patient with the Charles Bonnet syndrome (Lance, 1976). A third view suggests a psychologic cause.

Despite etiologic confusion, we know that some patients can be helped with particular treatments. Probably the most effective (as in the first patient of Rosenbaum and colleagues) is correction of decreased visual acuity. This is clearly applicable when cataracts are the cause of the syndrome, but is not feasible for the majority of patients.

Rosenbaum and associates (1987) recommended that the clinician communicate understanding and reassurance to the patient. Sometimes, in patients with progressive blindness, the physician can only point out that the hallucinations will probably end with end-stage blindness. There are no reports of neuroleptics helping these patients and overall treatment strategy will involve medication trials aimed at the hallucinations, support of the patient, and treatment of any complicating or developing psychiatric difficulty, such as depression. Predictable treatment approaches are not yet available.

DRUG TREATMENT OF PSYCHOSIS, RAGE, AND VIOLENCE

Neuroleptics

In the early 1950s, chlorpromazine (Thorazine) was introduced into the United States for clinical use. This was a major breakthrough because prior to its introduction, psychotic symptoms were managed by sedation only. The neuro-leptics were found to be capable of controlling many of the clinical signs and symptoms of psychosis such as aggressive and disordered behavior, hallucina-tions, delusions, paranoia, and disordered thinking.

All of the currently available neuroleptics have the ability to block dopa-mine and considerable clinical and laboratory evidence suggests that their clinical potency parallels their dopamine blocking power (Snyder et al, 1974; Bernstein, 1978). Antipsychotic effects are independent of their sedative potential.

Choosing a Neuroleptic

Neuroleptic agents have a wide range of potencies (Table 6–3) and can be roughly separated into three groups based on antipsychotic potency. As can be seen from Table 6–3, 2 mg of haloperidol (Haldol) is roughly equivalent to 100 mg of chlorpromazine. As with antidepressants, the various neuroleptics are generally considered to be equally effective and choice of medication should be based on predicted type of side effects.

Low-potency agents, such as chlorpromazine and thioridazine (Mellaril), produce significant sedation, orthostatic hypotension, and anticholinergic ef-fects (Jenike, 1985). On the other hand, high-potency drugs such as haloperidol and fluphenazine hydrochloride (Prolixin) are much more likely to cause extrapyramidal side effects such as dystonia, akathisia, and parkinsonism (Figure 6–1). Haloperidol produces negligible cardiovascular side effects even when used intravenously (Sos and Cassem, 1980).

Neuroleptics are also potent alpha-adrenergic blocking agents and produce peripheral vasodilatation and hypotension. Chlorpromazine and thioridazine (low-potency agents) are most likely to cause hypotension and this effect is so profound that chlorpromazine is even used to treat hypertensive crises induced by MAOI-tyramine interactions (see chapter 4). Haloperidol has the least alpha-adrenergic blocking ability of the currently available antipsychotic drugs and is the preferred agent in the very elderly or frail patient. Since falls are devastating in the very elderly, high-potency agents such as haloperidol, thiothixene (Navane), and fluphenazine (Prolixin) are safer because they are less likely to induce hypotensive episodes (Table 6–1).

Unfortunately, when administering the high-potency agents, which pro-duce fewer cardiovascular effects, the physician is more likely to induce extrapyramidal side effects. These can occasionally be very disabling espe-cially in patients with extrapyramidal illness such as Parkinson's disease. In patients with preexisting extrapyramidal illnesses, very low doses of chlor-promazine or thioridazine (ie, 10 mg twice daily initially) may produce the desired effect without further compromising motor status.

If the high-potency agents are used cautiously in low dosage (ie, haloperi-dol, 0.5 mg, or thiothixene, 1.0 mg once or twice daily initially), the possibility

Table 6–3
Equivalent Doses of Neuroleptics

| Generic Name | Trade Name | Side Effects | | | Approximate Equivalent Dose (mg) |
		Sedative	Anticholinergic	Extrapyramidal	
Low potency					
Chlorpromazine	Thorazine	High	High	Low	100
Thioridazine	Mellaril	High	High	Low	95
Intermediate potency					
Perphenazine	Trilafon	Moderate	Moderate	Moderate	10
Loxapine succinate	Loxitane	Moderate	Moderate	Moderate	15
Molindone HCl	Moban	Moderate	Moderate	Moderate	10
High potency					
Haloperidol	Haldol	Low	Low	High	2
Thiothixene	Navane	Low	Low	High	5
Fluphenazine HCl	Prolixin	Low	Low	High	2
Trifluoperazine HCl	Stelazine	Moderate	Low	Moderate	5

Reproduced with permission from Jenike MA: *Handbook of Geriatric Psychopharmacology.* Littleton, Mass, PSG Publishing, 1985.

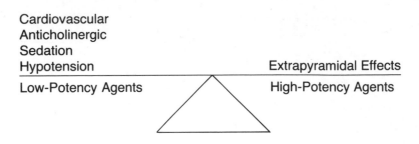

Cardiovascular
Anticholinergic
Sedation
Hypotension   Extrapyramidal Effects

Low-Potency Agents   High-Potency Agents

Figure 6–1 Balancing neuroleptic side effects. Reproduced with permission from Jenike MA: *Handbook of Geriatric Psychopharmacology*. Littleton, Mass, PSG Publishing, 1985, p 19.

of unwanted extrapyramidal effects can be minimized. Extrapyramidal reactions are uncommon at very low dosages but will regularly occur if doses must be increased to control symptoms. Extrapyramidal reactions, even if they do occur, are less likely than excessive drowsiness, cardiac effects, or severe hypotension to produce serious clinical problems in a geriatric patient.

At the time of preparation of this book, a novel antipsychotic, clozapine, is awaiting final approval from the Food and Drug Administration before coming on the market. A recent multicenter, random assignment, double-blind comparison trial of clozapine and chlorpromazine in 151 hospitalized schizophrenic patients who all had either tardive dyskinesia or hard-to-treat extrapyramidal reactions to other antipsychotic drugs showed that, even though the overall rate of adverse reactions did not vary significantly between clozapine and chlorpromazine, the types of reactions were different (Claghorn et al, 1987). Unexpectedly, clozapine appeared to have a more rapid onset of antipsychotic activity and as early as week 2, statistically significant differences favored use of clozapine to decrease psychopathologic behavior and these differences maintained over the eight weeks of this study. Clozapine was thus an effective antipsychotic agent without much tendency to provoke extrapyramidal reactions and furthermore, there are hopes that it may not cause tardive dyskinesia but may, instead, be palliative for that condition. In addition, clozapine has little tendency to elevate plasma prolactin levels, which is characteristic of other neuroleptic agents. It appears that clozapine may be a useful antipsychotic agent in patients who have been refractory to other drugs. One troublesome difficulty (Gelenberg, 1988) is the finding that clozapine is probably at least an order of magnitude more likely than other antipsychotic drugs to produce agranulocytosis (in as many as 2% of treated patients). It appears likely that when the Food and Drug Administration approves clozapine (Clozaril), it will require physicians to obtain weekly white blood cell counts on each patient before continuing that patient on the drug. The length of this intensive monitoring period is yet to be determined.

Neuroleptic Side Effects

Neuroleptics have a number of side effects which are reviewed briefly. In the elderly sedation, orthostatic hypotension, anticholinergic signs and symptoms, and extrapyramidal effects commonly develop. Some of the age-related metabolic changes were reviewed in chapter 2.

Anticholinergic side effects   Anticholinergic side effects, toxicity, diagnosis, and treatment are reviewed in chapter 9. The peripheral anticholinergic effects are generally less pronounced than those induced by the tricyclic antidepressants. In in vitro studies the least anticholinergic tricyclic, desipramine, is about equipotent to the most anticholinergic neuroleptic, thioridazine (see Table 9–5).

Physicians now know that the cholinergic system is intimately involved in memory (Drachman and Leavitt, 1974) and that in Alzheimer's disease there is a loss of cholinergic neurons and decrements in the enzyme choline acetyltransferase which is responsible for the production of central acetylcholine (Davies, 1979). The anticholinergic side effects of neuroleptic drugs in the presence of age-related decreases in cholinergic functioning can lead to serious problems in the elderly patient. When anticholinergic agents are given to treat neuroleptic-induced extrapyramidal problems, the likelihood of side effects increases. It is important that the clinician be aware of all medications that his or her elderly patient is taking, as anticholinergic effects are additive (see chapter 9).

Ophthalmologic side effects   The most serious eye problem related to neuroleptic usage is the irreversible degenerative pigmentary retinopathy caused by thioridazine in doses in excess of 800 mg/day (Baldessarini, 1977). In addition, reversible deposits of drug substances and pigment in the lens and cornea have been associated with long-term neuroleptic usage.

Photosensitivity   Patients taking neuroleptics are sometimes unusually sensitive to the sun. Maculopapular rashes occur on occasion and sometimes a blue-gray discoloration of the skin results, usually with prolonged high doses of chlorpromazine (Baldessarini, 1977). Photosensitivity is managed by decreased solar exposure and by sun screens.

Temperature regulation dysfunction   Neuroleptics may upset hypothalamic thermoregulatory mechanisms and make the elderly patient more vulnerable to either excessive heat or cold. This side effect is particularly dangerous in the south in the summer and in the north in the winter—where many elderly patients are surviving on low incomes and have to choose between food and heat or air conditioning.

Hematologic side effects   Hematologic complications of neuroleptic use are very rare. Frank agranulocytosis occurs infrequently (incidence of less than 0.01%) and has a peak incidence within the first two months of treatment (Baldessarini, 1977). Agranulocytosis is most common in elderly women and is almost always associated with the use of low-potency agents. It is virtually unknown with the use of haloperidol (Baldessarini, 1977). Agranulocytosis is a life-threatening medical emergency that can rarely be predicted from occasional white blood cell counts and must be suspected whenever fever, sore throat, or malaise occur early in the course of neuroleptic treatment. When agranulocytosis is diagnosed, the drug must be immediately discontinued and the patient hospitalized for reverse isolation. If a life-threatening infection does not supervene, agranulocytosis is usually reversible within a few weeks (Gelenberg, 1978).

Jaundice   Neuroleptic-induced jaundice is almost always an allergic type, is usually transient, and is usually caused by phenothiazines such as chlorpromazine. As modern technology has allowed for greater drug purity, this complication is exceedingly rare. Older patients with a history of obstructive jaundice or liver disease should probably not be treated with phenothiazines (Spira et al, 1984).

Weight gain   Weight gain is sometimes seen in association with neuroleptic use. This is particularly troublesome to some patients, particularly those who are already overweight. It is reported that molindone hydrochloride (Lidone, Moban) is less likely than other neuroleptics to induce an increase in body weight (Gelenberg, 1978).

Cardiovascular effects   Cardiac effects are rarely a problem with high-potency antipsychotic agents. Orthostatic hypotension can be induced by the less potent phenothiazines. Thioridazine is known to have the strongest effects of any of the antipsychotic drugs on cardiac conduction and repolarization (Gelenberg, 1978). Neuroleptic drugs, particularly thioridazine, can produce nonspecific changes of the T-wave on the ECG which are of no clinical significance. Because of its effect on cardiac conduction, thioridazine should probably not be used in patients with conduction defects or other cardiac disease, or in conjunction with drugs with similar cardiac actions such as the tricyclic antidepressants, quinidine, or procainamide (Gelenberg, 1978).

Seizures   Neuroleptics, especially low-potency agents, may increase the incidence of seizures in epileptic patients (Baldessarini, 1977) or in patients with preexisting CNS pathology (Spira et al, 1984). In the elderly, obtaining a careful history of seizures is mandatory and dosage increases in susceptible patients should be very slow. High-potency agents such as haloperidol may have less tendency to induce seizures (Baldessarini, 1977). Clinicians often find that these concerns are more theoretical than practical since it is very unusual for these agents to induce seizures, even in susceptible patients.

Sedation   Drowsiness is often seen early in therapy and is much more prominent with low-potency agents. Tolerance to sedation does appear to develop over a few weeks. Early in therapy, sedation can be advantageous for daytime calming or promoting sleep.

Syndrome of inappropriate secretion of antidiuretic hormone (SIADH)   Both high-potency and low-potency neuroleptics have been associated with SIADH (Matuk and Kalyanaraman, 1977; Rivera, 1975; Rao et al, 1975; Husband et al, 1981; Miller and Moses, 1976). Whenever patients taking neuroleptics show deterioration of their behavior, with irritability, personality changes, or progressive alteration of sensorium, SIADH must be considered in the differential diagnosis. This condition is not rare and can be easily diagnosed with simple tests of serum and urine osmolality.

Bartter (1973) outlined five criteria for the diagnosis of this syndrome: (a) hyponatremia and hypoosmolality of extracellular fluids, (b) persistence of sodium in the urine despite hyponatremia, (c) absence of signs of dehydration, (d) normal renal function, and (e) normal adrenal function. Simple water intoxication arising from a large intake of water may occur in psychotics (Raskind, 1974), but if antidiuretic hormone (ADH) secretion is appropriately suppressed, the urinary osmolality will be at the minimal possible value (Bartter, 1973).

Neuroleptic malignant syndrome Neuroleptic malignant syndrome (NMS) is an uncommon but life-threatening reaction to antipsychotic drugs that is characterized by hyperthermia, muscular rigidity, altered consciousness, and other disturbances of hypothalamic and neuromuscular function (Gelenberg, 1983; Caroff, 1980). The syndrome typically develops over a 24 to 72-hour period and can occur from hours to months after initial drug exposure (Gelenberg, 1982). A mortality rate of 14.3% has been reported (Cohen et al, 1985). An elevated level of creatine phosphokinase is a helpful diagnostic clue in patients who have not recently received intramuscular injections.

Guze and Baxter (1985) estimated that NMS occurs in 0.5% to 1.0% of patients exposed to neuroleptics, and retrospective surveys placed the annual rate between 0.4% and 1.4% (Pope et al, 1986; Shalev and Munitz, 1986). Gelenberg and colleagues (1988), in a survey of 1,470 patients treated with neuroleptic agents during a one-year period at a private psychiatric hospital, found only one patient in whom this syndrome developed—an annual frequency of 0.07%. They also reported six suspected cases of NMS that were ultimately diagnosed as other conditions. One was a catatonic reaction in a patient with bipolar illness. Two other patients had severe extrapyramidal reactions to neuroleptic drugs but no other evidence of NMS. Three patients had extrapyramidal reactions plus fever, which was attributed to coincident infections.

There is a hint that concomitant therapy with lithium and a neuroleptic might increase the patient's chances of developing NMS, but this is far from being confirmed (Keck et al, 1987).

Gelenberg's group (1988) noted that, despite the low prevalence of NMS, clinicians must remain aware of this serious condition, with its potentially lethal complications, and that attention is best focused on the differential diagnosis of fever, extrapyramidal reactions, and altered consciousness in patients taking antipsychotic medications. Their data would indicate that the majority of the neuroleptic-taking patients in whom fever develops do not, in fact, have NMS but some other treatable disorder.

Treatment of NMS itself generally involves medications or the use of

ECT. Fogel and Goldberg (1985) found it useful to think of the syndrome as a spectrum of extrapyramidal, cortical, and autonomic dysfunction related to neuroleptic drug therapy. They suggested titrating treatment to severity of the disorder; that is, managing milder manifestations, such as muscle rigidity and confusion without elevation of creatine phosphokinase levels or temperature, with amantadine (Symmetrel) and benzodiazepines. Dantrolene, bromocriptine, or the combination might be considered when confusion and rigidity are accompanied by elevated creatine phosphokinase, myoglobinuria, or markedly abnormal vital signs. Coons and associates (1982) reported effective treatment of one patient with dantrolene, 50 mg by mouth, and Goekoop and Carbaat (1982) reported another treated with dantrolene, 80 mg intravenously. Within two hours the patient's body temperature had dropped to 99.3° F from 102.4° F and the level of creatine phosphokinase decreased from 14,309 U/L to 4900 U/L. Muscle rigidity decreased over about four days.

More exotic treatments for NMS have been tried over the last few years. Sangal and Dimitrijevic (1985) used pancuronium (Pavulon) in a patient with severe muscle rigidity. They were reluctant to employ dantrolene because of a recent history of alcoholic liver disease, so they chose pancuronium for neuromuscular blockade. They intubated the patient and ventilated him mechanically during the treatment with diazepam administered for sedation. Blood pressure, heart rate, temperature, creatine phosphokinase level, and rigidity declined rapidly. After about a day, pancuronium was discontinued and rigidity did not recur.

Blue and colleagues (1986) reported the case of a patient with NMS who failed to improve with dantrolene but did respond well to the antihypertensive sodium nitroprusside (Nipride). Others reported successfully using ECT in patients with NMS (Lazarus, 1986). ECT is still controversial, however, as two of seven reported patients who received it for NMS had cardiac arrest associated with the ECT (Hughes, 1986; Lazarus, 1986).

Whether or not it is safe to rechallenge patients with neuroleptics after an episode of NMS is still unknown. If neuroleptics are absolutely required after an episode of NMS, agents structurally different from the offending drug should be used. We have seen a number of patients who recovered from NMS and in whom it did not develop on rechallenge with neuroleptics. On the other hand, Shalev and Munitz (1986) reported eight cases of patients with NMS who were later rechallenged with the same neuroleptic and six had recurrences. In the two who did not, the doses of the neuroleptics were raised very gradually. The authors found reports of six other patients who were rechallenged with other neuroleptics, but of the same potency as the drug that originally caused the NMS and in five the syndrome recurred and two of them died. Only two of 11 patients rechallenged with a low-potency neuroleptic, usually thioridazine (Mellaril), had recurrences, suggesting this drug as an alternative for the aftercare of patients who survive NMS (Gelenberg, 1986).

It may be that high-potency neuroleptics are more likely to produce NMS and also that higher doses are more dangerous (Cohen et al, 1985; Gelenberg,

1986). One may try to keep neuroleptic dosages as low as possible by concurrently administering a benzodiazepine (eg, lorazepam) when acutely excited patients require more sedation.

Extrapyramidal reactions and movement disorders A number of extrapyramidal reactions and movement disorders can occur with the use of neuroleptics; these are presumably due to the dopamine blocking power of these agents on the basal ganglia and the rest of the extrapyramidal motor system. For example, the frequently occurring drug-induced parkinsonian syndrome may reflect the ability of antipsychotic agents to block the action of dopamine as a synaptic neurotransmitter in the caudate nucleus, much as spontaneously occurring parkinsonism reflects the degeneration of the dopamine-mediated nigrostriatal pathway from midbrain to the caudate nucleus (Baldessarini, 1977). Clinicians must be aware of several discrete extrapyramidal syndromes that can be associated with the use of neuroleptic agents. These include acute dystonias, parkinsonism, akathisia, tardive dyskinesia, withdrawal dyskinesia, and catatonic reaction.

Dystonias The acute dystonias are exceedingly uncommon in the elderly (if they occur at all) but occur frequently in the young—particularly in males. These occur within the first few days of treatment and involve distressing tonic contractions of the muscles of the neck, mouth, and tongue. Opisthotonus and oculogyric crises also sometimes occur.

These reactions are frequently misdiagnosed as hysterical or as a psychotic symptom. Treatment is almost always rapidly effective and involves parenteral injection of an anticholinergic agent. Diphenhydramine hydrochloride (Benadryl), 25 mg administered intramuscularly or intravenously, or benztropine mesylate (Cogentin), 1 to 2 mg intravenously, will result in rapid relief.

Parkinsonism Drug-induced parkinsonism is commonly seen in the elderly and cannot be distinguished clinically from idiopathic Parkinson's disease. A history of neuroleptic intake must be obtained in order to make the diagnosis. The typical patient with drug-induced parkinsonism will exhibit slowed movements (bradykinesia) and muscular rigidity, stooped posture, shuffling gait, inexpressive mask-like face, tremor, and drooling (Figure 6–2).

This syndrome usually occurs from the first week to two months after neuroleptic treatment is begun. Tolerance probably develops to this symptom complex and the symptoms may fade over two to three months, allowing reduction and eventual discontinuation of antiparkinsonian agents. Besides anticholinergic agents, such as benztropine, diphenhydramine, and trihexyphenidyl hydrochloride (Artane), amantadine hydrochloride (Symmetrel) in doses of 100 to 300 mg daily is frequently effective in reversing parkinsonian side effects. Because of the dangers inherent in giving anticholinergic agents to the elderly (see chapter 9), amantadine is frequently used as the drug of first choice in treating such reactions in the elderly.

Akathisia Another neuroleptic-induced extrapyramidal side effect that is commonly seen in the elderly is akathisia. It involves motor restlessness, pacing, an inability to sit still, and a pressure to move about which is associated

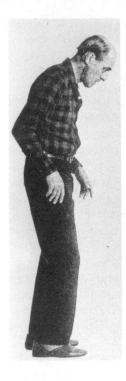

Figure 6–2 A patient with drug-induced parkinsonism, which is indistinguishable from the idiopathic form. A history of neuroleptic drug intake would be required to make the diagnosis.

with a subjective sensation of discomfort, often described as anxiety. Sleep is usually disturbed because the individual is unable to find a comfortable motionless position.

Sometimes this restlessness is misinterpreted as an increase in psychotic symptomatology and is inappropriately treated with an increase in neuroleptic dosage. It has been reported that the syndrome of neuroleptic-induced akathisia can even cause a worsening of the psychotic syndrome for which the neuroleptic treatment was initially being used (Van Putten et al, 1974; Van Putten, 1975).

One of the most effective treatments for akathisia has been lowering the dose of offending neuroleptic. Other treatments that have been reportedly successful include the administration of anticholinergic agents (Van Putten et al, 1974), benzodiazepines (Ekbom, 1965), and amantadine (DiMascio et al, 1976). These agents are, however, frequently ineffective.

Lipinski and colleagues (1984) performed an open trial of propranolol in 14 patients with neuroleptic-induced akathisia. Their decision to try propranolol for this disorder was based on an earlier report in which restless leg syndrome (an idiopathic disorder resembling akathisia) was reported to respond to treatment with propranolol (Ekbom, 1944; Strang, 1967). Lipinski and colleagues found that all 14 patients demonstrated substantial improvement of the akathisia; nine obtained complete relief. The maximum therapeutic result was often obtained within 24 hours after starting propranolol. Doses were quite low and ranged from 30 to 80 mg/day. It is noteworthy that patients experienced no improvement in symptoms of either parkinsonism or tardive dyskinesia. It seems very unlikely that improvement was due to a placebo effect, because 10 of the 14 patients previously received benztropine without result. On the basis of the results of this preliminary uncontrolled trial, it does appear that propranolol may be of considerable benefit in the treatment of neuroleptic-induced akathisia.

Catatonia   Rarely, elderly patients will become unresponsive and catatonic after very low doses of neuroleptic. This may respond rapidly to intravenous doses of diphenhydramine or benztropine. After resolution of the acute episode, anticholinergic agents or amantadine may be helpful in preventing recurrence.

Withdrawal dyskinesia   Another frequent extrapyramidal reaction is the induction of a withdrawal dyskinesia when neuroleptics, usually high doses, are tapered rapidly or discontinued. Abrupt withdrawal of large neuroleptic doses is very frequently complicated by acute choreoathetotic reactions, similar in appearance to tardive dyskinesia, but usually lasting for only a few days. Withdrawal dyskinesias require no treatment and probably represent a transient rebound increase in the activity of previously inhibited dopaminergic neurons in the basal ganglia (Baldessarini, 1977).

Meige's syndrome   Meige's syndrome, characterized by blepharospasm and involuntary movements of the lower face, neck, and jaw, has been reported with long-term use of neuroleptics (Ananth et al, 1988). Rarely, muscles of other areas are affected, but the typical feature is involvement of the orbicularis oculi muscles which produces, during the initial stages, an increased rate of blinking and, in later stages, uncontrollable eyelid spasms (Lees, 1985). This blepharospasm may last from several seconds to many minutes and can be triggered by an attempt to look upward or even by emotional stress (Figure 6–3).

The peak age of onset of the idiopathic form of the disorder is in the sixth decade of life and it is more common in females. It is likely that drug-induced forms of this disorder are frequently confused with tardive dyskinesia and the neurochemical pathophysiology may in fact be similar. It is also important to distinguish this disorder from an acute dystonia. This differential can be assisted by giving the patient anticholinergic medication (eg, intramuscular diphenhydramine or benztropine) which should rapidly improve an acute dystonia but not Meige's syndrome. Prompt recognition of the neuroleptic-induced form of Meige's syndrome is important as it can eventually obstruct vision, especially under stressful conditions such as driving, with dangerous consequences (Ananth et al, 1988). If it is recognized early, withdrawal of the offending neuroleptic may lead to recovery.

Tardive dyskinesia   Tardive dyskinesia is manifested by a wide variety of movements, including lip smacking, sucking, jaw movements, flycatcher's tongue, writhing tongue movements, chorea, athetosis, dystonia, tics, and

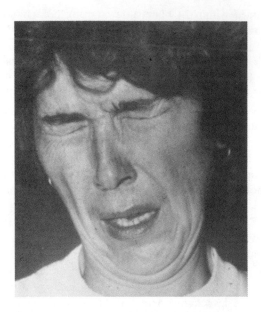

Figure 6–3 A patient with Meige's syndrome. Reproduced with permission from Lees AJ: *Tics and Related Disorders*. New York, Churchill Livingstone, 1985.

facial grimacing (Jenike, 1983). In severe cases, speech, eating, walking, and even breathing can be seriously impaired. The disorder usually has a gradual onset after long-term, high-dose administration of an antipsychotic drug, but on rare occasions it can occur in patients who have had short-term or low-dose administration (Baldessarini, 1977). It is becoming increasingly clear that elderly patients are at very high risk of developing tardive dyskinesia after neuroleptic use.

Many risk factors for tardive dyskinesia that have been studied include cumulative drug exposure, maximum neuroleptic dose, length of drug exposure, age, sex, drug type, polypharmacy, presence of organic mental disorder, prior use of anticholinergic antiparkinsonian drugs, presence or absence of drug-free intervals, and diagnosis of the patient.

Kane and Smith (1982) reviewed 56 studies comprising almost 35,000 patients who were treated with neuroleptics; they found a mean prevalence of tardive dyskinesia uncorrected for spontaneous dyskinesias of 20%. They also reviewed 19 studies involving 11,000 patients who were never treated with neuroleptics and found a 5% incidence of spontaneous dyskinesias. These figures suggest that abnormal involuntary movements may have developed in some treated persons for reasons other than neuroleptic exposure. A best estimate of true drug-induced tardive dyskinesia is about 15% (20% prevalence in neuroleptic-treated patients minus 5% incidence of spontaneous dyskinesias). Exposure to neuroleptics almost certainly plays a highly significant role in the production of abnormal involuntary movements. Of all the risk factors previously mentioned, only age and female sex have a relatively consistent effect in increasing the prevalence of tardive dyskinesia.

Smith and Baldessarini (1980) also found that advancing age correlated not only with increased prevalence but also with the severity of tardive dyskinesia. In addition, they observed diminishing rates of spontaneous remission of tardive dyskinesia after neuroleptics were discontinued in elderly patients. The correlation between age and the degree of remission after discontinuance of neuroleptics was highly significant. After cessation of neuroleptic therapy, the rate of improvement was 83% for patients younger than 60 but only 36% for those 60 years or older. In this study, the prevalence and severity of tardive dyskinesia increased only up to the age of 70; after that, there was no further increase with advancing age.

Mukherjee and co-workers (1982) examined 153 psychotic outpatients, receiving maintenance doses of neuroleptics, for tardive dyskinesia. Age, but not sex, was found to be significantly correlated with prevalence and severity of the disorder.

Perenyi and Arato (1980) studied 200 hospitalized schizophrenic patients, most of whom had received neuroleptic treatment for at least two years, and reported that the frequency and severity of tardive dyskinesia increased with age, and the more advanced the age was when the patient started taking neuroleptics, the more likely it was that tardive dyskinesia would develop. In patients less than 30 years old, when therapy with neuroleptics was begun, the incidence of tardive dyskinesia was approximately 18%, in those between 31 and 40 years old it was 22%, in those between 41 and 50 years old it was 28%, and in those older than 50 it was 50%.

Many elderly patients have been taking neuroleptics for longer periods of time than have their younger counterparts and one might consider whether increased prevalence and severity of tardive dyskinesia among older patients could be explained by their longer exposure to neuroleptics. Johnson and colleagues (1982) also considered whether the age differences in the prevalence of tardive dyskinesia are artifacts of differential exposure to neuroleptics. They studied 66 patients and, like other authors, reported that the incidence of tardive dyskinesia increased with age. In addition, the severity of tardive dyskinesia also increased with age. In order to distinguish the factor of cumulative dose from age, they separated their patients into four groups (33 years old or less, 34 to 45 years old, 46 to 56 years, over 57 years). They found that the mean length of neuroleptic regimens for the four groups was 2.9, 7.6, 8.3, and 8.4 years, respectively. Apart from the patients 33 years or younger, the duration of treatment with neuroleptic drugs did not seem to explain the differences in severity that were found. Unfortunately, Johnson and colleagues presented no data on cumulative neuroleptic doses, but because elderly patients are generally treated with lower doses of neuroleptics than their younger counterparts, it seems unlikely that the elderly patients would have received greater cumulative doses. These findings strongly suggested that increased prevalence and severity of tardive dyskinesia in older patients cannot be easily explained by longer exposure to neuroleptics.

There is overwhelming evidence that the aging brain is more susceptible to tardive dyskinesia. Neurotransmitter enzyme synthesis in the basal ganglia decreases with age (Granacher, 1981 ; McGreer et al, 1977). Some cell loss of dopaminergic tracts has been found in older patients, but most of the altered enzyme activity seems to be due to decreased function of remaining cells rather than to loss of neurons (McGreer et al, 1977).

Tardive dyskinesia frequently persists after discontinuation of neuroleptic drugs (Uhrbrand and Faurbye, 1960; Rodova and Nahunek, 1964; Hunter et al, 1964; Degwitz et al, 1967; Crane, 1968 and 1972) and this observation led investigators to search for permanent structural alteration in the brains of patients with tardive dyskinesia (Klawans et al, 1980).

Neuropathologic studies following acute or chronic administration of antipsychotic drugs in laboratory animals have not demonstrated specific or localized neuropathologic changes in the brain (Roizin et al, 1959; Julou et al, 1968). There is one report of reduced neuronal cell count in the basal ganglia of rats chronically receiving phenothiazines (Pakkenberg et al, 1972), but this is of uncertain importance because gliosis or degenerative changes were not observed. Postmortem neuropathologic changes in patients who received chronic phenothiazine treatment and did not have extrapyramidal movement disorders have usually consisted of scattered areas of neuronal degeneration and gliosis without specific localization (Roizin et al, 1959). Findings at autopsy of individual patients with drug-induced parkinsonism or tardive dyskinesia have been reported to show changes in the globus pallidus and putamen (Poursines et al, 1959), in the caudate nucleus and substantia nigra, and in the inferior olive (Gross and Kaltenbach, 1968). Other investigators, however, reported no significant neuropathologic abnormality in patients with tardive dyskinesia (Hunter et al, 1968).

One study (Christensen et al, 1970) reported the presence of neuronal degeneration and gliosis of the substantia nigra in 27 of 28 brains from patients with chronic oral dyskinesias; 21 of the cases were attributed to antipsychotic drugs. Only 7 of 28 matched control brains showed similar changes. Although these changes may represent a toxic effect of the drug, their occurrence in some elderly persons who did not have tardive dyskinesia raises the possibility that they may be events of aging, not directly related to the development of tardive dyskinesia.

The fact that no consistent anatomic alterations are associated with tardive dyskinesia has led investigators recently to give more attention to the neuro-chemistry and pharmacology of the disorder. The pathophysiology of tardive dyskinesia is therefore still unclear, and there is no sure explanation why elderly patients are vulnerable to this disorder.

The best way to prevent tardive dyskinesia is to avoid the use of neuroleptics. Obviously, these drugs are sometimes required, but they should not be used when indications are unclear or when less potentially toxic drugs may be as efficacious. As noted in chapter 1, Burke and associates (1982) reported the cases of 42 patients with tardive dyskinesia who were seen in movement disorder clinics in London, New York, and Houston and found that 19 had been inappropriately treated with neuroleptics. Of these, 6 patients have been treated for anxiety; 6, for depression; 4, for behavioral disturbances associated with mental retardation; and 3, for an acute psychotic episode precipitated by emotional stress. The therapeutic difficulties, the prolonged and possibly permanent nature of tardive dyskinesia in some cases, and the disability caused by the movements, all serve to emphasize the need to avoid unnecessary use of neuroleptic drugs to treat conditions that can be managed by alternative means.

It is important to make a baseline examination prior to starting neuroleptics and also to recognize the early signs of tardive dyskinesia. They include fine vermicular movements or restlessness of the tongue, mild choreiform finger or toe movements, and facial tics or frequent eye blinks (Gardos and Cole, 1980). Clinical recognition of early tardive dyskinesia involves systematic observation of patients in search for those signs. Crane (1972) recommended examination of drug-maintained patients every three months for signs of tardive dyskinesia. A more aggressive method of detecting the disorder may involve stopping the drug treatment for a few days or weeks. A drug-free period of less than three or four weeks is usually too short to precipitate psychotic relapse but long enough to uncover dyskinesia (Gardos and Cole, 1980).

It is important to remember that certain illnesses may cause dyskinesia, and causes of dyskinesias other than tardive dyskinesia should be ruled out. The differential diagnosis of tardive dyskinesia has been reviewed in depth elsewhere (Granacher, 1981). Indications for neuroleptics should be considered, and suitable alternatives should be tried; for example, lithium carbonate or carbamazepine (Ayd, 1982) for patients with schizoaffective or affective disorders (see chapter 4), benzodiazepines for anxiety (Jenike, 1982), and propranolol (Jenike, 1983a) or pindolol (Greendyke and Kanter, 1986) for aggressive or violent patients. In patients known to require antipsychotic drugs, attempts should be made to find the minimal effective dose.

The major classes of drugs used in the treatment of tardive dyskinesia include dopamine antagonists, cholinergic drugs, and gamma-aminobutyric acid (GABA) agonists (Gardos and Cole, 1980; Kobayashi, 1977). None of these has emerged as a satisfactory treatment, but nonspecific measures such as dose reduction may sometimes be helpful in the long term. In patients with very severe tardive dyskinesia, actually increasing the neuroleptic dosage may be the only effective treatment.

In view of the significant risk to the elderly patient and the ineffective treatment for tardive dyskinesia, physicians should avoid the use of neuroleptic drugs in elderly patients whenever possible.

Neuroleptic Overdose

Neuroleptics have a very high therapeutic index (ie, ratio of lethal dose to effective dose) and are unlikely to result in death when taken in large quantities. Patients have survived acute ingestions of many grams of these agents, and it is virtually impossible to commit suicide by an acute overdosage of an antipsychotic agent alone (Baldessarini, 1977).

Obviously, when neuroleptics are taken in combination with other toxic agents such as alcohol, barbiturates, or tricyclic antidepressants, death may result. Dialysis is not helpful in removing neuroleptics or antidepressants, but can be used to eliminate barbiturates from the body. Physostigmine, a centrally active anticholinesterase agent, can be used to reverse atropine-like anticholinergic symptoms (see chapter 9).

Beta-Blockers

Propranolol

Sometimes violent elderly patients do not respond to large doses of neuroleptics or benzodiazepines. Most of these patients have some type of organic brain disorder and many have a dementing illness.

Recently, findings in a few case reports suggested that propranolol may be useful in treating agitation and violent behavior in patients who have a variety of organic brain diseases, including senile dementia of the Alzheimer's type, stroke, postanoxic encephalopathy, gunshot wound to the head, closed-head trauma, and mental retardation (Jenike, 1983a and 1985; Ayd, 1981). In the reported cases, severely disabling rage and belligerent behavior of some previously unmanageable patients with CNS lesions or disease were controlled by the use of high doses of propranolol.

Although the total number of reported cases is small and no controlled studies have been performed yet, there is reason for optimism. At least half of the reported patients in whom propranolol produced positive behavioral changes involved elderly demented patients. Petrie and Ban (1981) reported on three patients, aged 54, 71, and 86 years, all with the diagnosis of primary dementia. Although no improvements in memory, cognition, or confusion were noted, propranolol did yield a therapeutic response within two weeks.

The first case was a 54-year-old man with presenile dementia who had a three-year history of progressive personality deterioration. He had been treated with numerous antipsychotics and benzodiazepines, all of which produced disabling side effects, including oversedation and extrapyramidal manifestations. Propranolol, 20 mg three times per day, produced control within two weeks. After a month, when the propranolol was discontinued, the behavior promptly relapsed, but remitted after propranolol was resumed.

The second case was a 71-year-old woman who had a severe lack of impulse control. Unable to sit still, she intermittently attacked other patients and wandered aimlessly. Haloperidol, as much as 20 mg/day, had no therapeutic effect. Following a 10-day course of propranolol in doses of 160 mg/day, the patient showed clear improvement with diminished agitation and she was also able to eat, dress, and communicate more effectively.

The third case involved an 86-year-old woman with a diagnosis of senile dementia who was unable to care for herself and exhibited rambling, destructive, and disorganized behavior. Despite a three-week course of haloperidol, 25 mg/day, she wandered constantly and destroyed furniture, ward furnishings, and even a water fountain. Propranolol, 60 mg/day, rapidly controlled her agitation and destructive behavior.

Yudofsky and colleagues (1981) reported on four patients with organic brain damage whose violent episodes responded to propranolol. Three of the patients were young; one had uncontrolled seizures and attacks of rage, another had Wilson's disease, and the third was mentally retarded. The fourth patient was a 63-year-old man who had been struck in the head by an exploding truck tire, resulting in diffuse, prefrontal cortical damage. After awakening from a three-week coma, he remained disoriented, agitated, and episodically violent and punched angrily and dangerously at family members and nursing staff. Antipsychotic medications did little to control the symptoms.

On transfer to a neuropsychiatric ward, he became furious, kicking and swinging his fists, and either spitting or shouting curses at staff members. Chlorpromazine, as much as 800 mg/day, was of little value in controlling the recurrent outbursts of rage and violence. Propranolol was administered at dosages of as much as 80 mg four times per day, and within three weeks the frequency, intensity, and duration of his rage and combativeness were markedly reduced. He was managed at home on 320 mg propranolol and 400 mg chlorpromazine daily. At 26-month follow-up, he remained at home without rehospitalization.

Greendyke and co-workers (1984) reported using as much as 520 mg/day of propranolol in eight patients who had organic brain disease characterized by violent and assaultive behavior refractory to conventional treatment. Improvement was demonstrated in the seven patients who were able to tolerate adequate drug dosages.

A few other case reports described younger patients with various types of brain injuries who responded similarly to propranolol (Mansheim, 1981; Schreier, 1979; Elliott, 1977). However, there appear to be no reports in the literature on non-brain-damaged patients exhibiting rageful and violent behaviors who were helped by the administration of propranolol.

In the case studies just described, bradycardia and hypotension were the most common side effects of propranolol. Propranolol causes myocardial depression, which can lead to congestive heart failure. Vital signs should be monitored frequently, particularly during early phases of treatment and when dosage is being increased (AMA Drug Evaluations, 1980). Propranolol is contraindicated in most patients with congestive heart failure, patients receiving most types of general anesthesia, patients with bronchial asthma or allergic or nonallergic bronchospasm (ie, emphysema), patients with severe sinus bradycardia, patients with ventricular failure or in cardiogenic shock, and many insulin-dependent diabetics and those prone to hypoglycemia (Yudofsky et al, 1981).

The mechanism by which propranolol exerts its effects on violent behavior in elderly patients is unknown at present. It is lipid-soluble, and thus passes through the blood-brain barrier; it also acts peripherally on beta-adrenergic receptors (Sheppard, 1979). Researchers speculate that it acts either on the brain to somehow mitigate the disinhibition of the response to rage caused by CNS lesions, or on the peripheral nervous system as beta-blocker to reduce somatic responses to frustration, fear, or panic that may trigger outbursts of rage (Yudofsky et al, 1981; Heiser and DeFrancisco, 1976; Cole et al, 1979).

Pindolol

Noting that all of the studies using high-dose propranolol reported a high incidence of bradycardia and hypotension, Greendyke and Kanter (1986) investigated a newer class of beta-blockers relative to their effects on brain-damaged patients. They chose to study pindolol because, unlike many other beta-blockers, pindolol exerts a partial agonist effect through intrinsic sympathomimetic activity. This effect provides slight stimulation of the blocked receptor and maintains better resting sympathetic tone. For these reasons, they expected that pindolol might bring about the same therapeutic benefits as propranolol without unwanted side effects.

In an attempt to ensure a therapeutic effect, Greendyke and Kanter selected subjects whose symptoms were dramatic and frequently demonstrated. All patients were, as a consequence of brain disease, pathologically impulsive, assaultive, openly hostile, and generally uncooperative. All were severely demented and unable to participate in interactive, conventional psychologic testing; none were psychotic, however. Eleven subjects who had proved refractory to conventional pharmacotherapy were identified, and all required frequent supplemental medication to preserve behavioral control.

During the study, each physical assault or attempted assault was documented by an incident report. At least two staff members closely monitored the study patients during waking hours to ensure that virtually all assaultive episodes would be recorded. Each administration of supplemental medication was also noted. In addition, daily behavioral ratings were conducted to assess lethargy, hostility, uncommunicativeness, uncooperativeness, and repetitive behaviors. All regular treatment with psychotropic medication was discontinued for two weeks before initiation of the study and a randomized, double-blind, placebo-controlled, crossover design was used.

Pindolol was started at 10 mg/day and was increased 10 mg/day every 3 to 4 days up to a daily dose of 60 mg. The active drug treatment group received pindolol at this dose for 10 days, then the dose was increased further to 100 mg/day to determine whether additional benefits could be gained at higher doses.

In general, the optimal clinical response appeared to occur with 40 to 60 mg/day. No additional therapeutic advantage was gained with dosage increases of more than 60 mg/day. In fact, as dosages were increased above this level, some patients appeared to be generally overstimulated and showed increased motor activity and agitation. Possible auditory hallucinations that occurred in one individual disappeared with dosage reductions. No patients became hypotensive while taking pindolol.

Greendyke and Kanter reported a significant reduction in assaultive episodes and hostility during pindolol treatment ($P<0.05$). Similarly, the need for supplemental medication was reduced significantly when patients received pindolol as compared with those who received placebo. Statistical analysis did not indicate an increase in lethargy while patients were taking pindolol. Improvements in patients' ability or willingness to communicate and in cooperativeness were also demonstrated and pindolol was associated also with a reduction of stereotyped repetitive behaviors.

After the completion of this study, these patients continued to receive treatment with pindolol at a dosage of 40 to 60 mg/day and four patients were substantially improved and were transferred to hospital units for patients who required lower levels of care. Two of the four were in a nursing home care unit; one was being prepared for discharge.

This study demonstrated in a controlled manner that beta-blockers improve a range of pathologic behaviors associated with brain damage. In contrast to earlier studies using propranolol, no bradycardia or hypotension was associated with the use of pindolol. The fact that pindolol brought about such dramatic behavioral improvements in this severely impaired and refractory sample of patients suggests its potential benefits for less impaired individuals as well.

Conclusions

Although beta-blockers have not been approved by the Food and Drug Administration for any psychiatric illness, possible psychiatric implications have been explored worldwide for more than 15 years (Cole et al, 1979; Ayd, 1981). The use of beta-blockers for an unapproved indication is not illegal, but it would be wise to advise patients and their families that it is an innovative form of therapy. Both the discussion with the patient and family and the rationale for using beta-blockers should be documented in the medical record (Gelenberg, 1981).

In summary, even though mechanisms remain speculative, it is clinically important to note that the severely disabling rage and belligerent behavior of some previously unmanageable patients with CNS lesions or disease have been controlled by the use of beta-blockers. In the cases reported thus far, a therapeutic response was noted between 10 days and 3 weeks, with doses ranging from 60 to 550 mg/day of propranolol and 40 to 60 mg/day of pindolol. There was no improvement in cognition, confusion levels, or memory proficiency with the use of beta-blockers in any of these patients.

Carbamazepine

There is growing evidence that carbamazepine (Tegretol) can help to control psychosis and agitation in patients with bipolar affective disorders acutely (Ballenger and Post, 1980; Post and Uhde, 1985; Nolen, 1983; Frankenburg, 1988). Its efficacy in the long term is not so convincing (Frankenburg, 1988) and it has been suggested that carbamazepine may only infrequently be useful in the long-term care of patients who fail to respond to standard treatment. In one extended study, two-thirds of patients with affective illnesses improved in the short term, but at longer follow-up, there was a marked decrease in the number of patients judged to be responders.

Carbamazepine may be helpful in treating some elderly patients who exhibit severely disabling rage and belligerent behavior. Carbamazepine has been advocated as an alternative to neuroleptics, based on reports that it decreased aggression, irritability, and impulsive behavior across a variety of clinical syndromes such as violent schizophrenia (Hokola and Laulumaa, 1982), episodic dyscontrol syndrome (Tunks, 1977), and violent interictal behavior (Dalby, 1971).

Two reports indicated that carbamazepine might be useful in the treatment of psychiatric patients who have EEG abnormalities (Hokola and Laulumaa, 1982; Neppe, 1983). From these reports, however, it was not clear whether this drug would help similar patients who had normal EEGs. To address this question, Luchins (1983) studied violent patients on two long-term psychiatric wards who had received carbamazepine for at least six weeks as an adjunct to neuroleptics. All of these patients (while not taking carbamazepine and without nasopharyngeal leads) had a normal EEG and did not have affective disorder. Luchins did not include patients with affective disorders as it was already known that such patients may respond to carbamazepine in the absence of EEG abnormality (Post, 1982) (see chapter 4). Luchins found seven appropriate study patients (five males); six met criteria for schizophrenia and the other for mixed personality disorder (DSM-III criteria).

Luchens retrospectively reviewed nursing notes of episodes of physical aggression during periods when these patients were taking and not taking carbamazepine. All were taking carbamazepine for a period of time; then it was discontinued for a six-week period and then begun again. The mean number of aggressive episodes while patients took carbamazepine was significantly less than that either before or after drug treatment. Six of the seven patients had fewer aggressive episodes during the carbamazepine period than either before or after treatment. All patients were receiving neuroleptics throughout the period of this study and there was no difference in mean neuroleptic dosage either before, during, or after carbamazepine administration. The mean carbamazepine dosage was 1,057 mg/day (range, 400 to 1,600 mg) with a mean serum concentration of 8.5 μ/mL (range, 6.3 to 13 μ/mL).

Luchin's findings need to be confirmed in a double-blind controlled trial. Furthermore, one cannot rule out the possibility that more extensive EEG studies would have detected an abnormality in these patients. Nevertheless, these cases do suggest that a normal clinical EEG in a violent elderly patient may not preclude a beneficial response to carbamazepine. In addition, these findings raise the possibility that carbamazepine's psychotropic effects may not be related to its anticonvulsive action. Moreover, because the drug's spectrum of psychotropic effects parallels that of lithium, with both being useful in aggressive patients (Sheard, 1975) as well as in the treatment and prophylaxis of affective disorders (Post, 1982), it would seem likely that some mechanism common to both drugs underlies their shared effects.

None of the patients in Luchin's study had dementia, but others studied carbamazepine's properties in agitated (Leibovici and Tariot, 1988) and assaultive (Patterson, 1988) dementing patients. Despite suggestions of the efficacy of carbamazepine for agitation in dementia, there is a dearth of case reports. McAllister (1985) reported the cases of five patients with frontal lobe syndrome who responded to carbamazepine, but the patients also had other major psychiatric illnesses.

Anton and associates (1986) treated one patient with bipolar disorder, cognitive impairment, and multiple cerebral infarcts with carbamazepine and reported reduced psychotic and manic symptoms along with some cognitive improvement. Essa (1986) reported the case of one patient with presenile dementia of the Alzheimer type with associated manic features and destructive behavior who responded to carbamazepine.

Leibovici and Tariot (1988) reported the cases of two patients (ages, 81 and 85 years) with agitation associated with dementia, but with no other psychiatric illness, who also responded to carbamazepine. One became paranoid, confused, angry, and dysphoric when placed in a nursing home. Trials of haloperidol, perphenazine, lorazepam, and nortriptyline did not produce sustained improvement. Within one week after obtaining "antiepileptic" levels of carbamazepine (taking 500 mg/day), the patient was less irritable, and within two weeks the patient was less agitated, less dysphoric, less confused, and better able to cooperate. Her sleep improved.

The second demented patient, an 85-year-old man, alternated between apathy and outbursts of rage which were triggered by minor changes in his daily routines. He frequently struck nursing staff while they were feeding or toileting him. Haloperidol and constant restraints were eventually required to control him. Carbamazepine was begun and raised to a blood level of 6.2 μ/mL (oral dose of 100 mg three times a day). His condition improved dramatically during the second week of treatment; hostility almost disappeared and restraints were removed.

Patterson (1988) administered carbamazepine in an open pilot study to 13 patients (ages, 40 to 69) with primary degenerative dementia characterized by aggressive and assaultive behavior refractory to conventional treatment. All of the 13 patients had histories of repeated physical attacks on the staff or other patients, with numerous episodes in which minor fractures and other injuries were inflicted on others or sustained by the patients. All were belligerent, uncooperative, and resistive with agitation and rage. Patterson attempted to get blood levels of carbamazepine into the standard antiepileptic range of 8 to 12 μ/mL, which usually took 7 to 10 days. Two patients complained of transient diplopia and ataxia, which cleared spontaneously and may have corresponded to peak absorption of carbamazepine. The frequency of assaultive behavior decreased after carbamazepine administration, with a subsequent return to baseline frequency after its discontinuation. Episodes of assaultive behavior decreased from a mean of 6.1 episodes per week before treatment to 3.3 per week during carbamazepine treatment and returned to 6.3 per week following discontinuation of carbamazepine.

Carbamazepine may be a reasonable drug to try in the demented patient when other agents have not been useful in controlling violent or aggressive behavior. One general approach (Leibovici and Tariot, 1988) is to use low doses initially and observe for reduction in carefully defined agitated behaviors. The dose can be gradually increased until beneficial effects are achieved and the drug is continued, or toxicity is encountered and the drug is stopped, or, in the absence of either benefit or toxicity, standard antiepileptic drug levels are achieved. Ongoing clinical monitoring for improvement or toxicity is always required.

From a practical standpoint, carbamazepine does not have hypotensive, anticholinergic, or extrapyramidal toxicity, nor is its use associated with tardive dyskinesia, all of which represent advantages over antipsychotic drugs. It has no potential for addiction or withdrawal, in contrast to benzodiazepines, and shows significantly less neurotoxicity in the elderly than does lithium. The major risk associated with its use is the rare occurrence of aplastic anemia or agranulocytosis. Increased levels of liver enzymes and mild hyponatremia are common with carbamazepine treatment, but clinically significant toxicity is rare. Even if patients improve acutely, there are no data on the long-term efficacy of carbamazepine in these patients.

In terms of carbamazepine's mechanism of action in controlling behavioral symptoms in demented patients, Leibovici and Tariot (1988) noted that carbamazepine has been postulated to have a variety of neurochemical effects apart from its antiseizure capabilities. Some of these may have particular relevance to dementia-associated clinical phenomena (Post, 1987). For example, there are known central cholinergic deficits in patients with dementia of the Alzheimer type that are related to some symptoms of the illness (Essa, 1986; see chapter 5), and carbamazepine administration produces at least regional increases in brain acetylcholine levels in rodents. Carbamazepine enhances the function of vasopressin, a peptide that is a putative neuromodulator that has memory and learning, and possible other psychotropic, effects in humans. Finally, carbamazepine also selectively increases plasma total and free tryptophan levels in humans, which may relate to some of its effects on impulsivity and aggression.

Lithium Carbonate

Since its introduction by Cade in 1949, lithium carbonate has become widely accepted as a treatment for manic-depressive illness (Cade, 1949; Sheard, 1975). Lithium is very effective at controlling hyperaggressiveness and hypersexuality, which are frequent concomitants of manic-depressive episodes. Lithium also plays an inhibitory role in animal aggressive behavior including that induced by hypothalamic stimulation in cats (Wasman and Flynn, 1972). In epileptic patients, lithium has reportedly produced interseizure behavioral improvements in patients who were impulsive, excited, and aggressive (Gershon and Trantner, 1956; Gershon, 1968; Glesinger, 1954; Williamson, 1966). On the other hand, one study (Jus et al, 1973) of 18 female patients with temporal lobe epilepsy showed that lithium worsened seizure activity. Other reports confirmed that lithium can induce grand mal seizures (Sheard, 1975) and thus the effect of lithium on convulsive disorders is still debated.

In brain-damaged children with periodic aggression (Annell, 1969), and in severely mentally retarded adolescents (Dostal and Zvoltsky, 1970), lithium reportedly has antiaggressive effects.

There are two reported trials of lithium in humans in whom abnormal aggressive behavior was the predominant manifestation and source of difficulty (Sheard, 1975). One studied 12 chronically assaultive males who were treated with lithium or placebo in a single-blind crossover trial. None of the subjects had overt evidence of brain damage or psychosis and all had IQs of more than 85. Lithium was maintained at blood levels of 0.8 to 1.2 mEq/L for one month, then placebo was given for one month, and finally lithium was given for another month. There was a significant reduction in the number of aggressive incidents during lithium periods as compared with placebo periods (Sheard, 1971).

The second study (Tupin et al, 1973) confirmed these findings in a longer trial involving 27 violent male convicts who were treated for as long as 18 months with lithium carbonate. Again, there was a significant reduction in the number of violent incidents, as compared with the number in the same length of time before treatment began. Many of these convicts were diagnosed as schizophrenic and some had brain damage.

There are no controlled trials of lithium in elderly brain-damaged patients who are violent; lithium, however, should be tried if other measures fail. Lithium is clearly indicated in elderly patients with preexisting manic-depressive illness (see chapter 4).

Serotonergic Agents

Trazodone and L-tryptophan

Some demented violent or assaultive patients as well as those who scream loudly or bang their heads are unresponsive to multiple therapeutic approaches. A few case reports of treatment with serotonergic agonists are worthy of note (Greenwald et al, 1986; O'Neil et al, 1986; Simpson and Foster, 1986). Greenwald and colleagues (1986) described the case of an 82-year-old woman with moderately advanced dementia who repetitively screamed and banged her head on the table and who responded to a combination of trazodone (Desyrel) and L-tryptophan (a precursor of serotonin). She was transferred from a skilled nursing facility after weeks of dysphoria, screaming, echolalia, and banging on the chair tray and sides of her head with both hands. Trials of thiothixene, haloperidol, oxazepam, and tranylcypromine failed to alter her symptoms and/or provoked unacceptable side effects. There was no mention of a trial using beta-blockers. The compulsive, stereotyped, and self-injurious nature of the banging movements, with seemingly involuntary and echolaic verbal productions, reminded the authors of behaviors observed in childhood autism and Gilles de la Tourettes syndrome. Noting that the brain serotonergic system had been implicated in these disorders, as well as in obsessive-compulsive disorder, depression (especially with self-aggressive features), and dementia, they decided to try trazodone, a preferential serotonin uptake inhibitor that has been safely and successfully used in psychogeriatric patients. The dose of trazodone was increased over a three-week period to 300 mg/day in divided doses, without side effects. Within three weeks, head-banging decreased, mood improved, and screaming was no longer constant. After the patient had been taking trazodone for six weeks, the banging ceased, though intermittent screaming and echolalia persisted. Adjunctive therapy was started with 1 g of the serotonergic precursor L-tryptophan, and titrated up to 2.5 g daily. Orthostatic hypotension developed, but blood pressure returned to normal with reduction of trazodone to a daily dose of 200 mg.

Within two weeks after addition of L-tryptophan, screaming and echolalia had almost stopped. Greenwald and associates thought that screaming and banging may have represented an unusual feature of depression in this demented patient and that the response to trazodone and L-tryptophan may reflect the antidepressant efficacy of these drugs. Just because a particular symptom responds to antidepressant medication does not mean that that symptom was related to depression. For example, low dosages of antidepressants often help pain patients despite the absence of clinical depression. Nevertheless, a diagnosis of depression may need to be considered in demented patients with similar presentations and even if no depressive symptoms are found, an empirical trial of serotonergic agents may improve the clinical situation. As noted, drugs with apparent serotonergic selectivity have been helpful in treating several neuropsychiatric conditions that may be characterized by brain serotonergic dysfunction; many of these conditions share features of impulsivity, aggressivity, and compulsivity.

Buspirone

A recent case report demonstrated the use of buspirone (Buspar), a novel drug with 5-HT_{1A} receptor agonist properties (ie, a partial serotonergic agonist), in the management of a patient with dementia and agitated behavior. Colenda (1988) reported the case of a 74-year-old woman with primary degenerative dementia, senile onset (Alzheimer's disease) for the past three years. Her MMSE score was 16 out of a possible 30 (see chapter 2). She had been followed in a dementia clinic and treated with varying amounts of haloperidol (0.5 mg four times daily at time of report). The family reported agitated behavior, characterized by constant rocking, vocal grunts, angry outbursts, oppositional behavior, and wandering. There was no concurrent depression. Her behavior pre-dated the use of haloperidol, and there were no signs of extrapyramidal symptoms, akathisia, dystonia, or anticholinergic side effects. She answered questions with nonverbal or yes-no responses. Buspirone, 10 mg three times daily, was begun and increased to 15 mg three times daily. Over a two-month period, rocking and vocal grunts stopped and there was less oppositional behavior. On interview she replied with well-formed simple sentences. Her daughter noted that the patient's management was easier and said that she could continue to manage her mother in her home.

This case indicates that buspirone may be a useful adjunct in managing the disruptive behavior of demented patients. Smith and Peroutka (1986) reported that in rats buspirone alters behaviors that are known to be mediated through serotonergic mechanisms. The reduction in rocking, oppositional, and restless behaviors in this one patient who was treated with buspirone suggests that these behaviors may be medicated by dysfunction of the serotonergic system. Hopefully, controlled clinical trials of buspirone alone and in combination with low-dose neuroleptics will determine the usefulness of this agent in reducing aggressive behavior in demented patients. Until more data are available, clinicians have little to lose by trying this apparently safe drug in these patients.

Conclusions

Even though mechanisms remain speculative, the clinical dilemmas faced by these physicians are common. Given the good outcome in these patients, other refractory demented patients whose behavior includes incessant screaming, violence, or head banging may respond to serotonergic agents. These agents, if effective, may well produce fewer side effects in elderly patients than neuroleptics which are usually used in an attempt to control these difficult patients.

Benzodiazepines

Benzodiazepines are generally of little use as a primary treatment for psychosis and may, in fact, exacerbate psychosis and agitation in some patients, especially those with dementing illnesses. Benzodiazepines are sometimes used as sedating adjuncts to neuroleptic agents in elderly patients (Bernstein, 1987) and this might allow the elderly agitated or psychotic patient to be controlled on a lower dosage of neuroleptic drug.

Dopaminergic Agents

Pathologic laughing and crying are defined as inappropriate laughing and crying unrelated to surrounding circumstances or stimulation, with no accompanying emotional feelings (Poeck, 1969). This has been reported in patients with cerebrovascular disease, brain trauma, brain tumor, amyotrophic lateral sclerosis, and other neurologic disorders (Udaka et al, 1984). These conditions can be very upsetting to patients, who fear loss of control, and to family members, who may feel that the patient either is depressed or is becoming psychotic (see chapter 4).

Wolf and associates (1979) reported that levodopa is effective in patients with pathologic laughing. Udaka and associates (1984) did a controlled trial during which they administered levodopa or amantadine hydrochloride to 25 patients with pathologic laughing or crying, or both. Levodopa showed remarkable effects in 10 of 25 patients and controlled the pathologic laughing and crying almost completely. Amantadine also improved the pathologic crying in four of eight patients. The effect appeared two to five days after drug administration and lasted for one to two weeks after the discontinuation of levodopa treatment. The symptoms were markedly improved in those patients who were devoid of cortical atrophy or periventricular lucency on CT scan and also devoid of severe dementia or a disturbance in activity of daily living. The concentration of homovanillic acid (a dopamine metabolite) in the cerebrospinal fluid of the patients was significantly decreased, whereas the concentration of 5-hydroxyindoleacetic acid (a serotonergic metabolite) remained within normal limits. The authors pointed out that because pathologic laughing and crying seem in part to be caused by decreased functioning of the dopaminergic neuron, levodopa or amantadine is worth trying. Perhaps in demented patients, lesions in other brain systems might prevent dopaminergic agents from being as helpful.

TREATING PSYCHOTIC SYMPTOMS
ASSOCIATED WITH DEMENTIA

Unfortunately, little data exist concerning the efficacy of treatments for psychotic symptoms associated with Alzheimer's disease (Barnes et al, 1982; Maletta, 1985; Helms, 1985; Jenike, 1985; Risse and Barnes, 1986; Rubin et al, 1988). If psychotic symptoms occur in patients with a medical illness (eg, hyperthyroidism or hypothyroidism), as a consequence of a medication (eg, digoxin), or as part of another psychiatric illness (eg, depression or schizophrenia), the principal treatment should be directed at that condition (Jenike, 1985). If psychosis or agitation occurs as the primary problem, medications and techniques outlined in this chapter and chapter 5 may be of help.

We have had considerable experience with patients who talk to their reflection in the mirror or who feel that whatever is occurring on television is actually taking place in their room; neuroleptic medications have been of no help. Mirror talking is generally a benign symptom and just explaining it to the family members is often treatment enough.

Patients who merge boundaries with the television generally must leave the room when other family members are watching television if the patient is troubled by the symptom. Medications are of little, if any, help with this troubling symptom.

SUMMARY

Violent, psychotic, or aggressive elderly patients are among the most difficult patients to manage. A number of medications are helpful to the clinician faced with such a patient. Neuroleptics have been the traditional treatment but have many potentially disabling side effects. They should be used at very low dosages to minimize unwanted effects. Haloperidol in doses of 0.5 mg or thiothixene administered as 1 mg once or twice daily are reasonable starting doses. In the very frail elderly, doses as low as 0.25 mg of haloperidol at bedtime may have a therapeutic effect.

Low-potency agents, such as chlorpromazine and thioridazine, have more associated sedation, orthostatic hypotension, anticholinergic effects, and cardiovascular problems, but have fewer extrapyramidal effects than high-potency agents. For this reason, they are preferred in patients with preexisting movement disorders such as Parkinson's disease. Doses as low as 10 mg twice daily should be tried initially.

Neuroleptic side effects have been reviewed and the use of alternative

242

medications such as beta-blockers, carbamazepine, serotonergic agents, benzodiazepines, and lithium carbonate is discussed. Neuroleptics should be avoided whenever possible. Indications for neuroleptic treatment should be reviewed periodically so that patients are exposed to risks and side effects for the minimum possible duration.

REFERENCES

AMA Drug Evaluations, ed 4. Chicago, American Medical Association, 1980, pp 533–535.

Ananth J, Edelmuth E, Dargan B: Meige's syndrome associated with neuroleptic treatment. *Am J Psychiatry* 145:513–515, 1988.

Annell AL: Lithium in the treatment of children and adolescents. *Acta Psychiatr Scand Suppl* 207:19–33, 1969.

Anton RF, Waid RL, Fossey M, et al: Case report of carbamazepine treatment of organic brain syndrome with psychotic features. *J Clin Psychopharmacol* 6:232, 1986.

Ayd FJ: Carbamazepine's acute and prophylactic effects in manic and depressive illness: An update. *Int Drug Ther Newsletter* 17:2,3,5, 1982.

Ayd FJ: Propranolol for rage and violence. *Int Drug Ther Newsletter* 16:19–20, 1981.

Baldessarini RJ: *Chemotherapy in Psychiatry*. Cambridge, Mass, Harvard University Press, 1977.

Ballenger JC, Post RM: Carbamazepine in manic-depressive illness: a new treatment. *Am J Psychiatry* 137:782–790, 1980.

Barnes R, Veith R, Okimoto J, et al: Efficacy of antipsychotic medications in behaviorally disturbed dementia patients. *Am J Psychiatry* 139:1170–1174, 1982.

Bartter FC: *The Syndrome of Inappropriate Secretion of Antidiuretic Hormone*. Chicago, Year Book Medical Publishers, 1973.

Bernstein JG: Chemotherapy of psychosis, in Bernstein JG (ed): *Clinical Psychopharmacology*. Littleton, Mass, PSG Publishing, 1978, pp 40–51.

Bernstein JG: Psychotropic drug prescribing, in Hackett TP, Cassem NH (eds): *Massachusetts General Hospital Handbook of General Hospital Psychiatry*. Littleton, Mass, PSG Publishing, 1987, pp 496–537.

Blue MG, Schneider SM, Noro S, et al: Successful treatment of neuroleptic malignant syndrome with sodium nitroprusside. *Ann Intern Med* 104:56–57, 1986.

Bonnet C: *Essai analytique sur les facultes de l'ane*. 2nd de, vol II. Copenhague & Geneve, 1769, 176–177.

Brooks SA: Folie a Deux in the aged: variations in psychopathology. *Can J Psychiatry* 32:61–63, 1987.

Burke RE, Fahn S, Janovic J, et al: Tardive dyskinesia and inappropriate use of neuroleptic drugs. *Lancet* 1:1299, 1982.

Cade JFJ: Lithium salts in the treatment of psychotic excitement. *Med J Aust* 36:349–352, 1949.

Caroff SN: The neuroleptic malignant syndrome. *J Clin Psychiatry* 41:79–83, 1980.

Casey DA, Wandzilak T: Senile macular degeneration and psychosis. *J Geriatr Psychiatry Neurol* 1:108–109, 1988.

Christensen E, Moller JE, Faurbye A: Neuropathological investigation of 28 brains from patients with dyskinesias. *Acta Psychiatr Scand* 46:14, 1970.

Christenson R, Blazer D: Epidemiology of persecutory ideation in an elderly population in the community. *Am J Psychiatry* 141:1088–1091, 1984.

Claghorn J, Honigfeld G, Abuzzahab FS Sr, et al: The risks and benefits of clozapine vs. chlorpromazine. *J Clin Psychopharmacol* 7:377–384, 1987.

Cohen BM, Baldessarini RJ, Pope HG Jr, et al: Neuroleptic malignant syndrome (letter). *N Engl J Med* 313:1293, 1985.

Cole JO, Altesman RI, Weingarten CH: Beta-blocking drugs in psychiatry. *McLean Hosp J* 4:40–68, 1979.

Colenda CC: Buspirone in treatment of agitated demented patient. *Lancet* 1:1169, 1988.

Coons DJ, Hillman FJ, Marshall RW: Treatment of neuroleptic malignant syndrome with dantrolene sodium: A case report. *Am J Psychiatry* 139:944–945, 1982.

Cooper AJ: Medroxyprogesterone acetate (MPA) treatment of sexual acting out in men suffering from dementia. *J Clin Psychiatry* 48:368–370, 1987.

Crane GE: Prevention and management of tardive dyskinesia. *Am J Psychiatry* 129:781, 1972.

Crane GE: Tardive dyskinesia in patients treated with neuroleptics: A review of the literature. *Am J Psychiatry* 124 (February Suppl):40, 1968.

Dalby MA: Antiepileptic and psychotropic effect of carbamazepine in the treatment of psychomotor epilepsy. *Epilepsia* 12:325, 1971.

Davies P: Neurotransmitter-related symptoms in SDAT. *Brain Res* 171:319, 1979.

Davies TS: Cyproterone acetate for male hypersexuality. *J Int Med Res* 2:159–163, 1974.

Degwitz R, Binsack KF, Herkert H: Zur Problem der persistierenden ex-trapyramidelen Hyperkinesen nach langfristiger Anwendung von Neuroleptica. *Nervenarzt* 38:170, 1967.

Diagnostic and Statistical Manual of Mental Disorders, ed 3, revised. (DSM-III-R). Washington DC, American Psychiatric Association Press, 1987.

DiMascio A, Bernardo DL, Greenblatt DJ, et al: A controlled trial of amantadine in drug-induced extrapyramidal disorders. *Arch Gen Psychiatry* 33:599–602, 1976.

Dostal T, Zvoltsky P: Antiaggressive effect of lithium salts in several mentally retarded adolescents. *Int Pharmacopsychiatry* 5.203–207, 1970.

Drachman DA, Leavitt J: Human memory and the cholinergic system. *Arch Neurol* 30:113–121, 1974.

Ekbom KA: Asthenia crurum paresthesia (irritable legs). *Acta Med Scand* 118:197, 1944.

Ekbom KA: Restless legs and akathisia. *J Swedish Med Assoc* 62:2376–2382, 1965.

Elliott FA: Propranolol for the control of belligerent behavior following acute brain damage. *Ann Neurol* 1:489–491, 1977.

Essa M: Carbamazepine in dementia. *J Clin Psychopharmacol* 6:234, 1986.

Fishbain DA: Folie a Deux in the aged. *Can J Psychiatry* 32:498–499, 1987.

Fogel BS, Goldberg RJ: Neuroleptic malignant syndrome (letter). *N Engl J Med* 313:1292, 1985.

Frankenburg FR, Tohen M, Cohen BM, et al: Long-term response to carbamazepine: A retrospective study. *J Clin Psychopharmacol* 8:130–132, 1988.

Gardos G, Cole JO: Overview: Public health issues in tardive dyskinesia. *Am J Psychiatry* 137:776, 1980.

Gelenberg AJ, Bellinghausen B, Wojick JD, et al: A prospective survey of neuroleptic malignant syndrome in a short-term psychiatric hospital. *Am J Psychiatry* 145:517–518, 1988.

Gelenberg AJ: Clozapine renascent. *Biol Ther Psychiatry* 11:25, 28, 1988.

Gelenberg AJ: Dantrolene (Dantrium;) for the treatment of neuroleptic malignant syndrome. *Biol Ther Psychiatry* 5:35–36, 1982.

Gelenberg AJ: Psychosis, in Bassuk EL, Schoonover SC, Gelenberg AJ (eds): *The Practitioners Guide to Psychoactive Drugs*, ed 2. New York, Plenum, 1983.

Gelenberg AJ: Return to NMS. *Biol Ther Psychiatry* 9:17, 20, 1986.

244

Gelenberg AJ: The long arm of propranolol: Extension to organic mental disorders. *Biol Ther Psychiatry* 4:13–14, 1981.

Gelenberg AJ: Treating the outpatient schizophrenic. *Postgrad Med* 64:48–55, 1978.

Gershon S, Trantner EM: The treatment of shock dependency by pharmacological agents. *Med J Aust* 43:783–787, 1956.

Gershon S: The use of lithium salts in psychiatric disorders. *Dis Nerv Syst* 29:51–62, 1968.

Glesinger B: Evaluation of lithium in the treatment of psychotic excitement. *Med J Aust* 41:277–283, 1954.

Goekoop JG, Carbaat PA: Treatment of neuroleptic malignant syndrome with dantrolene (letter). *Lancet* 2:49–50, 1982.

Goodman A, Gilman LS: *The Pharmacological Basis of Therapeutics*. Toronto, Macmillan, 1980.

Granacher RP: Differential diagnosis of tardive dyskinesia: An overview. *Am J Psychiatry* 138:1288, 1981.

Greendyke RM, Schuster DB, Wooten JA: Propranolol in the treatment of assaultive patients with organic brain disease. *J Clin Psychopharmacol* 4:282–285, 1984.

Greendyke RM, Kanter DR: Therapeutic effects of pindolol on behavioral disturbances associated with organic brain disease: A double-blind study. *J Clin Psychiatry* 47:423–426, 1986.

Greenwald BS, Marin DB, Silverman SM: Serotonergic treatment of screaming and banging in dementia. *Lancet* 2:1464–1465, 1986.

Gross H, Kaltenback E: Neuropathological findings in persistent dyskinesia after neuroleptic long term therapy, in Cerlett A, Boue FJ (eds): *The Present Status of Psychotropic Drugs*. Amsterdam, Excerpta Medica, 1968.

Guze BH, Baxter LR Jr: Neuroleptic malignant syndrome. *N Engl J Med* 313:163–166, 1985.

Halleck SL: The ethics of antiandrogen therapy. *Am J Psychiatry* 138:642–643, 1981.

Heiser JF, DeFrancisco D: The treatment of pathological panic states with propranolol. *Am J Psychiatry* 133:1389–1394, 1976.

Helms PM: Efficacy of antipsychotics in the treatment of the behavioral complications of dementia: A review of the literature. *J Am Geriatr Soc* 33:206–209, 1985.

Hoffet H: The treatment of sexual delinquents and psychiatric hospital patients with the testosterone blocker cyproterone acetate (SH 714). *Praxis* 577:221–230, 1968.

Hokola HPA, Laulumaa VA: Carbamazepine treatment of violent schizophrenics. *Lancet* 1:1358, 1982.

Hughes JR: ECT during and after the neuroleptic malignant syndrome: A case report. *J Clin Psychiatry* 47:42–43, 1986.

Hunter R, Blackwood W, Smith MC, et al: Neuropathological findings in 3 cases of persistent dyskinesias following phenothiazine medication. *J Neurol Sci* 7:763, 1968.

Hunter R, Earl CJ, Janz D: A syndrome of abnormal movements and dementia in leukotomized patients treated with phenothiazines. *J Neurol Neurosurg Psychiatry* 27:219, 1964.

Husband C, Mal FM, Carruthers G: Syndrome of inappropriate secretion of antidiuretic hormone in a patient treated with haloperidol. *Can J Psychiatry* 26:197, 1981.

Jenike MA: *Handbook of Geriatric Psychopharmacology*. Littleton, Mass, PSG Publishing, 1985.

Jenike MA: Tardive dyskinesia: Special risk in the elderly. *J Am Geriatr Soc* 31:71–73, 1983.

Jenike MA: Treatment of rage and violence in elderly patients with propranolol. *Geriatrics* 38:29–34, 1983a.

Jenike MA: Using sedative drugs in the elderly. *Drug Ther* 12:184–190, 1982.

Johnson GFS, Hunt GE, Rey JM: Incidence and severity of tardive dyskinesia with age. *Arch Gen Psychiatry* 39:486, 1982.

Julou L, Ducrot R, Ganter P, et al: Chronic toxicity, side effects and metabolism of neuroleptics of the phenothiazine group, in *Proceedings of the European Society for Study of Drug Toxicity*. Amsterdam, Excerpta Medica, 1968, vol 9: Toxicity and Side Effects of Psychotropic Drugs, International Congress Series 145.

Jus A, Villeneuve A, Goutier J, et al: Some remarks on the influence of lithium carbonate on patients with temporal epilepsy. *Int J Clin Pharmacol Ther Toxicol* 7:67–74, 1973.

Kane JM, Smith JM: Tardive dyskinesia. *Arch Gen Psychiatry* 39:473, 1982.

Keck PE Jr, Pope HG Jr, McElroy EL: Frequency and presentation of neuroleptic malignant syndrome: a prospective study. *Am J Psychiatry* 144:1344–1346, 1987.

Klawans HL, Goetz CG, Perliks S: Tardive dyskinesia: Review and update. *Am J Psychiatry* 137:900, 1980.

Kobayashi RM: Drug therapy of tardive dyskinesia. *N Engl J Med* 296:259, 1977.

Kolmel HW: Complex visual hallucinations in the hemianopic field. *J Neurol Neurosurg Psychiatry* 48:29–38, 1985.

Lance JW: Simple formed hallucinations confined to the area of a specific visual field defect. *Brain* 99:719–731, 1976.

Layman WA, Cohen L: A modern concept of Folie a Deux. *J Nerv Ment Dis* 125:412–419, 1957.

Lazarus A: Treatment of neuroleptic malignant syndrome with electroconvulsive therapy. *J Nerv Ment Dis* 174:47–49, 1986.

Lees AJ: *Tics and Related Disorders*. New York, Churchill Livingstone, 1985.

Leibovici A, Tariot PN: Carbamazepine treatment of agitation associated with dementia. *J Geriatr Psychiatry Neurol* 1:110–112, 1988.

Lipinski JF, Zubenko GS, Cohen BM, et al: Propranolol and the treatment of neuroleptic-induced akathisia. *Am J Psychiatry* 141:412–415, 1984.

Luchins DJ: Carbamazepine for the violent psychiatric patient. *Lancet* 1:766, 1983.

Maletta GJ: Medications to modify at-home behavior of Alzheimer's patients. *Geriatrics* 40:31–42, 1985.

Mansheim P: Treatment with propranolol of the behavioral sequelae of brain damage. *J Clin Psychiatry* 42:132, 1981.

Matuk F, Kalyanaraman K: Syndrome of inappropriate secretion of antidiuretic hormone in patients treated with psychotropic drugs. *Arch Neurol* 34:375, 1977.

Mayeux R, Stern Y, Suno M: Psychosis in patients with dementia of the Alzheimer type (abstract). *Ann Neurol* 18:144, 1987.

McAllister TW: Carbamazepine in mixed frontal lobe and psychiatric disorders. *J Clin Psychiatry* 46:393, 1985.

McGreer PL, McGreer EG, Suzoki JS: Aging and extrapyramidal function. *Arch Neurol* 34:33, 1977.

McNamara ME, Heros RC, Boller F: Visual hallucinations in blindness: The Charles Bonnet syndrome. *Int J Neurosci* 17:13–15, 1982.

McNeil J, Verwoert A, Peak D: Folie a Deux in the aged: review and case report of role reversal. *J Am Geriatr Soc* 20:316–323, 1972.

Miller M, Moses AM: Drug-induced states of impaired water excretion. *Kidney Int* 10:96–103, 1976.

Mukherjee S, Rosen AM, Cardemas C, et al: Tardive dyskinesia in psychiatric outpatients. *Arch Gen Psychiatry* 39:466, 1982.

Neppe VM: Carbamazepine in the psychiatric outpatient. *Lancet* 1:766, 1983.

Nolen WA: Carbamazepine, a possible adjunct or alternative to lithium in bipolar disorder. *Acta Psychiatr Scand* 67:218–225, 1983.

O'Neil M, Page N, Adkins WN, et al: Tryptophan-trazodone treatment of aggressive behavior. *Lancet* 2:859–860, 1986.

Pakkenberg H, Fog R, Nilakantan B: The long term effect of perphenazine enanthate on the rat brain: Some metabolic and anatomical observations. *Psychopharmacologia* 29:329, 1972.

Patterson JF: A preliminary study of carbamazepine in the treatment of assaultive patients with dementia. *J Geriatr Psychiatry Neurol* 1:21–23, 1988.

Perenyi A, Arato M: Tardive dyskinesia on Hungarian psychiatric wards. *Psychosomatics* 21:904, 1980.

Petrie WM, Ban TA: Propranolol in organic agitation. *Lancet* 1:324, 1981.

Poeck K: Pathophysiology of emotional disorders associated with brain damage, in Vinken PJ, Bruyn GW (eds): *Handbook of Clinical Neurology*. Amsterdam, North-Holland Publishing Co, 1969, vol 3, pp 343–367.

Pope HG Jr, Keck PE Jr, McElroy SL: Frequency and presentation of neuroleptic malignant syndrome in a large psychiatric hospital. *Am J Psychiatry* 143:1227, 1233, 1986.

Post RM, Uhde TW: Carbamazepine in bipolar illness. *Psychopharmacol Bull* 21:10–17, 1985.

Post RM: Mechanisms of action of carbamazepine and related anticonvulsants in affective illness, in *Psychopharmacology: A Generation of Progress*. New York, Raven Press, 1987.

Post RM: Use of the anticonvulsant carbamazepine in primary and secondary affective illness: Clinical and theoretical implications. *Psychol Med* 12:701–704, 1982.

Poursines Y, Alliez J, Toga M: Syndrome parkinsonian consecutif a la prise prolongee de chlorpromazine avec ictus mortel intercurrent. *Rev Neurol (Paris)* 100:745, 1959.

Rao KJ, Miller M, Moses A: Water intoxication and thioridazine (Mellaril). *Ann Intern Med* 82:61, 1975.

Raskind M: Psychosis, polydipsia and water intoxication. *Arch Gen Psychiatry* 30:112–114, 1974.

Risse SC, Barnes R: Pharmacologic treatment of agitation associated with dementia. *J Am Geriatr Soc* 34:368–376, 1986.

Rivera JLGD: Inappropriate secretion of antidiuretic hormone from fluphenazine therapy. *Ann Intern Med* 82:811–812, 1975.

Rodova A, Nahunek R: Persistent dyskinesia after phenothiazines. *Cesk Psychiatr* 60:250, 1964.

Roizin L, True C, Kuigut M: Structural effects of tranquilizers. *Res Pubi Assoc Res Nerv Ment Dis* 37:285, 1959.

Rosenbaum F, Harati Y, Freedman M: Visual hallucinations in sane people: Charles Bonnet syndrome. *J Am Geriatr Soc* 35:66–68, 1987.

Rosenfield A, Maine D, Rochat, R, et al: The Food and Drug Administration and medroxyprogesterone acetate. *JAMA* 249:2922–2928, 1983.

Rubin EH, Drevets WC, Burke WJ: The nature of psychotic symptoms in senile dementia of the Alzheimer type. *J Geriatr Psychiatry Neurol* 1:16–20, 1988.

Rubin EH, Drevets WC: The progression of personality changes in senile dementia of the Alzheimer type (SDAT). *J Am Geriatr Soc* 13: 1629, 1987.

Rubin EH, Morris JC, Berg L: The progression of personality changes in senile dementia of the Alzheimer type (SDAT). *J Am Geriatr Soc* 35:721–725, 1987a.

Rubin EH, Morris JC, Storandt M, et al: Behavior changes in patients with mild senile dementia of the Alzheimer's type. *Psychiatry Res* 21:55–62, 1987.

Sangal R, Dimitrijevic R: Neuroleptic malignant syndrome: successful treatment with pancuronium. *JAMA* 154:2795–2796, 1985.

Schreier HA: Use of propranolol in the treatment of postencephalitic psychosis. *Am J Psychiatry* 136:840–841, 1979.

Shalev A, Munitz H: The neuroleptic malignant syndrome: agent and host interaction. *Acta Psychiatr Scand* 73:337–347, 1986.

Sheard MH: Effect of lithium in human aggression. *Nature* 230:113–114, 1971.

Sheard MH: Lithium in the treatment of aggression. *J Nerv Ment Dis* 160:108–118, 1975.

Sheppard GP: High dose propranolol in schizophrenia. *Br J Psychiatry* 134:470–476, 1979.

Simpson DN, Foster D: Improvement in organically disturbed behaviour with trazodone treatment. *Gen Clin Psychiatry* 47:192–193, 1986.

Smith JM, Baldessarini RJ: Changes in prevalence, severity, and recovery in tardive dyskinesia with age. *Arch Gen Psychiatry* 37:1368, 1980.

Smith LM, Peroutka SJ: Differential effects of 5-hydroxytryptamine 1A selective drugs on the 5-HT behavioral syndrome. *Pharmacol Biochem Behav* 24:1513–1519, 1986.

Snyder SH, Banerjee SP, Yamamura HI, et al: Drugs, neurotransmitters and schizophrenia. *Science* 184:1234–1253, 1974.

Sos J, Cassem NH: Intravenous use of haloperidol for acute delirium in intensive care settings, in Speidel H, Rodewald G (eds): *Psychic and Neurological Dysfunctions after Open-Heart Surgery*. Stuttgart, Georg Thieme Verlag, 1980, pp 196–199.

Spira N, Dysken MW, Lazarus LW, et al: Treatment of agitation and psychosis, in Salzman C (ed): *Clinical Geriatric Psychopharmacology*. New York, McGraw-Hill Book, 1984, pp 49–76.

Strang RR: The symptoms of restless legs. *Med J Aust* (24):1211–1213, 1967.

Teri L, Larson EB, Reifler BV: Behavioral disturbance in dementia of the Alzheimer's type. *J Am Geriatr Soc* 36:1–6, 1988.

Tunks ER: Carbamazepine in the dyscontrol syndrome associated with limbic system dysfunction. *J Nerv Ment Dis* 164:56, 1977.

Tupin JP, Smith DB, Classon TL, et al: Long-term use of lithium in aggressive prisoners. *Compr Psychiatry* 14:311–317, 1973.

Udaka F, Yamao S, Nagata H, et al: Pathologic laughing and crying treated with levodopa. *Arch Neurol* 41:1095–1096, 1984.

Uhrbrand L, Faurbye A: Reversible and irreversible dyskinesia after treatment with perphenazine, chlorpromazine, reserpine, ECT therapy. *Psychopharmacologia* 1:408, 1960.

Van Putten T, Mutalipassi LR, Malkin MD: Phenothiazine-induced decompensation. *Arch Gen Psychiatry* 30:102–105, 1974.

Van Putten T: The many faces of akathisia. *Compr Psychiatry* 16:43–47, 1975.

Wasman M, Flynn JP: Direct attack elicited from hypothalamus. *Arch Neurol* 6:220–227, 1972.

White NJ: Complex visual hallucinations in partial blindness due to eye disease. *Br J Psychiatry* 136:284–286, 1980.

Williamson B: Psychiatry since lithium. *Dis Nerv Syst* 27:775–782, 1966.

Winograd CH, Jarvik LF: Physician management of the demented patient. *J Am Geriatr Soc* 34:295–308, 1986.

Wolf JK, Santana JB, Thorpy M: Treatment of emotional incontinence with levodopa. *Neurology* 29:1435–1436, 1979.

Yudofsky S, Williams D, Gorman J: Propranolol in the treatment of rage and violent behavior in patients with chronic brain syndrome. *Am J Psychiatry* 138:218–220, 1981.

7

Anxiety Disorders of Old Age

OVERVIEW

Results of older studies (Shepherd and Gruenberg, 1957) indicated that the prevalence of anxiety disorders peaked during early adulthood and was followed by a rapid decline in prevalence from middle age onward; it was generally believed that anxiety states were not a major problem in older age (Lader, 1982). Findings of more recent studies, however, indicated otherwise (Lader, 1982; Primrose, 1962; Kessel and Shepherd, 1962). An estimated 10% to 15% of women over the age of 65 experience anxiety sufficiently severe to warrant medical intervention (Turnbull and Turnbull, 1985).

Results from the Epidemiologic Catchment Area (ECA) study by the National Institute of Mental Health (Myers et al, 1984) indicated that, for the elderly, the prevalence of panic disorder, obsessive-compulsive disorder, and phobias combined ranged between 5.7% and 33% for the three investigation sites. Phobias were the most common psychiatric disorder in elderly women and the second most common in elderly men.

Unfortunately, the presence of anxiety symptoms alone often does not serve as a sufficient impetus to seek help; Shader and associates (1982), for example, revealed that even patients with severe anxiety symptoms wait to seek treatment for 12 years, on the average, after the onset of symptoms. Another difficulty is that elderly patients with anxiety disorders often may present with physical complaints that mask the underlying disorder.

Even though roughly 11% of the population is over the age of 65, this group uses about 25% of all prescription and over-the-counter drugs sold, a large proportion of which are aimed at the alleviation of anxiety. For these reasons, physicians who care for the elderly should be aware of a number of special considerations (Jenike, 1982 and 1983; Altesman and Cole, 1983).

The prudent clinician, when evaluating an anxious elderly patient will perform a careful mental status evaluation of cognition, affect, and psychotic symptoms (CAP, see chapter 2). Anxiety states in a depressed, or demented, or psychotic patient may require quite different interventions. Anxiety and agitation are sometimes prominent symptoms of both dementia and depression, which often creates diagnostic confusion.

DIFFERENTIAL DIAGNOSIS

Anxiety is a universal human experience and generally should not be regarded as an indication for medication. It can, however, reach disabling proportions and can also be associated with phobias and panic attacks. The elderly, in fact, may present with any of the DSM-III-R (1987) anxiety disorders. New onset panic attacks occur in the elderly but are rarely discussed in the medical literature. As noted, phobic anxiety is also more common than is generally appreciated (Lader, 1982) since the elderly may be embarrassed by their symptoms and conceal them behind protestations of physical illness or debility. Social phobias, on the other hand, seem relatively uncommon in the elderly. Numerous factors, such as loss of friends and loved ones, failing health, intellectual decline, feelings of helplessness and worthlessness, and loss of control over the immediate environment, make the elderly particularly susceptible to anxiety states.

The essential features of panic disorder are recurrent panic attacks which are characterized by discrete periods of intense fear or discomfort, with at least four characteristic associated symptoms (Table 7–1). Such attacks usually last a few minutes, but can occasionally last for a few hours. This diagnosis is made only when no organic factor is thought to be involved etiologically.

Panic attacks typically start suddenly with feelings of apprehension, fear, or terror, often with a feeling of impending death or disaster. Most patients who have repeated panic attacks have at least some symptoms of agoraphobia (Table 7–2), the fear of being in public places from which escape might be difficult or embarrassing or in which help might not be available in the event of a panic attack. Agoraphobia usually results in either travel restrictions or need for a companion when away from home. Common agoraphobic situations include being outside the home alone; being in a crowd or standing in a line; being on a bridge; and traveling in a bus, train, or car (DSM-III-R, 1987).

Elderly patients also occasionally present with generalized anxiety disorder (Table 7–3), social phobia (Table 7–4), simple phobias (Table 7–5), and posttraumatic stress disorder (Table 7–6). Obsessive-compulsive disorders, also included in DSM-III-R under anxiety disorders, are covered in detail in chapter 11 and are not reviewed here.

The elderly patient who presents with an anxiety disorder should receive a thorough physical examination and pertinent laboratory tests, and a careful history must be obtained. Before drug treatment for anxiety is considered, the possibility of organicity, drug reactions, or nondrug toxicity must be taken into account.

Table 7–1
Diagnostic Criteria for Panic Disorder

A. At some time during the disturbance, one or more panic attacks (discrete periods of intense fear or discomfort) have occurred that were (1) unexpected, ie, did not occur immediately before or on exposure to a situation that almost always caused anxiety, and (2) not triggered by situations in which the person was the focus of others' attention.
B. Either four attacks, as defined in criterion A, have occurred within a four-week period, or one or more attacks have been followed by a period of at least a month of persistent fear of having another attack.
C. At least four of the following symptoms developed during at least one of the attacks:
    (1) shortness of breath (dyspnea) or smothering sensations
    (2) dizziness, unsteady feelings, or faintness
    (3) palpitations or accelerated heart rate (tachycardia)
    (4) trembling or shaking
    (5) sweating
    (6) choking
    (7) nausea or abdominal distress
    (8) depersonalization or derealization
    (9) numbness or tingling sensations (paresthesias)
    (10) flushes (hot flashes) or chills
    (11) chest pain or discomfort
    (12) fear of dying
    (13) fear of going crazy or doing something uncontrolled
Note: Attacks involving four or more symptoms are panic attacks; attacks involving fewer than four symptoms are limited symptom attacks.
D. During at least some of the attacks, at least four of the C symptoms developed suddenly and increased in intensity within ten minutes of the beginning of the first C symptom noticed in the attack.
E. It cannot be established that an organic factor initiated and maintained the disturbance, eg, amphetamine or caffeine intoxication, hyperthyroidism.
Note: Mitral valve prolapse may be an associated condition, but does not preclude a diagnosis of panic disorder.

Reprinted with permission from the *Diagnostic and Statistical Manual of Mental Disorders, third edition, revised.* Copyright 1987. American Psychiatric Association.

The clinician must determine whether the anxiety condition in an elderly patient represents a persistence of earlier patterns into old age or whether it has recently arisen (Lader, 1982). Although many social factors can play a role in either type of anxiety, new onset illness requires particularly careful evaluation of physical as well as mental factors (see Table 7–7). There is a close association between physical illness and anxiety disorders in old age.

When anxious patients with long-standing symptoms are compared with those with late-onset anxiety, the latter group had less childhood maladjustment and fewer premorbid neurotic symptoms, had experienced more social deprivation in old age, and had more physical illness, particularly cardiac disease (Bergmann, 1971). Depression was more characteristic than anxiety in most

Table 7–2
Diagnostic Criteria for Agoraphobia

Agoraphobia: Fear of being in places or situations from which escape might be difficult (or embarrassing) or in which help might not be available in the event of a panic attack. (Includes cases in which persistent avoidance behavior originated during an active phase of panic disorder, even if the person does not attribute the avoidance behavior to fear of having a panic attack.) As a result of this fear, the person either restricts travel or needs a companion when away from home, or else endures agoraphobic situations despite intense anxiety. Common agoraphobic situations include being outside the home alone, being in a crowd or standing in a line, being on a bridge, and traveling in a bus, train, or car.

Specify current severity of agoraphobic avoidance:
Mild: Some avoidance (or endurance with distress), but relatively normal life-style, eg, travels unaccompanied when necessary, such as to work or to shop; otherwise avoids traveling alone.
Moderate: Avoidance results in constricted life-style, eg, the person is able to leave the house alone, but not to go more than a few miles unaccompanied.
Severe: Avoidance results in being nearly or completely housebound or unable to leave the house unaccompanied.
In Partial Remission: No current agoraphobic avoidance, but some agoraphobic avoidance during the past six months.
In Full Remission: No current agoraphobic avoidance and none during the past six months.

Specify current severity of panic attacks:
Mild: During the past month, either all attacks have been limited symptom attacks (ie, fewer than four symptoms), or there has been no more than one panic attack.
Moderate: During the past month attacks have been intermediate between "mild" and "severe."
Severe: During the past month, there have been at least eight panic attacks.
In Partial Remission: The condition has been intermediate between "In Full Remission" and "Mild."
In Full Remission: During the past six months, there have been no panic or limited symptom attacks.

Reprinted with permission from the *Diagnostic and Statistical Manual of Mental Disorders, third editon, revised.* Copyright 1987. American Psychiatric Association.

patients with late-onset anxiety, whereas anxiety alone was more common in patients whose symptoms had persisted from early life.

In addition to dementing illnesses and toxic states, a few well-delineated physical conditions may be characterized by symptoms of anxiety (Lader, 1982; Shader and Greenblatt, 1982). The most important of these conditions is hyperthyroidism which often presents in the elderly in an atypical way, with few of the classic physical signs. Sweating, tachycardia, cardiac arrhythmias, or frank heart failure that responds poorly to conventional treatment can be the presenting symptoms (Lader, 1982). Anxiety or restlessness without recognizable cause can also occur. Detailed thyroid tests are necessary.

Table 7–3
Diagnostic Criteria for 300.02 Generalized
Anxiety Disorder

A. Unrealistic or excessive anxiety and worry (apprehensive expectation) about two or more life circumstances, eg, worry about possible misfortune to one's child (who is in no danger) and worry about finances (for no good reason), for a period of six months or longer, during which the person has been bothered more days than not by these concerns. In children and adolescents,this may take the form of anxiety and worry about academic, athletic, and social performance.

B. If another Axis I disorder is present, the focus of the anxiety and worry in A is unrelated to it, eg, the anxiety or worry is not about having a panic attack (as in panic disorder), being embarrassed in public (as in social phobia), being contaminated (as in obsessive-compulsive disorder), or gaining weight (as in anorexia nervosa).

C. The disturbance does not occur only during the course of a mood disorder or a psychotic disorder.

D. At least 6 of the following 18 symptoms are often present when anxious (do not include symptoms present only during panic attacks):

Motor tension
(1) trembling, twitching, or feeling shaky
(2) muscle tension, aches, or soreness
(3) restlessness
(4) easy fatigability

Autonomic hyperactivity
(5) shortness of breath or smothering sensations
(6) palpitations or accelerated heart rate (tachycardia)
(7) sweating, or cold clammy hands
(8) dry mouth
(9) dizziness or lightheadedness
(10) nausea, diarrhea, or other abdominal distress
(11) flushes (not flashes) or chills
(12) frequent urination
(13) trouble swallowing or "lump in throat"

Vigilance and scanning
(14) feeling keyed up or on edge
(15) exaggerated startle response
(16) difficulty concentrating or "mind going blank" because of anxiety
(17) trouble falling or staying asleep
(18) irritability

E. It cannot be established that an organic factor initiated and maintained the disturbance, eg, hyperthyroidism, caffeine intoxication.

Reprinted with permission from the *Diagnostic and Statistical Manual of Mental Disorders, third edition, revised*. Copyright 1987. American Psychiatric Association.

Also, amine-secreting tumors, such as pheochromocytoma, can present with anxiety, and the possibility of amine secretion from a secondary tumor should be borne in mind. Usually, however, blood pressure is markedly raised, either episodically or continuously, which is atypical of simple anxiety states.

Ingestion of a number of drugs can closely mimic an anxiety state. Caffeinism may occur in the elderly, even without increased intake of coffee,

Table 7–4
Diagnostic Criteria for 300.23 Social Phobia

A. A persistent fear of one or more situations (the social phobic situations) in which the person is exposed to possible scrutiny by others and fears that he or she may do something or act in a way that will be humiliating or embarrassing. Examples include: being unable to continue talking while speaking in public, choking on food when eating in front of others, being unable to urinate in a public lavatory, hand-trembling when writing in the presence of others, and saying foolish things or not being able to answer questions in social situations.
B. If an Axis III or Axis I disorder is present, the fear in A is unrelated to it, eg, the fear is not of having a panic attack (panic disorder), stuttering (stuttering), trembling (Parkinson's disease), or exhibiting abnormal eating behavior (anorexia nervosa or bulimia nervosa).
C. During some phase of the disturbance, exposure to the specific phobic stimulus (or stimuli) almost invariably provokes an immediate anxiety response.
D. The phobic situation(s) is avoided, or is endured with intense anxiety.
E. The avoidant behavior interferes with occupational functioning or with usual social activities or relationships with others, or there is marked distress about having the fear.
F. The person recognizes that his or her fear is excessive or unreasonable.
G. If the person is under 18, the disturbance does not meet the criteria for avoidant disorder of childhood or adolescence.

Specify generalized type if the phobic situation includes most social situations, and also consider the additional diagnosis of avoidant personality disorder.

Reprinted with permission from the *Diagnostic and Statistical Manual of Mental Disorders, third edition, revised.* Copyright 1987. American Psychiatric Association.

because of increased sensitivity to stimulants. Other drugs associated with anxiety include amphetamines and other sympathomimetics, such as ephedrine, appetite suppressants, and corticosteroids (Lader, 1982). Patients should be questioned about coffee and tea drinking habits and about the use of other medications and over-the-counter agents.

Withdrawal from prescribed sedatives and tranquilizers, particularly barbiturates and benzodiazepines, but sometimes also antidepressants, is often associated with anxiety.

Sometimes hospitalization, even for a relatively benign condition, can produce marked anxiety, particularly because of prevalent fears of undetected underlying cancer or because dependency, further isolation, or changes in routine can be destabilizing (Shader and Greenblatt, 1982).

It is also reported that individuals of below-average intelligence are particularly at risk for the development of anxiety late in life (Lader, 1982).

Before pharmacologic treatment is started, it is important to rule out medical causes of anxiety (Table 7–7) and to discuss possible precipitating factors with the patient. Occasionally, treatment of a medical condition will resolve superimposed anxious feelings. For example, the patient with hypoxia secondary to congestive heart failure may feel much less anxious after treatment with digitalis and a diuretic (Dietch, 1981).

Table 7–5
Diagnostic Criteria for 300.29 Simple Phobia

A. A persistent fear of a circumscribed stimulus (object or situation) other than fear of having a panic attack (as in panic disorder) or of humiliation or embarrassment in certain social situations (as in social phobia).
   Note: Do not include fears that are part of panic disorder with agoraphobia or agoraphobia without history of panic disorder.
B. During some phase of the disturbance, exposure to the specific phobic stimulus (or stimuli) almost invariably provokes an immediate anxiety response.
C. The object or situation is avoided, or endured with intense anxiety.
D. The fear or the avoidant behavior significantly interferes with the person's normal routine or with usual social activities or relationships with others, or there is marked distress about having the fear.
E. The person recognizes that his or her fear is excessive or unreasonable.
F. The phobic stimulus is unrelated to the content of the obsessions of obsessive-compulsive disorder or the trauma of post-traumatic stress disorder.

Reprinted with permission from the *Diagnostic and Statistical Manual of Mental Disorders, third edition, revised.* Copyright 1987. American Psychiatric Association.

When there is a clear precipitating event, discussion of the problem or suggestion of an alternative solution may be adequate. If an elderly person in a nursing home is anxious, for example, because the patient in the next bed died last evening, it would be inappropriate to treat such anxiety initially with medication. Occasionally, anxiety can be alleviated by environmental manipulation or by discussion of the patient's problems in a direct manner (see chapter 11). When medical causes have been ruled out and when no precipitating factor for the anxiety can be identified, antianxiety drugs may be useful.

CONSEQUENCES OF ALTERED PHYSIOLOGY IN THE ELDERLY

The clinically significant physiologic concomitants of aging, as reviewed in chapter 3, must be considered before antianxiety agents are prescribed. These include changes in absorption, distribution, protein binding, hepatic metabolism, and renal excretion of drugs. Some of these changes, as they pertain to antianxiety agents, are briefly reviewed.

There are several age-related changes in the gut of the elderly, but these seem to have little, if any, effect on drug absorption (Shader and Greenblatt, 1982). Splanchnic blood flow decreases and gastric pH increases with age. Both active absorption processes and passive transport, which is important in drug absorption, are altered in the elderly (Omslander, 1981).

The proportion of total body fat generally increases with age, especially in women, and this increases the volume of distribution of lipid soluble drugs, such as diazepam (Valium), and greatly prolongs drug half-life. In addition, body water may decrease in the same period; thus, water-soluble drugs, such

Table 7–6
Diagnostic Criteria for 309.89 Post-traumatic
Stress Disorder

A. The person has experienced an event that is outside the range of usual human experience and that would be markedly distressing to almost anyone, eg, serious threat to one's life or physical integrity; serious threat or harm to one's children, spouse, or other close relatives and friends; sudden destruction of one's home or community; or seeing another person who has recently been, or is being, seriously injured or killed as the result of an accident or physical violence.

B. The traumatic event is persistently reexperienced in at least one of the following ways:
   (1) recurrent and intrusive distressing recollections of the event (in young children, repetitive play in which themes or aspects of the trauma are expressed)
   (2) recurrent distressing dreams of the event
   (3) sudden acting or feeling as if the traumatic event were recurring (includes a sense of reliving the experience, illusions, hallucinations, and dissociative [flashback] episodes, even those that occur upon awakening or when intoxicated)
   (4) intense psychological distress at exposure to events that symbolize or resemble an aspect of the traumatic event, including anniversaries of the trauma

C. Persistent avoidance of stimuli associated with the trauma or numbing of general responsiveness (not present before the trauma), as indicated by at least three of the following:
   (1) efforts to avoid thoughts or feelings associated with the trauma
   (2) efforts to avoid activities or situations that arouse recollections of the trauma
   (3) inability to recall an important aspect of the trauma (psychogenic amnesia)
   (4) markedly diminished interest in significant activities (in young children, loss of recently acquired developmental skills such as toilet training or language skills)
   (5) feeling of detachment or estrangement from others
   (6) restricted range of affect, eg, unable to have loving feelings
   (7) sense of a foreshortened future, eg, does not expect to have a career, marriage, or children, or a long life

D. Persistent symptoms of increased arousal (not present before the trauma), as indicated by at least two of the following:
   (1) difficulty falling or staying asleep
   (2) irritability or outbursts of anger
   (3) difficulty concentrating
   (4) hypervigilance
   (5) exaggerated startle response
   (6) physiologic reactivity upon exposure to events that symbolize or resemble an aspect of the traumatic event (eg, a woman who was raped in an elevator breaks out in a sweat when entering any elevator)

E. Duration of the disturbance (symptoms B, C, and D) of at least one month.

Specify delayed onset if the onset of symptoms was at least six months after the trauma.

Table 7–7
Physical Disorders Often Presenting with Anxiety

Cardiovascular	*Endocrinologic* (continued)
Myocardial infarction	Carcinoid syndrome
Paroxysmal atrial tachycardia	Hypothermia
Mitral valve prolapse	Cushing's disease
	Hyperkalemia
Dietary	
Caffeine	*Hematologic*
Vitamin deficiencies	Anemia
Drug-Related	*Immunologic*
Akathisia	Systemic lupus erythematosus
Anticholinergic toxicity	
Antihypertensive side effects	*Neurologic*
Digitalis toxicity	CNS infections
Withdrawal syndromes:	CNS masses
alcohol, sedative-hypnotics	Toxins
	Temporal lobe epilepsy
Endocrinologic	Postconcussion syndrome
Insulinoma	
Hypoglycemia	*Pulmonary*
Hypo- or hyperthyroidism	Chronic obstructive lung disease
Hypo- or hypercalcemia	Pneumonia
Pheochromocytoma	Hypoxia

Reproduced with permission from Jenike MA: *Handbook of Geriatric Psychopharmacology.* Littleton, Mass, PSG Publishing, 1985, p 98.

as ethanol, will have higher concentrations in the elderly because of an apparent decrease in the size of their reservoir (Crook and Cohen, 1981).

A number of studies have demonstrated a 15% to 25% reduction in serum albumin levels in patients over the age of 60 years, as compared with persons under the age of 40 (Schumacher, 1980; Bender et al, 1975; Hayes et al, 1975; Wallace et al, 1976; Greenblatt, 1979). Because most sedatives are highly protein-bound, this decrease in protein-binding sites in the elderly liberates more free active drug into the circulation and increases the risk of toxicity. Activity of hepatic cytochrome P-450 may decrease with age, and demethylation slows, leading to higher levels of unmetabolized drug. Other factors, such as cigarette smoking, alcohol consumption, and administration of other drugs, also influence the rate of hepatic clearance.

After the age of 40, the glomerular filtration rate (GFR) and renal plasma flow normally decline progressively, by approximately 50% by the age of 70 (Papper, 1978). This results in a longer duration of drug action and increases the likelihood of toxicity if dosage is not adjusted.

In addition to these pharmacokinetic changes in the elderly, decreased CNS dopamine and acetylcholine levels can lead to increased sensitivity to extrapyramidal and anticholinergic side effects, respectively. An increased tendency to CNS disinhibition increases the likelihood of drug-associated confusion, sedation, and paradoxical reactions.

EARLY ANTIANXIETY AGENTS

In the early part of the twentieth century, bromides were used as antianxiety drugs. In the 1930s, however, they were implicated as the cause of a toxic delirium, which resulted from their accumulation with chronic use. Until the early 1950s, phenobarbital was also commonly used as an antianxiety agent, and shorter-acting barbiturates, such as secobarbital and amobarbital, were used as hypnotics. However, the potential for tolerance, physical dependence, and the development of a life-threatening withdrawal syndrome with these drugs made them far from ideal.

After meprobamate (Miltown) was introduced, it became so popular that manufacturers could not keep up with the demand, even though it differed only slightly from barbiturates (Hollister, 1978). The structure of meprobamate was manipulated to produce numerous similar drugs such as glutethimide and methyprylon (Noludar). As dissatisfaction with the barbiturates increased, other drugs, such as ethchlorvynol (Placidyl), enjoyed a brief period of popularity. The enthusiasm for these drugs dwindled, however, as clinicians realized that they had many of the same drawbacks as the barbiturates. Meprobamate, for example, carries an unacceptable risk of addiction and fatality on overdose; in fact, the addicting dose overlaps with the therapeutic range. Although the therapeutic range is 1,200 to 2,400 mg/d (Baldessarini, 1977), physical signs of withdrawal can occur with the discontinuation of doses as low as 1,200 mg/day; severe withdrawal signs and seizures can be expected at doses above 3,200 mg/day.

Although these drugs are still on the market, with the advent of safer and more effective medications, such as the benzodiazepines, they no longer have a place in the treatment of anxiety in the elderly.

ANTIDEPRESSANTS

Antidepressant medications are currently the cornerstone of treatment of panic disorder (Griest and Jefferson, 1988), as they have been shown to substantially reduce the frequency and severity of spontaneous panic attacks and often block them altogether (see chapter 4 for guidelines on usage). Antidepressants will also likely improve anxious feelings associated with depressed states in the elderly.

When elderly patients are both depressed and markedly anxious both an antidepressant and low doses of a short-acting benzodiazepine can be started together, with the benzodiazepine discontinued gradually as the symptoms improve.

BENZODIAZEPINES

Overview

Introduced in 1960, chlordiazepoxide (Librium) was the first benzodiazepine to come on the market. Many others soon followed, including diazepam, flurazepam (Dalmane), clorazepate dipotassium (Tranxene), oxazepam (Serax), lorazepam (Ativan), and prazepam (Centrax). The benzodiazepines have been shown to be superior to placebo, barbiturates, meprobamate, and the sedative-type antihistamines in most clinical trials of anxious patients (Cole, 1978; Davies et al, 1977; Douglas, 1975; Bernstein, 1979; Salzman, 1981), although no one benzodiazepine has been shown to be superior to any other in relieving anxiety.

In the elderly, benzodiazepines are closer to the ideal sedative-hypnotic than other drugs currently available. They are less addicting than the antianxiety drugs typically used in earlier years, and are unlikely to cause lethal overdosage when they are taken alone. Most of the fatalities associated with benzodiazepine overdosage have occurred when other respiratory depressants, such as alcohol, were also ingested.

Each of the benzodiazepines produces more sedation as dosage is increased, but antianxiety effects are exhibited at lower doses. This has been attributed to their primary action on the limbic system, which is believed to control anxiety, fear, and rage. As no benzodiazepine has been shown to be better at relieving anxiety than any other (Baldessarini, 1977; Cole, 1978; Davies et al, 1977; Douglas, 1975), the choice of an individual drug for an elderly patient should be based on the potential for serious side effects.

Although there are many similarities among benzodiazepines, there are interdrug differences that are clinically significant in elderly patients (Table 7–8). Benzodiazepines can be divided into two groups on the basis of metabolism.

Short-Acting Agents

One group consists of relatively short-acting drugs that are simply conjugated to glucuronide in the liver and then eliminated in the urine (Greenblatt, 1980). Lorazepam and oxazepam, two drugs in this category, are especially attractive choices in the elderly because they have a short half-life and no active metabolites, and their metabolism is affected only slightly, if at all, by the physiologic changes that accompany aging (Koepke et al, 1982). The main disadvantage of these drugs is that they may have to be given more than once a day. Initial dosage should be 10 mg of oxazepam or 0.5 mg of lorazepam two or three times daily. Lorazepam is the only benzodiazepine that is well absorbed intramuscularly (Schuckit, 1983 and 1984) and may be particularly useful when oral dosing is impossible.

Table 7-8
Comparison of Benzodiazepine Anxiolytics

Drug	Rate of Onset	Half-Life (h)	Active Metabolites	Half-Life of Metabolites (h)	Doses (mg/d) Adult	Elderly	Route of Administration
Oxazepam (Serax)	Intermediate to slow	5–15	None	—	10–60	10–30	Oral
Lorazepam (Ativan)	Intermediate	10–20	None	—	1–4	0.5–4.0	Oral, IM, IV
Diazepam (Valium)	Fastest	26–53	Yes	36–200	5–30	2–10	Oral, IM, IV†
Chlordiazepoxide HCl (Librium)	Intermediate	8–28	Yes	36–200	10–100	5–30	Oral, IM, IV†
Prazepam (Centrax)	Slow	30–200	Yes	36–200	20–60	10–15	Oral
Clorazepate dipotassium (Tranxene)	Fast	30–200	Yes	36–200	15–60	7.5–15	Oral
Alprazolam (Xanax)	Intermediate	6–15	Yes	*	0.25–2.0	0.125–0.5	Oral
Halazepam (Paxipam)	Intermediate to slow	14	Yes	36–200	20–120		Oral
Triazolam (Halcion)	Fast	2–5	—	—	0.25–0.5	0.25–0.5	Oral
Temazepam (Restoril)	Intermediate to slow	12–24	—	—	15–30	15–30	Oral

*Unknown; probably about the same as the parent drug.
†IM doses unreliably absorbed.
Reproduced with permission from Jenike MA: *Handbook of Geriatric Psychopharmacology.* Littleton, Mass, PSG Publishing, 1985, p 101.

Long-Acting Agents

Drugs in the other category, such as diazepam, flurazepam, chlordiazepoxide, clorazepate, and prazepam, have a long duration of action, have long-acting active metabolites, and are slowly eliminated from the body. Their metabolism is profoundly affected by the physiologic concomitants of aging. For example, the mean half-life of diazepam's metabolites, which is 20 hours at the age of 20 years, increases to 90 hours at the age of 80 (Rosenbaum, 1979). The long half-lives of these drugs in the elderly can lead to accumulation with deleterious clinical effects. Their advantage, however, is that they can be given once a day or even every other day. Initial dosages of these drugs should be in the range of 2 to 5 mg/day of diazepam or its equivalent. Dosage should be increased cautiously, because it may take more than a week for steady-state levels to be reached with the longer-acting drugs.

Alprazolam (Xanax) is a benzodiazepine that is metabolized extensively in the liver. A number of metabolites have been identified but, because of their rapid clearance, none is known to exert significant biologic action (Abernathy et al, 1983). The elimination half-life of alprazolam increases significantly with age in men but not in women. The mean half-life in young males is 11 hours and this increases to 19 hours in elderly men (Greenblatt et al, 1983).

Benzodiazepine Withdrawal

The physical manifestations of withdrawal syndromes due to abrupt discontinuation of any of the benzodiazepines are similar (Jenike, 1984). However, drugs with longer half-lives tend to produce onset of withdrawal syndromes later than those with shorter half-lives (Hollister et al, 1961; Pevnick et al, 1978; Einarson, 1980; Khan et al, 1980; Jenike, 1984). Minor withdrawal symptoms include elevated pulse and respiration rates, postural hypotension, coarse rhythmic intention tremors, hyperreflexia, muscular weakness and aching, apprehension, anorexia, insomnia, and profuse sweating. Severe withdrawal symptoms can include hyperthermia, delirium, generalized convulsions, and psychosis that can include paranoia with visual and auditory hallucinations.

Because withdrawal seizures are thought to be due to a rapid drop in blood level, patients who have been taking large doses for a long time should be very slowly weaned off the drug. Addicting doses of diazepam have been estimated at 80 to 120 mg for 40 to 50 days; for chlordiazepoxide, 300 to 600 mg for 60 to 180 days (Jenike, 1984). Addicting doses of the shorter-acting agents are more difficult to estimate, but there was one report of a patient who took 12 mg of lorazepam daily who had a grand mal seizure 72 hours after stopping the drug (Einarson, 1980).

Memory Impairment with Benzodiazepines

There are a number of anecdotal reports that various benzodiazepines can interfere with memory (Angus and Romney, 1984; Scharf et al, 1983; Pandit et al, 1976; Bixler et al, 1979; Roth et al, 1980; McKay and Dundee, 1980; Petersen and Ghoneim, 1980; Barclay, 1982; George and Dundee, 1977; Kothary et al, 1981). Some authors believe that benzodiazepines interfere with both short-term and long-term memory, and most think that they interfere with the memory consolidation process.

There is some new evidence that the new short-acting benzodiazepine triazolam (Halcion) produces an anterograde amnestic effect while it does not interfere with immediate recall (Scharf et al, 1988; Bixler et al, 1987). In young adults, triazolam and also lorazepam were demonstrated to have similar effects on memory while a longer-acting agent, clorazepate (Tranxene), did not cause such effects (Scharf et al, 1983 and 1985).

On the other hand, some investigators found that benzodiazepines actually enhance recall in patients who have generalized anxiety disorder (Brown et al, 1978; Liljequist, 1978; Hartley, 1980; Fabre and Putman, 1988), and others found that, in a sample of normal student volunteers, a low dose of diazepam (5 mg) impaired short-term memory of low-anxiety subjects but actually improved memory in high-anxiety subjects (Barnett et al, 1981).

The bulk of the evidence indicates that the short-term benzodiazepines are more likely to induce memory deficits, mainly in tests of delayed recall, which appear to be dose related (Scharf et al, 1988). Clinically, at dosages recommended in this book, one does not frequently see isolated memory deficits in elderly patients who are not oversedated.

Dyscontrol in Patients Treated with Benzodiazepines

Periodic reports have suggested that benzodiazepines may be associated with a loss of control over aggressive impulses with manifestations ranging from irritability to increased verbal hostility to frank assaultiveness. After reviewing data from case reports, experimental studies, and incidence reports, Dietch and Jennings (1988) estimated the incidence of clinically adverse sequelae to be less than 1% and did not find any consistent predictive factors. Clinical experience, however, indicates that dementing patients treated with benzodiazepines may be at higher risk for developing such reactions (see later section in this chapter).

Benzodiazepines in Patients with Liver Disease

Since the benzodiazepines are metabolized by the liver, special considerations apply when using these agents in patients with hepatic disease. Cirrhosis produces a twofold to threefold increase in the half-life of both diazepam and chlordiazepoxide relative to age-matched controls (Wilkinson and Schenker, 1975; Klotz et al, 1975; Ochs et al, 1983). Acute viral hepatitis has a similar but slightly smaller effect on plasma clearance, which is reversible on clinical recovery. Neither of these diseases has a significant effect on the disposition of oxazepam and lorazepam (Wilkinson and Schenker, 1975).

Ochs and colleagues (1983) clearly demonstrated that when given diazepam cirrhotic patients had more self-rated daytime sedation than normal control subjects. Sedation strongly correlated with total levels of diazepam and its major metabolite, desmethyldiazepam (Ochs et al, 1983). They concluded that reduced hepatic clearance of diazepam in cirrhotics leads to increased accumulation during long-term dosing, and recommended that diazepam could probably be given to cirrhotics safely provided daily dosage is reduced by approximately 50%.

In elderly patients with liver disease, it is probably wisest to use lorazepam or oxazepam as their metabolism is not significantly altered by such disease.

Benzodiazepines in Patients with Lung Disease

In general, benzodiazepines are thought to be safer drugs than barbiturates in terms of respiratory depression associated with overdosage (Cohn, 1983). A number of studies have shown that the longer-acting benzodiazepines do, however, have significant respiratory depressant effects (Utting and Pleuvry, 1975; Cohn, 1983; Rao et al, 1973; Huch and Huch, 1974; Catchlove and Kafer, 1971; Kronenberg et al, 1975). In contrast, short-acting agents seem to be much less likely to depress respiration. Steen and colleagues (1966) gave intravenous oxazepam (only approved for oral use) to four volunteers and could not show statistically significant change in the response to breathing elevated carbon dioxide levels. Others reported actual respiratory stimulation after oral doses of lorazepam (Dodson et al, 1976) and triazolam (Elliott et al, 1975). Temazepam, in oral doses of 40 mg, but not 20 mg, significantly depressed the ventilatory response to carbon dioxide in 12 healthy volunteers (Pleuvry et al, 1980).

Denaut and colleagues (1975) compared the respiratory effects of lorazepam and diazepam in 20 patients with chronic obstructive lung disease. Both drugs induced a respiratory depression with slight respiratory acidosis, but lorazepam caused no significant hypoxemia. They concluded that the respiratory depressant effects of both lorazepam and diazepam are modest; nevertheless, preference should be given to lorazepam because of its less prolonged duration of action with no modification of the arterial partial pressure of oxygen (PaO_2). At the present time, the bulk of the data supports lorazepam as the drug of first choice in the anxious elderly patient who has significant lung disease.

Benzodiazepine Overdose

Overall, benzodiazepines seem to be extremely safe when taken alone in overdose. Of deaths reported to the American Association of Poison Control

Table 7–9
Nonbenzodiazepine Anxiolytes

Type	Representative Drugs	Dose (mg)	Side Effects
Antihistamines	Diphenhydramine	25	Anticholinergic
	Hydroxyzine	25	Sedation
Neuroleptics	*High-potency*		
	Haloperidol	0.5 bid	Extrapyramidal
			Dystonia
	Thiothixene	1 bid	Akathesia
	Fluphenazine	1 bid	Tardive dyskinesia
	Low-potency		
	Chlorpromazine	10 bid	Orthostatic hypotension
	Thioridazine	10 bid	Sedation
			Tardive dyskinesia
β-Blockers*	Propranolol	40 qid*	Contraindications
	Atenolol	50–100	Asthma
			Sinus bradycardia
			Congestive heart failure
Serotonergic	Buspirone	5–15 tid	Nausea
			Dizziness
			Spacey feelings

*Kathol et al (1980).
Adapted with permission from Jenike MA: *Handbook of Geriatric Psychopharmacology*. Littleton, Mass, PSG Publishing, 1985, p 105.

Centers (Litovitz, 1987) over a four-year period, 66 involved benzodiazepines; however, only in five cases was the benzodiazepine the only drug ingested. Three deaths were associated with alprazolam (Xanax); one, with temazepam (Restoril); and one, with triazolam (Halcion). In only one of these five cases was a postmortem examination done, and in no case was the benzodiazepine level reported.

Two of the fatalities were in patients with profound underlying medical conditions that limited the extent of resuscitation: one had end-stage renal failure from severely complicated diabetes mellitus; the other had cancer and chronic obstructive pulmonary disease.

In general, clinical impressions of the safety of the benzodiazepines, even in the elderly, seem to hold true.

OTHER ANTIANXIETY AGENTS

Other drugs that have been used to treat anxiety are listed in Table 7–9.

Buspirone

Buspirone (Buspar) is a nonbenzodiazepine antianxiety agent, with partial serotonergic agonist properties, which has been demonstrated in a controlled trial to be as efficacious as diazepam in the treatment of anxiety states (Rickels et al, 1982). Preliminary data (Eison and Temple, 1986) indicated that buspirone is a 5-HT$_{1A}$ receptor agonist but not a "full" agonist (eg, it has no effect on type 2 serotonergic receptors). In a small open trial (n=14), it was not effective (see chapter 13) either for obsessive-compulsive symptoms or for the anxiety associated with such symptoms (Jenike and Baer, 1988).

Buspirone appears, however, to be well tolerated by elderly patients and has a large margin of safety. It is slowly acting and may take more than a week to have a full effect, so elderly patients should be cautioned not to expect rapid relief of symptoms.

Buspirone does not exhibit crosstolerance with benzodiazepines, and thus caution is required in switching from a benzodiazepine to buspirone so as not to produce a benzodiazepine withdrawal syndrome; that is; buspirone will not cover benzodiazepine withdrawal. There is at least one case report (Jerkovich and Preskorn, 1987) of an elderly man (age, 74 years) who was being treated with lorazepam, 1 mg three times a day, which was abruptly stopped as buspirone was initiated at a dose of 10 mg three times a day. Over several days the patient became more anxious, restless, and dysphoric, and he then became disorganized and confused. He eventually had two grand mal seizures before his symptoms were recognized as being due to benzodiazepine withdrawal; symptoms resolved within 36 hours after restarting lorazepam. Later, when lorazepam was discontinued over two weeks, the patient did well. This case indicates that when switching from a benzodiazepine to buspirone, gradual withdrawal of the benzodiazepine is important to avoid producing an abstinence syndrome.

Antihistamines

Antihistamines such as diphenhydramine (Benadryl) and hydroxyzine (Atarax, Vistaril) are sometimes prescribed for anxiety or insomnia, and they are also common ingredients in over-the-counter agents. Although they are frequently effective, antihistamines have many potential side effects, including disturbed coordination, weakness, inability to concentrate, urinary frequency, palpitations, and hypotension. In addition, their anticholinergic properties make them poor choices for patients taking other anticholinergic agents, such as tricyclic antidepressants, neuroleptics, and antiarrhythmic agents. An acute toxic delirium can result when antihistamines are coadministered with these agents, with such classic anticholinergic signs as blurred vision, dryness of the mouth, urinary retention, tachycardia, and constipation.

Antihistamines may be most useful in elderly patients with severe chronic obstructive lung disease, whose respiration may be easily depressed by other antianxiety agents. Antihistamines are much less likely to depress respiratory drive than most other drugs, except perhaps the high-potency neuroleptics. In patients with severe lung disease, sedatives could worsen respiratory depression and thereby, paradoxically, increase anxiety. If increasing anxiety is treated by an increase in medication, a lethal spiral may result (Shader and Greenblatt, 1977).

Neuroleptics

Neuroleptics are sometimes used in the treatment of severe anxiety and agitation. Low doses of a high-potency neuroleptic, such as haloperidol (Haldol), thiothixene (Navane), or fluphenazine (Permitil, Prolixin), are preferred in the elderly. Low-potency neuroleptics, such as chlorpromazine (Thorazine) and thioridazine (Mellaril), have more associated hypotensive, cardiovascular, and anticholinergic side effects. The low-potency agents may be preferred in patients who have movement disorders such as Parkinson's disease where they will be less likely to exacerbate extrapyramidal symptoms (see chapter 6).

Patients with organic brain disease may feel much better and exhibit less agitation, paranoia, antisocial behavior, and insomnia with doses as low as 0.5 mg of haloperidol (Haldol) or 1 mg of thiothixene (Navane) once or twice daily. Chlorpromazine and thioridazine should be used with initial doses as low as 10 mg once or twice daily (Jenike, 1985).

Neuroleptics should be used with caution, because elderly patients are much more sensitive to side effects such as tardive dyskinesia (Jenike, 1983a) (see chapter 6).

Beta-Blockers

Because anxiety often has both psychological and somatic components—palpitations, diaphoresis, tremulousness, urinary frequency, and tachycardia, which are mediated by the sympathetic nervous system—it is occasionally recommended that beta-blockers be used to alleviate this type of anxiety (Omslander, 1981; James, 1909; Pitts and McClure, 1967). Some investigators even believe that sometimes anxiety is the subjective feeling resulting primarily from the somatic manifestations (James, 1909); that is, one feels anxious because his or her heart beats fast, rather than tachycardia being a result of the anxiety. Others reproduced panic attacks by infusing lactate into susceptible patients (Pitts and McClure, 1967).

Agents such as propranolol hydrochloride (Inderal) can be used to block peripheral sympathetic concomitants of anxiety. One study (Kathol et al, 1980) reported that propranolol, 40 mg four times daily, not only reduced the somatic concomitants of anxiety, but also improved the psychological symptoms, such as apprehension and irritability. Propranolol may be helpful in patients who have clear-cut somatic concomitants to anxiety. Contraindications such as asthma, sinus bradycardia, and heart failure must be heeded.

Antidepressants

The depressed patient who is also anxious may respond best to a tricyclic antidepressant or, in more extreme cases, to ECT (see chapter 4). In fact, antianxiety drugs alone may make the depressed patient feel worse. Prescribing anxiolytic medication for an anxious individual whose primary diagnosis is depression might relieve the anxiety but will usually have no effect on the depressive symptomatology. This fact should also be kept in mind when a benzodiazepine is being considered for the treatment of insomnia, because sleep difficulties are frequently symptomatic of depression. The differential diagnosis can be difficult when the patient has symptoms of both anxiety and depression; a history of depressive illness and/or the absence of clear episodes of anxiety in the past suggest a diagnosis of depression (Crook, 1982).

Many depressed elderly patients show such classic signs of depression as decreased appetite and sleeplessness (or increased appetite and somnolence), inability to concentrate, fatigue, guilt, suicidal ideation, and psychomotor retardation or agitation. Some patients, however, appear more demented than depressed. A rapidly progressive dementia, especially in a previously depressed elderly patient, should alert the clinician to the possibility of pseudodementia secondary to depression (Wells, 1979; Jenike, 1985).

ANXIETY AND AGITATION IN DEMENTIA

Moderate anxiety is a natural reaction to the fear engendered by gradual deterioration of intellectual function and the realization of impending loss of control over one's life. Occasionally, extreme agitation and even overt aggression occur in patients with senile dementia, particularly in the later stages of the disease (see chapter 5). Possible causes of acute, severe agitation other than dementia, such as toxic drug reactions or withdrawal, metabolic or endocrine disorders, should be considered.

Despite having little to treat the primary illness, the clinician can usually alleviate severe agitation with medication and environmental manipulations. In early dementia, anxiety may be ameliorated simply by inducing the patient to reduce daily demands that can no longer be met and by providing, whenever possible, stable companionship. For example, an individual who is still attempting, in the face of progressive intellectual impairment, to hold a job or operate a business might be persuaded to retire. More severe patients who are living alone with some occasional support can become less anxious or agitated when given more care and attention in a nursing home. Sometimes even psychotic symptoms can be relieved nonpharmacologically by increasing the level of care of a decompensating patient.

Sedative-hypnotic agents sometimes disinhibit older patients or can increase irritability and thereby aggravate anxiety (Shader and Greenblatt, 1982). In such patients, low dosages of a high-potency antipsychotic drug might alleviate symptoms (see chapter 5).

DRUG INTERACTIONS

Since elderly patients frequently have medical problems, they often take several medications concomitantly. Among the drugs commonly used in the elderly that have CNS depressant effects are antihypertensive medications (eg, methyldopa, reserpine, or clonidine), other sedative-hypnotics, analgesics, tricyclic antidepressants, MAOIs, and neuroleptics. It is therefore crucial to remember that, when these medications are combined with antianxiety medication, these CNS depressant effects are additive. Such effects may be manifested by a variety of symptoms, including dysarthria, diplopia, ataxia, blurred vision, confusion, dizziness, vertigo, nystagmus, muscle weakness, lack of coordination, and somnolence (Shader and Greenblatt, 1977; Byck, 1975). Patients with underlying organic brain disease are more prone to such effects from benzodiazepines alone, or in combination with other drugs.

Blood levels of most of the benzodiazepines (including alprazolam) are increased by more than one-third when cimetidine is used concomitantly (Klotz and Reimann, 1980 and 1980a; Desmond et al, 1980; Abernathy et al, 1983a). Cimetidine does not, however, interfere with the metabolism of the short-acting benzodiazepines, such as lorazepam and oxazepam, which are eliminated exclusively after conjugation as glucuronide (Patwardhan et al, 1980; Jenike, 1982a).

TREATMENT GUIDELINES

The following guidelines are suggested for managing anxiety in the elderly:

—Look for a clear-cut precipitating factor for the anxiety and consider possible organic causes of anxiety.

—Before prescribing medication, try to alleviate anxiety by manipulating environmental factors or discussing the patient's problems. Psychotherapy, alone or in combination with drug therapy, should always be considered when an elderly individual presents with anxiety. Many older patients respond to counseling techniques, which are preferable to pharmacotherapies whenever a choice exists.

—Use benzodiazepines as first-line drugs. Lorazepam and oxazepam are the safest benzodiazepines to use in the elderly, because they have relatively short half-lives and because their metabolism is not altered appreciably in the elderly or by the concomitant use of other drugs.

—If longer-acting benzodiazepines, such as diazepam, chlordiazepoxide, or prazepam, are chosen, use very low doses once daily or even every other day. More than a week of therapy will be required to reach a steady state, so increase doses cautiously.

—Abrupt stopping of long-term benzodiazepine usage can precipitate a withdrawal syndrome. Discontinue such usage gradually.

—Oxazepam and lorazepam are probably safest in patients with liver disease. Lorazepam seems the best drug for patients with severe lung disease.

—Antihistamines may be useful in patients with severe chronic obstructive lung disease. Be aware of their anticholinergic side effects.

—Neuroleptics are most useful in severely agitated or psychotic patients. Low doses of high-potency neuroleptics are preferred unless patients have a preexisting movement disorder.

—Beta-blockers, such as propranolol, may occasionally be helpful when anxiety is accompanied by signs of sympathetic overstimulation. Be aware of contraindications to these agents.

—Antidepressants may be useful if the patient is clinically depressed or pseudodemented. They are not as effective as benzodiazepines in treating primary anxiety.

—If anxiety persists despite adequate treatment, reevaluate the patient for possible organic causes.

REFERENCES

Abernathy DR, Greenblatt DJ, Divoll M, et al: Pharmacokinetics of alprazolam. *J Clin Psychiatry* 44:45–47, 1983.

Abernathy DR, Greenblatt DJ, Divoll M, et al: Differential effects of cimetidine on drug oxidation vs. conjugation. *J Pharmacol Exp Ther* 224:508–513, 1983a.

Altesman RI, Cole JO: Psychopharmacologic treatment of anxiety. *J Clin Psychiatry* 44:12–18, 1983.

Angus WR, Romney DM: The effect of diazepam on patients' memory. *J Clin Psychopharmacol* 4:203–206, 1984.

Baldessarini RJ: *Chemotherapy in Psychiatry*. Cambridge, Mass, Harvard University Press, 1977.

Barclay J: Variations in amnesia with intravenous diazepam. *Oral Surg* 53:329–334, 1982.

Barnett DB, Taylor-Davies A, Desai H: Differential effect of diazepam on short-term memory in subjects with high or low level anxiety. *Br J Clin Pharmacol* 11:411–412, 1981.

Bender AD, Post A, Meier JP, et al: Plasma protein binding of drugs as a function of age in adult human subjects. *J Pharm Sci* 64:1711–1713, 1975.

Bergmann K: The neuroses of old age, in Kay DWK, Walk A (eds): *Recent Developments in Psychogeriatrics*. Psychiatry Special Publication No 6. Ashford, Headley Bros, 1971.

Bernstein JG: Psychotropic drugs in the elderly, in Manschreck T (ed): *Psychiatric Medicine Update*. New York, Elsevier-North Holland, 1979, pp 75–89.

Bixler EO, Scharf MB, Soldatos CR, et al: Effects of hypnotic drugs on memory. *Life Sci* 25:1379–1388, 1979.

Bixler EO, Kales A, Brubaker BH, et al: Adverse reactions to benzodiazepine hypnotics: Spontaneous reporting system. *Pharmacology* 35:286–300, 1987.

Brown J, Lewis V, Brown M, et al: Amnesic effects of intravenous diazepam and lorazepam. *Experientia* 34:501–502, 1978.

Byck R: Drugs and the treatment of psychiatric disorders, in Goodman LS, Gilman A (eds): *The Pharmacological Basis of Therapeutics*. New York, Macmillan, 1975, pp 152–200.

Catchlove RFH, Kafer ER: The effects of diazepam on respiration in patients with obstructive pulmonary disease. *Anesthesiology* 34:14–18, 1971.

Cohn MA: Hypnotics and the control of breathing: A review. *Br J Clin Pharmacol* 16:2455–2505, 1983.

Cole JD: Clinical use of antianxiety drugs, in Bernstein JD (ed): *Clinical Psychopharmacology*. Littleton, Mass, PSG Publishing, 1978, pp 14–26.

Crook T, Cohen G (eds): *Physician's Handbook on Psychotherapeutic Drug Use in the Aged*. New Canaan, Conn, Mark Powley Associates, 1981.

Crook T: Diagnosis and treatment of mixed anxiety-depression in the elderly. *J Clin Psychiatry* 43:35–43, 1982.

Davies B, et al: Effects on the heart of different tricyclic antidepressants, in Medela J (ed): *Sinequan (Doxepin HCl): A Monograph of Recent Clinical Studies*. Princeton, NJ, Excerpta Medica, 1977, pp 54–58.

Denaut M, Yernault JC, DeCoster A: Double-blind comparison of the respiratory effects of parenteral lorazepam and diazepam in patients with chronic obstructive lung disease. *Curr Med Res Opin* 2:611–615, 1975.

Desmond PV, Patwardhen RV, Schenker S, et al: Cimetidine impairs elimination of chlordiazepoxide in man. *Ann Intern Med* 93:266–268, 1980.

Diagnostic and Statistical Manual of Mental Disorders, ed 3, revised. (DSM-III-R.) Washington DC, American Psychiatric Association Press, 1987.

Dietch JT: Diagnosis of organic anxiety disorders. *Psychosomatics* 22:661–669, 1981.

Dietch JT, Jennings RK: Aggressive dyscontrol in patients treated with benzodiazepines. *J Clin Psychiatry* 49:184–188, 1988.

Dodson ME, Yousseff Y, Maddison S, et al: Respiratory effects of lorazepam. *Br J Anaesth* 48:611–612, 1976.

Douglas WW: Histamine and antihistamines: 5-hydroxytryptamine and antagonists, in Goodman LS, Gilman A (eds): *The Pharmacological Basis of Therapeutics*. New York, Macmillan, 1975, pp 590–629.

Einarson TR: Lorazepam withdrawal seizures. *Lancet* 1:151, 1980.

Eison AS, Temple DL Jr: Buspirone: review of its pharmacology and current perspectives on its mechanism of action. *Am J Med* 80(3B):1–9, 1986.

Elliott HW, Navarro G, Kokka N, et al: Early phase I evaluation of sedatives hypnotics or minor tranquilizers, in *Hypnotics, Methods of Development and Evaluation*. New York, Spectrum Publications, 1975, pp 87–108.

Fabre LF, Putman P: Depressive symptoms and intellectual functioning in anxiety patients treated with clorazepate. *J Clin Psychiatry* 49:189–192, 1988.

George K, Dundee J: Relative amnesic actions of diazepam, flunitrazepam and lorazepam in man. *Br J Psychopharmacol* 4:45–50, 1977.

Greenblatt DJ: Reduced serum albumin concentration in the elderly: A report from the Boston Collaborative Drug Surveillance Program. *J Am Geriatr Soc* 27:20–22, 1979.

Greenblatt DJ: Pharmacokinetic comparisons. Benzodiazepines 1980: Current Update. *Psychosomatics* 21(suppl):9–14, 1980.

Greenblatt DJ, Divoll M, Abernathy DR, et al: Alprazolam kinetics in the elderly: Relation to antipyrine disposition. *Arch Gen Psychiatry* 40:287–290, 1983.

Greist JH, Jefferson JW: Anxiety disorders, in *Review of General Psychiatry*, ed 2. Norwalk, Conn, Appleton and Lange, 1988, pp 349–364.

Hartley L: Diazepam: Human learning of different material. *Prog Neuropsychopharmacol* 4:193–197, 1980.

Hayes MJ, et al: Changes in drug metabolism with increasing age: Phenytoin clearance and protein binding. *Br J Clin Pharmacol* 2:73–79, 1975.

Hollister LE: *Clinical Pharmacology of Psychotherapeutic Drugs*. New York, Churchill Livingstone, 1978.

Hollister LE, Motzenbecker FP, Degan FO: Withdrawal reactions from chlordiazepoxide. *Pharmacologia* 2:63–68, 1961.

Huch R, Huch A: Respiratory depression after tranquilizers. *Lancet* 1:1267, 1974.

James W: *Psychology.* New York, Holt, 1909.

Jenike MA, Baer L: An open trial of buspirone in obsessive-compulsive disorder. *Am J Psychiatry* 145:1285–1286, 1988.

Jenike MA: Using sedative drugs in the elderly. *Drug Ther* 12:186–190, 1982.

Jenike MA: Cimetidine in elderly patients: Review of uses and risks. *J Am Geriatr Soc* 30:170–173, 1982a.

Jenike MA: Treatment of anxiety in elderly patients. *Geriatrics* 38:115–120, 1983.

Jenike MA: Tardive dyskinesia: Special risk in the elderly. *J Am Geriatr Soc* 31:71–73, 1983a.

Jenike MA: Drug abuse. *Sci Am Med* 7:1–8, 1984.

Jenike MA: Use of psychopharmacologic agents in the elderly, in Goroll AH, May L, Mulley A (eds): *Primary Care Medicine.* Philadelphia, JB Lippincott, 1985.

Jerkovich GS, Preskorn SH: Failure of buspirone to protect against lorazepam withdrawal symptoms. *JAMA* 258:204–205, 1987.

Kathol RG, et al: Propranolol in chronic anxiety disorders. *Arch Gen Psychiatry* 37:1361–1365, 1980.

Kessel N, Shepherd M: Neurosis in hospital and general practice. *J Ment Sci* 108:159–166, 1962.

Khan A, Joyce P, Jones AV: Benzodiazepine withdrawal syndromes. *NZ Med J* 92:94–96, Aug 13, 1980.

Klotz U, Avant GR, Hoyumpa A, et al: The effects of age and liver disease on the disposition and elimination of diazepam in man. *J Clin Invest* 55:347–359, 1975.

Klotz U, Reimann I: Delayed clearance of diazepam due to cimetidine. *N Engl J Med* 302:1012–1014, 1980.

Klotz U, Reimann I: Influence of cimetidine on the pharmacokinetics of desmethyldiazepam and oxazepam. *Eur J Clin Pharmacol* 18:517–520, 1980a.

Koepke HH, Gold RL, Linden ME, et al: Multicenter controlled study of oxazepam in anxious elderly outpatients. *Psychosomatics* 23:641–645, 1982.

Kothary S, Braun A, Pandit U, et al: Time course of antirecall effect of diazepam and lorazepam following oral administration. *Anesthesiology* 55:641–644, 1981.

Kronenberg RS, Cosio MG, Stevenson JE, et al: The use of oral diazepam in patients with obstructive lung disease and hypercapnia. *Ann Intern Med* 83:83–84, 1975.

Lader M: Differential diagnosis of anxiety in the elderly. *J Clin Psychiatry* 43:4–7, 1982.

Liljequist R, Linnoila M, Mattila M: Effect of diazepam and chlorpromazine on memory functions in man. *Eur J Clin Pharmacol* 13:339–343, 1978.

Litovitz T: Fatal benzodiazepine toxicity? (The author replies, letter to editor.) *Am J Emerg Med* 5:472–473, 1987.

McKay AC, Dundee JV: Effect of oral benzodiazepines on memory. *Br J Anaesth* 52:1247–1257, 1980.

Myers JK, Weissman MM, Tischler GL, et al: Six month prevalence of psychiatric disorders in three commitments. *Arch Gen Psychiatry* 41:949–958, 1984.

Ochs HR, Greenblatt DJ, Eckardt B, et al: Repeated diazepam dosing in cirrhotic patients: Cumulation and sedation. *Clin Pharmacol Ther* 33:471–476, 1983.

Omslander JG: Drug therapy in the elderly. *Ann Intern Med* 94:711–722, 1981.

Pandit SK, Heisterkamp DV, Cohen PJ: Further studies of the antirecall effect of lorazepam. *Anesthesiology* 45:495–500, 1976.

Papper S: *Clinical Nephrology.* Boston, Little, Brown, 1978.

Patwardhan RV, et al: Cimetidine spares the glucuronidation of lorazepam and oxazepam. *Gastroenterology* 79:912–916, 1980.

Petersen R, Ghoneim M: Diazepam and human memory: Influence on acquisition, retrieval, and state-dependent learning. *Prog Neuropsychopharmacol* 4:81–89, 1980.

Pevnick JS, Jasinski DR, Haertzen CA: Abrupt withdrawal from therapeutically administered diazepam: Report of a case. *Arch Gen Psychiatry* 35:995–998, 1978.

Pitts FN, McClure JN: Lactate metabolism in anxiety neurosis. *N Engl J Med* 277:1329–1336, 1967.

Pleuvry BJ, Maddison SE, Odeh RB, et al: Respiratory and psychological effects of oral temazepam in volunteers. *Br J Anaesth* 52:901–905, 1980.

Primrose EJR: Psychological illness: A community study. Mind and Medicine Monographs. London, Tavistock, 1962.

Rao S, Sherbaniuk RW, Prasad K, et al: Cardiopulmonary effects of diazepam. *Clin Pharmacol Ther* 14:182–189, 1973.

Rickels K, Weisman K, Norstad N, et al: Buspirone and diazepam in anxiety: a controlled study. *J Clin Psychiatry* 43:81–86, 1982.

Rosenbaum J: Anxiety, in Lazare A (ed): *Outpatient Psychiatry*. Baltimore, Williams & Wilkins, 1979, pp 252–256.

Roth T, Hartse KM, Saal PG, et al: The effects of flurazepam lorazepam and triazolam on sleep and memory. *Psychopharmacology (Berlin)* 1980.

Salzman C: Antianxiety agents, in Crook T, Cohen G (eds): *Physicians' Handbook on Psychotherapeutic Drug Use in the Aged*. New Canaan, Conn, Mark Powley Associates, 1981.

Scharf MB, Khosla N, Lysaght R, et al: Anterograde amnesia with oral lorazepam. *J Clin Psychiatry* 44:362–364, 1983.

Scharf MB, Hirschowitz J, Woods M, et al: Lack of amnestic effects of clorazepate on geriatric recall. *J Clin Psychiatry* 46:518–520, 1985.

Scharf MB, Fletcher K, Graham JP: Comparative amnestic effects of benzodiazepine hypnotic agents. *J Clin Psychiatry* 49:134–137, 1988.

Schuckit MA: The diagnosis and treatment of panic and phobic states. *Fam Prac Recertification* 5:29–38, 1983.

Schuckit MA: Anxiety treatment: A commonsense approach. *Postgrad Med* 75:52–63, 1984.

Schumacher GE: Using pharmacokinetics in drug therapy. VII: Pharmacokinetic factors influencing drug therapy in the aged. *Am J Pharmacol* 37:559–562, 1980.

Shader RI, Greenblatt DJ: Clinical implications of benzodiazepine pharmacokinetics. *Am J Psychiatry* 134:652–655, 1977.

Shader RI, Goodman M, Gever J: Panic disorders: Current perspectives. *J Clin Psychopharmacol* 2(suppl 6):2–10, 1982.

Shader RI, Greenblatt DJ: Management of anxiety in the elderly: The balance between therapeutic and adverse effects. *J Clin Psychiatry* 43:8–16, 1982.

Shepherd M, Gruenberg EM: The age for neuroses. *Milbank Mem Fund* 35:258–265, 1957.

Steen SM, Amaha K, Martinez LR: Effect of oxazepam on respiratory response to carbon dioxide. *Curr Res Anaesth Analg* 45:455–458, 1966.

Turnbull JM, Turnbull SK: Management of specific anxiety disorders in the elderly. *Geriatrics* 8:75–82, 1985.

Utting HG, Pleuvry BJ: Benzoctamine—A study of the respiratory effects of oral doses in human volunteers and interactions with morphine in mice. *Br J Anaesth* 47:987–992, 1975.

Wallace S, et al: Factors affecting drug binding in plasma of elderly patients. *Br J Pharmacol* 3:327–330, 1976.

Wells CE: Pseudodementia. *Am J Psychiatry* 136:895–900, 1979.

Wilkinson GR, Schenker S: Drug disposition in liver disease. *Drug Metab Rev* 4:139–175, 1975.

8

Sleep Disorders in the Elderly

CHANGES IN SLEEP WITH INCREASING AGE

Each year, approximately 30% of the US population reports having difficulty with sleep that is sufficiently severe that they take prescription sleep medication. Awakenings in the middle of the night are about twice as common as inability to fall asleep or awakening too early in the morning; combinations of these are common (Evans, 1987). People older than 65 are about six times more likely to have these complaints than those younger than 45. In fact, difficulties with sleep are one of the most common complaints of elderly patients.

With aging there are natural changes in sleep architecture which must be considered normal and are not altered significantly by medication. Infants sleep most of the day; with age the lengthy deep sleep of childhood naturally evolves into the lighter, shorter, and interrupted sleep of old age. As people age, they tend to spend more time in bed although actual sleep time tends to decline (Regestein, 1984).

Sleep latency (the time it takes to get to sleep) lengthens, and sleep is normally interrupted by an increased number of awakenings (Miles and Dement, 1980). Clinicians must be aware of these normal changes with aging so that unnecessary drugs are avoided (Coleman et al, 1981; Greenblatt, 1978). There is a relationship between REM sleep deprivation and depression, and because the elderly sleep less and dream less frequently, this could predispose them to depression.

DSM-III-R CRITERIA

DSM-III-R (1987) classifies disorders of sleep that are chronic (of more than one month's duration) and not the transient disturbances of sleep that are a

272

Table 8–1
Diagnostic Criteria for Insomnia Disorders

A. The predominant complaint is of difficulty in initiating or maintaining sleep, or of nonrestorative sleep (sleep that is apparently adequate in amount, but leaves the person feeling unrested).
B. The disturbance in A occurs at least three times a week for at least one month and is sufficiently severe to result in either a complaint of significant daytime fatigue or the observation by others of some symptom that is attributable to the sleep disturbance, eg, irritability or impaired daytime functioning.
C. Occurrence not exclusively during the course of sleep-wake schedule disorder or a parasomnia.

Reprinted with permission from the *Diagnostic and Statistical Manual of Mental Disorders, third edition, revised*. Copyright 1987. American Psychiatric Association.

normal part of everyday life. Thus, insomnia for a few nights, apparently caused by a psychosocial stressor, would not be diagnosed as a disorder. The sleep disorders are divided into two major subgroups: the dyssomnias (disturbance in the amount, quality, or timing of sleep) and the parasomnias (an abnormal event occurring during sleep).

Dyssomnias

The dyssomnias include three groups of disorders: insomnia disorders, hypersomnia disorders, and sleep-wake schedule disorder. In the insomnia disorders, sleep is deficient in the quality or quantity necessary for normal daytime functioning. In the hypersomnia disorders, the patient feels excessively sleepy when awake, despite sleep of normal length. In sleep-wake schedule disorder, there is a mismatch between the person's sleep-wake pattern and that which is normal for his or her environment.

Insomnia Disorders
The essential feature of insomnia disorders is a predominant complaint of difficulty in initiating or maintaining sleep, or of not feeling rested after sleep that is apparently adequate in amount (Table 8–1). These are common afflictions of elderly patients and are often associated with complaints of disturbances in mood, memory, and concentration. The sleep disorder occurs at least three times a week for at least one month and is sufficiently severe to result in either a complaint of significant daytime fatigue or the observation by others of some symptom that is attributable to the sleep disturbance such as irritability or impaired daytime functioning. Thus the elderly person who complains of insomnia and is functioning normally does not meet criteria for this disorder and may normally require little sleep. Although these disorders can begin at any age, they become increasingly common in people of advanced age.

If insomnia is not secondary to another mental or organic factor, it is called primary insomnia in DSM-III-R (1987).

Hypersomnia Disorders

The essential feature of these disorders (Table 8–2) is either excessive daytime sleepiness or sleep attacks or, more rarely, a prolonged transition to the fully awake state on awakening (sleep drunkenness). The disturbance occurs nearly every day for at least one month, or episodically for longer periods of time, and is sufficiently severe to result in impaired occupational functioning or impairment in usual social activities or relationships with others. As with insomnia disorders, it can be related to another mental disorder or to a known organic factor; or it can be classified as primary hypersomnia.

Usually the hypersomnia is present every day, as when related to sleep apnea or narcolepsy; more rarely, the hypersomnia is episodic as in atypical forms of major depression.

Sleep-Wake Schedule Disorder

The essential feature of sleep-wake schedule disorder is a mismatch between the normal sleep-wake schedule that is demanded by the person's environment and the person's biological rhythm (Table 8–3). Even when people live in environments in which cues about the time of day have been removed, most biologic functions still follow a rhythm with a period that lasts about 24 hours (circadian rhythm). Patients with this disorder complain of either insomnia or hypersomnia; however, if early in the development of the disorder the person is allowed to follow his or her own sleep-wake schedule, the insomnia or hypersomnia disappears.

Transient sleep-wake schedule mismatches commonly occur when people change time zones rapidly or occasionally stay up late for several days.

A number of subtypes of this disorder include frequently changing type, advanced or delayed type, and disorganized type. In the advanced or delayed type, the onset and offset of sleep are considerably advanced or delayed in relation to what the person desires, usually the conventional schedule for the particular society. Patients will have to go to bed much earlier than others or will need to sleep much later each morning and go to bed much later than others.

Table 8–2
Diagnostic Criteria for Hypersomnia Disorders

A. The predominant complaint is either (1) or (2):
   (1) excessive daytime sleepiness or sleep attacks not accounted for by an inadequate amount of sleep
   (2) prolonged transition to the fully awake state on awakening (sleep drunkenness)
B. The disturbance in A occurs nearly every day for at least one month, or episodically for longer periods of time, and is sufficiently severe to result in impaired occupational functioning or impairment in usual social activities or relationships with others.
C. Occurrence not exclusively during the course of sleep-wake schedule disorder.

Reprinted with permission from the *Diagnostic and Statistical Manual of Mental Disorders, third edition, revised.* Copyright 1987. American Psychiatric Association.

Table 8-3
Diagnostic Criteria for Sleep-Wake Schedule Disorder

Mismatch between the normal sleep-wake schedule for a person's environment and his or her circadian sleep-wake pattern, resulting in a complaint of either insomnia (criteria A and B of insomnia disorder) or hypersomnia (criteria A and B of hypersomnia disorder).

Specify Type:

Advanced or Delayed Type: Sleep-wake schedule disorder with onset and offset of sleep considerably advanced or delayed (if sleep-wake schedule is not interfered with by medication or environmental demands) in relation to what the person desires (usually the conventional societal sleep-wake schedule).

Disorganized Type: Sleep-wake schedule disorder apparently due to disorganized and variable sleep and waking times, resulting in absence of a daily major sleep period.

Frequently Changing Type: Sleep-wake schedule disorder apparently due to frequently changing sleep and waking times, such as recurrent changes in work shifts or time zones.

Reprinted with permission from the *Diagnostic and Statistical Manual of Mental Disorders, third edition, revised*. Copyright 1987. American Psychiatric Association.

The advanced pattern is often observed among older people. Because it also frequently results in early morning awakening, depression has to be differentiated from the advanced type of sleep by the presence of the SIG E CAPS criteria (see chapter 4).

In the frequently changing type, the essential feature is a sleep-wake schedule disorder apparently the result of recurring changes in sleep and waking times. This is often associated with frequent airplane flights involving time-zone changes or with changing work schedules (shift work). In general older people, especially those with early-stage dementing illnesses, have more difficulty adjusting to frequent schedule changes.

Other Sleep Disorders
DSM-III-R has a category called "dyssomnia not otherwise specified" for insomnias, hypersomnias, or sleep-wake schedule disturbances that do not fit one of the categories just described.

Parasomnias

The essential feature of this group of disorders is an abnormal event that occurs either during sleep or at the threshold between wakefulness and sleep, with the predominant complaint focusing on this disturbance rather than on its effect on sleeping or wakefulness. These disorders occasionally occur in the elderly.

Dream Anxiety Disorder (Nightmare Disorder)
These disorders are reportedly more common in people with frequent physical and mental health problems and are occasionally primary complaints of elderly patients. The essential feature is repeated awakenings from sleep with detailed recall of frightening dreams. Similar themes may recur and patients are generally quite distressed. Dream anxiety episodes occur during periods of REM sleep and certain drugs that have been reported to be associated with nightmares include: reserpine, thioridazine, mesoridazine, tricyclic antidepressants, and benzodiazepines. Abrupt withdrawal from REM-suppressant drugs (eg, tricyclics) generally induces REM rebound, which may be associated with increased intensity of dreaming and with the possible occurrence of nightmares.

Sleep Terror Disorder
The essential features of this disorder are repeated episodes of abrupt awakening from sleep, usually beginning with a panicky scream. During a typical episode, the person abruptly sits up in bed and has a frightened expression and signs of intense anxiety, dilated pupils, profuse perspiration, piloerection, rapid breathing, and a quick pulse and the person in this state is unresponsive to efforts of others to comfort him or her until the agitation and confusion subside. Morning amnesia for the entire episode is the rule. This disorder rarely has onset after the age of 40 years.

Sleepwalking Disorder
The essential features of this disorder are repeated episodes of a sequence of complex behaviors that progress to leaving the bed and walking about, without the person's being conscious of the episode or later remembering it. Patients may even get dressed, walk about, open doors, eat, and go to the bathroom. Childhood-onset disorder usually resolves by the age of 20, but the adult-onset form may persist into older age.

EVALUATION OF THE PATIENT WITH A SLEEP COMPLAINT

The term insomnia refers to a symptom, not a diagnosis (Addy, 1988), and suggests that an evaluation is in order. Symptomatic treatment without an attempt to identify the cause of the symptom may be poor medical practice.

A look at data across age groups shows that one-third to one-half of the patients with chronic insomnia have an underlying psychiatric disorder, with affective disorders constituting a major portion (Coleman et al, 1982; Addy, 1988). Also, psychophysiologic insomnia and drug and alcohol dependence or abuse are other relatively common causes of insomnia seen in specialized sleep centers. In addition to drug-alcohol dependence, the other common organic causes are periodic leg movements during sleep and sleep apnea syndrome, especially of the central type (Addy, 1988).

In view of this information, it is clear that the evaluation of insomnia should include more than just questions about sleep habits. Knowledge about the patient's daytime functioning is important. A careful history to identify the presence of a medical condition, such as painful arthritis, which may be responsible for the patient's disrupted sleep, should be obtained. A complete mental status examination may reveal a psychiatric disorder or evidence of an early dementing process.

Interviewing the patient's bed partner is often helpful in obtaining a history of sleep apneic episodes, snoring (often associated with obstructive sleep apnea), or periodic leg movements during sleep. The prevalence of both periodic leg movements and central sleep apnea increases with age (Addy, 1988).

In refractory or unusual patients, a nocturnal polysomnogram performed at a sleep center may be helpful. Controversy exists, however, on the role of polysomnography in the evaluation of insomnia. Some have found these examinations to be of major importance in diagnosing unsuspected causes of insomnia, such as periodic leg movements.

DRUGS AND ILLNESSES ASSOCIATED WITH INSOMNIA

A number of drugs alter sleep patterns. One of the most common offenders is caffeine (also found in tea and soft drinks as well as coffee), whose stimulant action in an elderly patient may last more than 12 hours after a single cup of coffee (Brezinova, 1974). In chronic alcohol abusers, sleep is uniformly impaired, both during abstinence and while drinking (Wagmen and Allen, 1975).

Smoking is well documented as a cause of lighter sleep (Myrsten et al, 1977) and smokers obtain significantly improved sleep within a week after they stop (Regestein, 1984). Over-the-counter agents like cold tablets, nasal decongestants, stimulants, and appetite suppressants frequently interrupt sleep patterns of the elderly.

Many prescription drugs, including antiarrhythmic agents, methysergide, thyroid hormones, steroids, methyldopa, epinephrine, and theophylline commonly produce some stimulation and can reduce sleep depth or onset.

Numerous medical illnesses are associated with sleep difficulty. Common offenders include arthritis or other pain-inducing diseases, restless-leg syndrome, itching, diabetes mellitus, hyperthyroidism, respiratory disease and sleep apnea, angina, and paroxysmal nocturnal dyspnea. Dementing illnesses such as Alzheimer's disease, multi-infarct dementia, parkinsonian dementia, and normal pressure hydrocephalus are associated with increased sleep difficulty.

In sleep apnea, the patient fails to exchange air for many prolonged episodes each night, reflexively awakening momentarily to regain respiratory function. The patient's sleep becomes fragmented and light. Although breathing when awake is normal, mini-naps during the day are common because of the permanent debilitating sleep deprivation. The prolonged oxygen deficits can produce serious heart failure and cognitive impairment, often mistaken for Alzheimer's disease. It is most common in older men and loud intermittent snoring punctuated by long silence is a key diagnostic sign (Evans, 1987).

Psychological causes of sleep difficulty are myriad—ranging from simple worries to severe endogenous depression. Sometimes boredom and lack of daytime stimulation lead to frequent naps during the day with resultant nighttime awakening. Many elderly patients go to bed at 7 or 8 PM and wake at 2 or 3 AM and do actually get enough sleep even though they may complain vigorously of insomnia. In all elderly patients complaining of insomnia, especially if early morning awakening is present, clinical depression should be sought by inquiring about the SIG E CAPS criteria (see chapter 4).

SLEEP RECORDS

Because of the variety of sleep difficulties, it is mandatory that the clinician carefully outline the patient's individual problem. Sleep logs are used commonly by sleep researchers. Patients are asked to document when they go to bed, when they fall asleep, the number and time of awakenings during the night, why they awoke (eg, pain, short of breath, urination), time of morning awakening, and time of getting out of bed. This information will aid the clinician in differentiating problems of sleep latency, interrupted sleep, or early morning awakening and will assist both diagnostically and therapeutically. Also such logs are of help in following the patient's response to treatment intervention.

NONPHARMACOLOGIC TREATMENT OF INSOMNIA

General Guidelines

The treatment should, if possible, primarily be aimed at any underlying causes. Medications should be avoided if at all feasible; physicians should use drugs only as a last resort.

A number of simple manipulations may improve the quality of sleep in many patients (Table 8–4). If a patient is expecting that his or her sleep will not change with age, education may be extremely beneficial. If interrupted lighter sleep can be redefined as normal, many elderly patients will seem relieved and be less concerned with forcing themselves to sleep. Once the pressure is off, some patients will be more relaxed and sleep quality will improve.

Daytime napping should generally be discouraged and activities should

Table 8–4
Nonpharmacologic Treatment of Insomnia

Education: The elderly sleep lighter, waken more often, and sleep fewer hours. This is normal.
Evening fluid restriction decreases nocturia.
Discourage daytime napping.
Exercise regularly when permissible: Avoid evening exercise.
Avoid caffeine, nicotine, and alcohol.
Avoid prescription drugs that are stimulatory or attempt to give them early in the day.
Optimally manage medical illnesses, especially heart and lung disease.
Control nighttime pain.
Recommend regular times for going to bed and arising.
Use behavioral modification techniques.

become part of the daily routine of all elderly patients, particularly those who are institutionalized. When it can be safely recommended, exercise is usually beneficial when not done late in the evening. Evening exercise may lead to increased arousal and difficulty getting to sleep.

Patients with severe insomnia should be advised to discontinue caffeine and alcohol intake and cigarette smoking. As previously noted, even one morning cup of coffee can contribute to nighttime sleep problems. Prescription medications should be adjusted so that nighttime stimulating side effects are minimized.

Patients should set regular times for going to bed and for getting up in the morning. They should stay in bed a preset amount of time which should be based on the average daily amount of sleep time (Regestein, 1984).

Not infrequently the elderly awaken many times in the night to urinate. Urinary system problems should be evaluated and treated (eg, enlarged prostate). If no pathology is found, evening fluid restriction may decrease the frequency of nocturia.

Medical problems such as congestive heart failure, emphysema, and arthritis should be under optimal medical control to minimize nighttime symptoms.

Behavioral Interventions

A number of behavioral interventions may be of use in treating insomnia in geriatric patients (Borkovec, 1982; Bootzin et al, 1983; Moran and Rapp, 1987):

Optimize Sleep Environment
Environmental factors such as temperature, light, noise, and mattress comfort should be considered, especially in nursing home environments.

Moran and Rapp (1987) made a number of practical suggestions. Strategic placement of curtains or changing lighting from global to spot can reduce undesired illumination. The use of background noise from a fan or white noise from a radio can mask disruptive sounds; ear plugs may help. Blankets, fans, and air-conditioning can be used. By placing boards beneath it, an excessively soft mattress can be firmed although it may be necessary to replace it all together.

Educational Intervention

Frequently, elderly persons entertain unrealistic expectations regarding the amount and pattern of sleep that is appropriate; for example, they often believe that they must have the same 8 hours of uninterrupted sleep as when they were younger and become anxious or upset with the shorter duration of sleep that occurs with age (Moran and Rapp, 1987). As noted, correction of these misconceptions may improve or solve the patient's difficulties.

Stimulus Control Treatment

These techniques involve strengthening the associations between bed/bedroom and sleep behavior and weakening associations between this area and nonsleeping behaviors (Bootzin et al, 1983). This is generally achieved by curtailing sleep-incompatible behaviors and regulating wake-sleep schedule.

Morin and Rapp (1987) recommended that a short educational session be devoted to explaining to the patient the rationale for the tasks at hand. Ample time should be spent explaining how people learn to respond to environmental cues developed through association even though they are unaware of the process; analogies are helpful. For example, some people develop a preference for reading in a specific location, reporting that they seem to read best there. This is because that particular room, chair, position, sounds, and smells gradually become associated with reading behaviors. In a similar way people can learn to sleep in a certain location by associating a bedroom with sleeping behavior. These authors outlined a number of these stimulus control procedures which may be helpful in dealing with elderly insomniacs:

1. Go to bed only when sleepy and only at night.
2. When unable to get to sleep or return to sleep within 20 minutes, get out of bed, go to another room, and engage in quiet, nonarousing activity.
3. Return to bed only when sleepy again and repeat this procedure as often as necessary throughout the night.
4. Avoid the use of the bed/bedroom for nonsleep activities (ie, reading, eating, TV, etc).
5. Arise at the same time every morning regardless of the amount of sleep obtained on the previous night.
6. Avoid daytime napping.

7. Adhere to a standard pre-bedtime routine (eg, reading, washing face, brushing teeth).

These techniques have produced improvement rates of 60% for sleep onset difficulties and 50% for duration of awakenings, in outcome studies that addressed the management of sleep onset (Pruder et al, 1983) and insomnia (Morin and Azrin, in press).

Morin and Rapp (1987) noted that it is common to encounter reluctance by an individual to comply with these behavioral guidelines and that offering a time-limited contract whereby the person agrees to comply for two weeks is sometimes sufficient to produce clinical benefits and motivate further compliance if necessary. Another suggestion is to allow the person to select the behavioral procedure(s) that they prefer after hearing about each. Finally, if daytime napping is unavoidable, naps taken in the morning do not disrupt night sleep as much as those taken in late afternoon or early evening.

Life-style Changes
With age, especially in the context of retirement, several life-style changes can interfere with sleep. These include reduced activity and performance demands, increased daytime napping and resting, and changes in sleep schedules. Some data indicate that elderly insomniacs, when compared with good sleepers, are more sedentary, less involved in work, worry more about themselves and their problems, and more frequently engage in solitary activities (Marchini et al, 1983; Morin and Rapp, 1987). Thus, increasing daytime physical activity, involvement with others, and engagement in pleasant events can be beneficial to sleep.

As noted, attention to eating and drinking habits can affect sleep. Reducing or stopping caffeine, alcohol, and nicotine intake may help. While a light snack can induce sleep, spicy and high-protein foods make the digestive system more active and should be avoided at night.

Stress management procedures such as muscle relaxation and imagery training can be particularly beneficial at bedtime for reducing physical tension and for controlling intrusive worries (Morin and Rapp, 1987; Kirmil-Gray et al, 1985). It is best not to engage in problem-solving just prior to bedtime since it is physiologically arousing and therefore incompatible with sleep. A more fruitful strategy would be to set aside a specific time and place, other than at bedtime and in the bedroom, to engage in problem-solving.

DRUG TREATMENT OF INSOMNIA

Overview

Most researchers believe that sedative-hypnotic drugs have only a minor role, if any, in the treatment of chronic insomnia; when sleep disturbances are severe

282

Table 8–5
Drugs Used To Treat Insomnia

Drug	Dosage	Problems
L-Tryptophan	500 mg–4 g	None
Chloral Hydrate	500 mg–2 g	Gastric irritation
		Induces liver enzymes
Diphenhydramine	25–50 mg	Anticholinergic
Benzodiazepines		
Short-acting		
Oxazepam	10–30 mg	
Lorazepam	0.5–2 mg	Amnesia very rare
Alprazolam	0.125–0.5 mg	Occasional daytime
Triazolam	0.25–0.5 mg	sedation
Temazepam	15–30 mg	
Long-acting		
Flurazepam	15 mg	Active metabolites
		Very long-acting
		Daytime drowsiness, lethargy, ataxia
Sedating Antidepressants		
Trazodone	50–400 mg	Only when depressed
Nortriptyline	50–200 mg	

Reproduced with permission from Jenike MA: *Handbook of Geriatric Psychopharmacology.* Littleton, Mass, PSG Publishing, 1985, p 146.

and do not respond to nonpharmacologic approaches, however, a number of drugs might be at least transiently helpful (Table 8–5).

Neuroleptics (see chapter 6) and antidepressants (see chapter 4) should be avoided in nonpsychotic and nondepressed patients. However, major depression or other affective or nonaffective psychiatric disorders should be appropriately treated with pharmacotherapy or psychotherapy, or both, as indicated.

Many of the antianxiety agents (see chapter 7) are also helpful for treating insomnia. For the treatment of anxiety or insomnia, it seems reasonable to avoid using barbiturates and older agents such as meprobamate (Miltown) and ethchlorvynol (Placidyl) as first-line agents. Tolerance develops rapidly to these agents and they are very addicting (Ewing and Bakewell, 1967; Kales et al, 1974).

The treatment of periodic leg movements is primarily pharmacologic, with the drug of choice being clonazepam (Clonopin) taken at bedtime, although other benzodiazepines are also reported to be of benefit (Addy, 1988). Baclofen and opiates have also been used. Although the medication used may not decrease the number of periodic movements, it often improves sleep continuity and thus decreases the subjective complaint of insomnia.

The successful treatment of central sleep apnea syndrome is difficult, but acetazolamide has been shown to be helpful in some patients (Addy, 1988). Continuous nasal-positive airway pressure (CPAP) ventilation has also been used for central sleep apnea treatment. CPAP ventilation is, however, more clearly indicated and helpful in patients who have obstructive sleep apnea syndrome, a condition in which tricyclic antidepressant medications may also be helpful (Addy, 1988). Highlighting the importance of differential diagnosis, benzodiazepines may make sleep apnea syndrome worse.

L-Tryptophan

L-Tryptophan is an amino acid that is metabolized to serotonin and is thought to be involved in the regulation of deep sleep. It has been shown to significantly reduce sleep latency in normal volunteers. Smith and Prockop (1962) reported that drowsiness was one of the CNS effects when tryptophan was injected in normal subjects, a finding that was later confirmed by a number of studies.

Oswald and associates (1966) were the first to look at the effect of tryptophan on sleep and they found that tryptophan (5 to 10 g orally) could shorten the time before onset of REM sleep, and that this effect was prevented by prior administration of the 5-HT blocker methysergide. Since then more than 40 studies on tryptophan's effect on sleep have been published (Wurtman and Wurtman, 1986; Cole et al, 1980 and 1980a).

L-Tryptophan is probably worth trying in those elderly patients whose primary difficulty is falling asleep (Hartman et al, 1971 and 1974; Bernstein, 1983). Dosage seems to be important; while doses of more than 1 g seem to decrease sleep latency with equal efficiency, doses of 0.25 and 0.5 g showed a trend toward decreased latency, but the effect was not statistically significant (Wurtman and Wurtman, 1986). Also, the effect of age on dosage has not been studied.

Another important variable is time of administration. Tryptophan has a definite effect in producing sleepiness, but its effect becomes significantly different from that of placebo only starting at 45 minutes after administration (Hartmann et al, 1976). Wurtman and Wurtman (1986) suggested that it may take that long for brain levels of 5-HT to rise sufficiently to influence arousal.

Certain patients seem to respond better than others. Tryptophan, given at an adequate dose, was invariably found to decrease sleep latency in subjects with mild insomnia or in subjects with a long sleep latency who did not complain of insomnia. In studies on normal subjects or patients with chronic or severe insomnia, however, positive results occurred only sometimes (Wurtman and Wurtman, 1986).

When tryptophan is compared in a controlled fashion, although better than placebo, it does not appear to be as effective as benzodiazepines or chloral hydrate, especially in the more severe insomniacs (Hartmann et al, 1983; Linnoila et al, 1980). Also, in several studies of patients who improved with tryptophan treatment, ingestion of tryptophan at bedtime for several nights was followed by ingestion of placebo for several nights, with continuing improvement during the placebo period. This has led to the tentative suggestion that interval therapy might be useful. It has been hypothesized that tryptophan works through increasing pineal melatonin with resultant entrainment of the diurnal sleep rhythm (Wurtman and Wurtman, 1986).

L-Tryptophan can be purchased as 500-mg tablets in most so-called health food stores. Since it is not approved by the Food and Drug Administration, it is not available at this time in pharmacies. Initially, 1 g should be prescribed 45 minutes to one hour before bedtime. If not effective at that dose, it may be increased to as much as 4 g; larger doses are not likely to be helpful if this dose is not effective. L-Tryptophan, although relatively expensive, is apparently safe (liver ultrastructural changes develop in rats, however) and should be tried initially if sleep latency difficulties are part of the clinical picture (Cole et al, 1980).

Chloral Hydrate

Chloral hydrate is a time-tested, safe medication that is often effective in the elderly. It exerts a rapid hypnotic effect and has a relatively short elimination half-life of approximately eight hours (Regestein, 1984). Drug interactions with chloral hydrate are uncommon (Greenblatt, 1981) and it is less likely to induce dependence and distort sleep patterns than barbiturates and related drugs (Regestein, 1984). Its main drawbacks are that it sometimes produces GI discomfort and excessive bowel flatus and that it induces hepatic enzymes and therefore increases the rate of metabolism of other drugs such as the anticoagulants. It also can irritate the gastric mucosa and is therefore not recommended for patients with gastritis or peptic ulcer.

Although doses of 500 mg are frequently effective, as much as 2 g may be needed. It is supplied either as rather large 500-mg pills or as a syrup and it is one of the cheapest hypnotics available (Linnoila et al, 1980).

Antihistamines

Sedating antihistamines, such as diphenhydramine hydrochloride (Benadryl), are sometimes effective in speeding the onset of sleep in a patient who has an otherwise relatively normal sleep pattern. Tolerance to their sedative effects develops after several weeks (Regestein, 1984). At a dose of 25 to 50 mg given orally about a half hour before bedtime, these agents are relatively safe. They do, however, have fairly potent anticholinergic effects and can on their own produce central or peripheral anticholinergic symptoms (see chapter 9). These effects are additive with other anticholinergic drugs.

These agents are probably not the best choice for patients with Alzheimer's disease because the cholinergic system is already not functioning optimally and even a mild anticholinergic load can precipitate clinical deterioration (see chapter 5). Antihistamines are the most common ingredients in over-the-counter sleep-inducing aids.

Benzodiazepines

Benzodiazepines are widely used as hypnotic agents and are considered to be very safe drugs in the elderly. The same considerations outlined in chapter 7 for use as antianxiety agents apply here. These drugs do not induce production of hepatic enzymes and are unlikely to be lethal on overdose when taken alone.

When long-acting agents, such as flurazepam (Dalmane), diazepam (Valium), or clorazepate (Tranxene), are used, there is a significant danger of a gradual buildup of long-acting metabolites with resulting daytime drowsiness and lethargy. Even though flurazepam is marketed as a hypnotic agent, it is apparently no better at inducing sleep than other benzodiazepines. It does, however, have one of the longest half-lives (Greenblatt et al, 1981) and when used in the elderly should be used briefly in low doses (15 mg) (Roth et al, 1979 and 1980).

The short-acting benzodiazepines have fewer or no active metabolites and are rapidly eliminated. These shorter half-lives may be an advantage to older patients because the drugs are not likely to accumulate and produce daytime sedation (Merlis and Koepke, 1975).

Benzodiazepines are not helpful in preventing early morning awakening and have even been reported to produce early morning insomnia when used continuously for a couple of weeks (Kales et al, 1983). For this reason, they should not be used on a daily basis for long periods.

In addition, some of the short-acting agents have been reported to be associated with retrograde and anterograde amnesia (Regestein, 1984) (see chapter 7). Clinically, however, this must be very rare as a number of experienced geriatricians have never seen this.

Lorazepam (Ativan) and oxazepam (Serax) have been around for many years and are generally very safe and effective for brief periods. These agents are relatively slowly absorbed and should be given about an hour prior to going to bed. Dosages range from 10 to 30 mg for oxazepam and from 0.5 to 2.0 mg for lorazepam. Triazolam (Halcion), temazepam (Restoril), and alprazolam (Xanax) are newer agents that may be as safe and effective as the older agents.

Alcohol

Small doses of alcohol are sometimes effective sleep aids. This may be best prescribed in carefully controlled environments such as nursing homes. Not all patients will respond and the dangers of dependence, addiction, and morning hangover are important (Regestein, 1984; Mishara and Kastenbaum, 1974; Stone, 1980).

SUMMARY

1. Carefully diagnose the specific problem. Difficulties are typically with sleep latency, interrupted sleep, or early morning awakening. Sleep logs may be helpful.
2. Normal elderly patients require less sleep and their sleep is typically lighter with more awakenings. Advising the patient of this is often therapeutic in and of itself.
3. A careful medical and drug history can illuminate potential causes of insomnia. Caffeine, nicotine, and alcohol intake should be temporarily discontinued. Discontinue offending drugs or adjust dosing schedule to minimize evening stimulation. Optimally control medical illnesses.
4. Carefully rule out depression. When depression is present, a sedating antidepressant is the most effective medication. Early morning awakening is very common with depression.
5. Avoid hypnotic medications initially and try to get the patient to avoid daytime naps and to get regular exercise when possible. Other behavioral techniques are reviewed.
6. Advise patients to set regular times for going to bed and awakening.
7. If nocturia is a problem, rule out urinary system pathology and have the patient avoid drinking fluids in the evening.
8. If nonpharmacologic approaches fail, a relatively brief trial of medication should be considered. L-Tryptophan is a reasonable, but relatively expensive, agent to try initially if the patient has trouble getting to sleep.
9. Chloral hydrate is safe and effective with minimal side effects.
10. Antihistamines can be prescribed and are common ingredients in over-the-counter preparations. They have anticholinergic effects that will be additive with other drugs, however.
11. Benzodiazepines are the most commonly used hypnotics. Long-acting agents have active metabolites and are best avoided in the elderly. Short-acting drugs, such as lorazepam and oxazepam, are helpful for relatively short periods of time. Newer agents which may be as safe and effective are available.
12. Alcohol may be effective in some patients under carefully controlled situations.

REFERENCES

Addy RO: The causes and management of chronic insomnia. *Clinical Advances in the Treatment of Psychiatric Disorders*. Roerig Publication. 99:1–3, July/August 1988.

Bernstein JG: *Drug Therapy in Psychiatry*. Boston, Wright-PSG, 1983.

Bootzin RR, Engle-Friedman M, Hazelwood L: Insomnia, in Lewinsohn PM, Teri L (eds): *Clinical Geropsychology: New Directions in Assessment and Treatment*. New York, Pergamon Press, 1983.

Borkovec TD: Insomnia. *J Consult Clin Psychol* 50:880–895, 1982.

Brezinova V: Effect of caffeine on sleep: EEG study in late middle age. *Br J Clin Pharmacol* 1:203–208, 1974.

Cole JO, Hartmann E, Brigham P: L-Tryptophan: Clinical studies, in Cole JO (ed): *Psychopharmacology Update*. Lexington, Mass, The Collamore Press, 1980.

Cole JO, Hartmann E, Brigham P: L-Tryptophan: Clinical studies. *McLean Hosp J* 5:37–71, 1980a.

Coleman RM, Miles LE, Guilleminault C, et al: Sleep-wake disorders in the elderly: A polysomnograhic analysis. *J Am Geriatr Soc* 29:289–296, 1981.

Coleman RM, Roffwarg HP, Kennedy SJ, et al: Sleep-wake disorders based on a polysomnographic diagnosis. A national cooperative study. *JAMA* 247(7):997–1003, 1982.

Diagnostic and Statistical Manual of Mental Disorders, ed 3, revised. (DSM-III-R) Washington DC, American Psychiatric Association Press, 1987.

Evans FJ: Sleep disorders and insomnia: Causes and cures. *Carrier Foundation Letter* #129, November 1987.

Ewing JA, Bakewell WE: Diagnosis and management of depressant drug dependence. *Am J Psychiatry* 123:909–917, 1967.

Greenblatt DJ, Divoll M, Harmatz JS, et al: Kinetics and clinical effects of flurazepam in young and elderly insomniacs. *Clin Pharmacol Ther* 30:475–486, 1981.

Greenblatt DJ: Drug therapy of insomnia, in Bernstein JG (ed): *Clinical Psychopharmacology*. Littleton, Mass, PSG Publishing, 1978, pp 27–39.

Greenblatt DJ: Sedative-hypnotics: Sleep disorders in the elderly, in Crook T, Cohen G (eds): *Physician's Handbook on Psychotherapeutic Drug Use in the Elderly*. New Canaan, Conn, Mark Powley Associates, 1981, pp 59–65.

Hartmann E, Chung R, Chien C: L-Tryptophan and sleep. *Psychopharmacologia* 19:114–127, 1971.

Hartmann E, Cravens J, List S: Hypnotic effects of L-tryptophan. *Arch Gen Psychiatry* 31:394–397, 1974.

Hartmann E, Lindsley JG, Spinweber CL: Chronic insomnia: Effects of tryptophan, flurazepam, secobarbital, and placebo. *Psychopharmacology* 80:138–142, 1983.

Hartmann E, Spinweber CL, Ware C: L-Tryptophan, L-leucine, and placebo: Effects on subjective alertness. *Sleep Res* 5:57, 1976.

Kales A, Bixler EO, Tan TL, et al: Chronic hypnotic drug use. *JAMA* 227:513–517, 1974.

Kales A, Soldatos CR, Bixler EO, et al: Early morning insomnia with rapidly eliminated benzodiazepines. *Science* 220:95–97, 1983.

Kirmil-Gray K, Eaglelston JR, Thoresen CE, et al: Brief consultation and stress management treatments for drug-dependent insomnia: Effects on sleep quality, self-efficacy, and daytime stress. *J Behav Med* 8:19–99, 1985.

Linnoila M, Viukari M, Numminen A, et al: Efficacy and side effects of chloral hydrate and tryptophan as sleeping aids in psychogeriatric patients. *Pharmacopsychiatry* 15:124–128, 1980.

Marchini EJ, Coates TJ, Magistad JG, et al: What do insomniacs do, think, and feel during the day? A preliminary study. *Sleep* 6:147–155, 1983.

Merlis S, Koepke HH: The use of oxazepam in elderly patients. *Dis Nerv Syst* 36:27–29, 1975.

Miles LE, Dement WC: Sleep and aging. *Sleep* 3:119–220, 1980.

Mishara BL, Kastenbaum R: Wine in the treatment of long-term geriatric patients in mental institutions. *J Am Geriatr Soc* 22:88–94, 1974.

Morin C, Azrin NH: Stimulus control and imagery training in treating sleep-maintenance-insomnia. *J Consult Clin Psychol,* in press.

Morin C, Rapp SR: Behavioral management of geriatric insomnia. *Clin Gerontologist* 6 (4): 15–23, 1987.

Myrsten AL, Elgerot A, Edgren B: Effects of abstinence from tobacco smoking on physiological and psychological arousal levels in habitual smokers. *Psychosom Med* 39:25–38, 1977.

Oswald I, Ashcroft GW, Berger RJ, et al: Some experiments in the chemistry of normal sleep. *Br J Psychiatry* 112:391–399, 1966.

Pruder R, Lacks P, Bertelson AD, et al: Short term stimulus control treatment of insomnia in older adults. *Behav Ther* 14:424–429, 1983.

Regestein QR: Treatment of insomnia in the elderly, in Salzman C (ed): *Clinical Geriatric Psychopharmacology.* New York, McGraw-Hill Book, 1984, pp 149–170.

Roth T, Hartze KM, Zorick FJ, et al: The differential effects of short- and long-acting benzodiazepines upon nocturnal sleep and daytime performance. *Drug Res* 30:891–894, 1980.

Roth T, Piccione P, Salis P, et al: Effects of temazepam, flurazepam, and quinalbarbitone on sleep: Psychomotor and cognitive function. *Br J Clin Pharmacol* 8:47S–54S, 1979.

Smith P, Prockop DJ: Central-nervous-system effects of ingestion of L-tryptophan by normal subjects. *N Engl J Med* 267:1338–1341, 1962.

Stone BM: Sleep and low doses of alcohol. *Electroencephalogr Clin Neurophysiol* 48:706–709, 1980.

Wagmen AM, Allen RP: Effects of alcohol ingestion and abstinence on slow wave sleep of alcoholics. *Adv Exp Med Biol* 59:453–466, 1975.

Wurtman RJ, Wurtman JJ (eds): *Nutrition and the Brain.* New York, Raven Press, 1986.

9

Delirium in Elderly Patients

OVERVIEW

Delirium is an organic psychiatric syndrome characterized by acute onset and impairment in cognition, perception, and behavior (Beresin, 1988). A number of reports indicated that delirium occurs in as many as 10% to 15% of all hospitalized medical and surgical patients (Lipowski, 1980; DeVaul, 1976; Engel, 1967; Beresin, 1988). Because many delirious patients are hypoactive, it is likely that many cases of delirium do not come to medical attention (Lipowski, 1980). Lipowski (1980a) estimated that between one-third and one-half of hospitalized geriatric patients are likely to become delirious during an admission.

Delirium may be most prevalent in patients undergoing open heart surgery, among severely burned patients, and in patients on intensive care units (Beresin, 1988) and delirium is often found in patients who have numerous medical problems. Despite the seriousness and prevalence of delirium, only one book in the English language (Lipowski, 1980) is devoted to delirium and researchers have largely ignored it.

Delirium is a grave prognostic sign in the elderly; as many as 15% to 30% of delirious patients will progress to stupor, coma, and death (Liston, 1982). One group reported that 25% of delirious elderly patients admitted to a general hospital died within one month after entry (Simon and Cahan, 1963).

Delirium is usually underdiagnosed; in one study, researchers found that 79% of cognitive deficits were missed by the examining physicians and in only 4 of 395 examinations were mental status evaluations reported in the medical record (McCartney and Palmateer, 1985).

When optimally diagnosed and treated, delirium is often a completely reversible syndrome. In one large study (Bedford, 1959) of 4,000 geriatric patients with delirium, 80% recovered within one month. Rapid assessment, differential diagnosis, and treatment are essential to reverse and prevent serious

Table 9–1
DSM-III-R Diagnostic Criteria for Delirium

Reduced ability to maintain attention to external stimuli and to appropriately shift attention to new external stimuli

Disorganized thinking as indicated by rambling, irrelevant, or incoherent speech

At least two of the following:
1. Reduced level of consciousness
2. Perceptual disturbances: misinterpretations, illusions, or hallucinations
3. Disturbance of sleep-wake cycle with insomnia or daytime sleepiness
4. Increased or decreased psychomotor activity
5. Disorientation to time, place, or person
6. Memory impairment (eg, new material or past material)

Clinical features that develop acutely (hours to days) and fluctuate over the course of a day

Either 1 or 2
1. Evidence from the history, physical examination, or laboratory tests of an organic etiology
2. In absence of such evidence, an etiologic organic factor can be presumed if the disturbance cannot be accounted for by an nonorganic mental disorder

Reproduced with permission from Beresin EV: Delirium in the elderly. *J Geriatr Psychiatry Neurol* 1:128, 1988.

consequences of the underlying medical disorder and control behavior that may be life-threatening.

DIAGNOSTIC CRITERIA

The diagnostic criteria for delirium, according to DSM-III-R, are listed in Table 9–1. The clinical presentations can be manifested in many ways and variability in symptoms is a hallmark of the disorder. Mental status may vary over hours from completely lucid to total disorientation. Symptoms are often worse in the evening and at night.

Because of the potentially serious and sometimes life-threatening nature of delirium, rapid diagnosis and treatment are imperative. Beresin (1988) noted that the diagnostic process has two components: (1) identifying the syndrome and differentiating it from other psychiatric syndromes and (2) determining the organic cause (Lipowski, 1980). For instance, if a clinician is called to evaluate a patient with "dementia" and the patient does indeed appear demented on clinical interview, but when the spouse is consulted it turns out that he was working in his law office without deficit only two weeks ago, it is most likely that this patient has a potentially reversible delirium and not dementia. As this case points out, since a hallmark of both delirium and dementia is altered cognitive status, it is imperative for the clinician to gather information from multiple sources who have had recent contact with the patient.

The clinician should do a complete mental status examination as outlined in chapter 2. Also ask about delusions, paranoid ideation, mood changes, perceptual disturbances, and suicide. Some delirious patients will be very embarrassed and secretive about cognitive deficits, and one should proceed very gently after building some alliance with the patient. Beresin (1988) discussed tips for alliance building with a delirious patient and he suggested meeting with the patient during a lucid interval and explaining clearly and directly that he is not "going crazy" but that a medical problem is causing a disturbance in the nervous system producing bizarre experiences. Even when the patient is floridly delirious, the words "medical" or "neurologic" should be used and any reference to "psychiatric" should be avoided because of the common connotations that are associated with psychiatric disorders in our society.

Because the diagnosis is largely based on the presence of cognitive dysfunction, cognitive evaluation is key. The MMSE (Folstein et al, 1975), which takes less than 10 minutes to administer, is a reliable and valid tool for such evaluation (see chapter 2). It should be used routinely throughout an elderly patient's hospitalization and placed in the medical record to chart the patient's progress.

To establish a medical cause, a thorough history that focuses on medical history, medication (prescription and over-the-counter) use, and a complete review of systems is required. Physical and neurologic examinations as well as laboratory tests (see Table 9–2) are required.

CLINICAL FEATURES

The early signs of delirium include feelings of uneasiness, malaise, headache, fatigue, decreased concentration, irritability, restlessness, anxiety, depression, or decreased interests. Sometimes disorientation, impaired recent memory, and perceptual disturbances appear (Beresin, 1988). Deficits in retention result in diminished new learning, a good indicator of delirium in its early stages (Lishman, 1978). As in early dementia, deficits in remote memory are less frequent. Commonly, daytime somnolence and nighttime insomnia with vivid dreams or nightmares occur with a reversal of sleep-wake cycles. In nursing homes, the night nurses may be the first to notice that something is amiss. Symptoms may be mild but patients know something is wrong and may react in a number of ways depending on their personalities and usual ways of handling stress (Beresin, 1988). Patients may try to act as if nothing is wrong and may refuse cognitive testing.

If delirium progresses, attention is reduced and distractibility and concentration problems follow. Thinking is disorganized and the patient may exhibit rambling or incoherent speech. Sense of time becomes unclear and patients may have trouble distinguishing dreams from reality. Thinking abnormalities

Table 9–2
Laboratory Tests To Evaluate Delirium

Routine procedures
    Complete blood count
    Blood chemistries: electrolytes (Na, K, Cl, CO_2) calcium, phosphate, glucose, blood
        urea nitrogen, liver enzymes
    Serologic test for syphilis
    Urinalysis
    Erythrocyte sedimentation rate
    Chest x-ray
    Electrocardiogram
    Electroencephalogram
    CAT scan

Special procedures
    Blood chemistries: creatinine, magnesium, B_{12}, folate, thyroxine, ammonia, serum
        proteins, osmolality, arterial blood gases
    Blood levels of medications
    Blood and urine toxic screens (drugs and poisons)
    Blood cultures
    LE-preparation and ANA levels
    Cerebrospinal fluid exam: cells, protein, glucose, culture, serology, pressures
    Urine: osmolality, porphobilinogen
    Skull films
    Positron-emission tomographic scan
    Sodium amobarbital interview (functional vs organic differential)

Reproduced with permission from Beresin EV: Delirium in the elderly. *J Geriatr Psychiatry Neurol* 1:137, 1988.

are prominent and patients may appear illogical, tangential, and incoherent. Simple tasks cannot be accomplished. The content of thinking (as opposed to patients with dementia where impoverishment and stereotypy are the rule in later stages) tends to abound with rich imagery and fantasies that are a reflection of the individual's experiences. For example, one delirious gentleman, who was quite conservative in manner and expression when he was well, had had great difficulty urinating after a surgical procedure and there had been much discussion at bedside throughout the day about this problem. After many hours of inability to urinate, he finally was able to void. About 10 minutes later the neurologist was making his rounds and asked the patient what his name was and he replied, much to the shock of his wife and son, "I'm the big pisser."

    Persecutory delusions and suspicions are common but these are quite different from schizophrenic delusions by being vague, transient, poorly systematized, easily forgotten, inconsistently reported, and highly influenced by the environment (Beresin, 1988).

    Language functions are always abnormal in delirium and speech may be tangential, circumstantial, or slurred. Word-finding difficulties are common. Chedur and Geschwind (1972 and 1972a) reported that dysgraphia, when patients draw letters poorly and misalign them, was the most sensitive indicator of delirium. Syntactical and spelling errors are also common. Often patients resist writing tasks.

Confabulation occurs sometimes (in 8% to 15% of patients) and usually involves activities that never took place (Wolff and Curran, 1935). Patients mistake the unfamiliar for the familiar (Levin, 1954). Frank hallucinations of a visual (eg, bugs or snakes on the floor), auditory (eg, sounds, music, voices), or tactile (eg, crawling insects on skin) nature might be reported. Illusions that are misinterpretations of external sensory experiences (eg, loud noise in hall is a gunshot) can occur.

Violent behavior has been reported in about 10% of elderly delirious patients (Simon and Cahan, 1963; Beresin, 1988). Patients commonly express fear and sadness as well as anxiety, anger, and embarrassment.

MECHANISM OF DELIRIUM

Delirium appears to be a common final pathway which can be reached by a number of ways. By definition, a biological stressor must be present for delirium to occur, but psychological or environmental factors are often involved. It appears that the elderly are intrinsically more vulnerable to delirium secondary to changes associated with aging, such as vision and hearing impairment, metabolic changes, and presence of multiple medical illnesses and medication use. Cell loss occurs with age in many brain centers such as the hypothalamic nuclei, frontal cortex, hippocampus, and locus ceruleus. In addition, decreased acetylcholine synthesis, cerebral blood flow, and glucose metabolism predispose to vulnerability to delirium.

In one study (Purdie et al, 1981) of elderly subjects admitted to a general hospital, 44% of the patients had an underlying chronic brain disease with a superimposed insult that caused the decompensation; infection was involved in 23% and an environmental change, in 17%. In patients who did not have underlying brain disease, the most common cause for the delirium was drug related.

The pathologic mechanisms underlying delirium remain a mystery, but recently Lipowski (1980 and 1980a) hypothesized that there might be an imbalance between acetylcholine and norepinephrine, with effects on the reticular activating system along with its hypocampal and frontal circuits which are involved in arousal, attention, and wakefulness.

Kral (1975) postulated that increased vulnerability in the elderly to stress might be secondary to the release of corticosteroids, which are more slowly degraded, along with increased sensitivity of the hypothalamus to the effects of corticosteroids. Other authors pointed to possible structural pathology in the left superior temporal and inferior parietal regions of the brain (Swigar et al, 1985), and still others attributed delirium to sensory deprivation (NIA Task Force, 1980).

Table 9–3
Organic Causes of Delirium

Intoxication
    Medications: anticholinergics, tricyclic antidepressants, lithium, sedative-hypnotics,
        antihypertensive agents, antiarrhythmic drugs, digitalis, anticonvulsants, anti-
        parkinsonian agents, steroids and anti-inflammatory drugs, analgesics (opiates
        and non-narcotic), disulfiram, antibiotics, antineoplastic drugs, cimetidine
    Drugs of abuse: phencyclidine and hallucinogenic agents
    Alcohol
    Poisons: heavy metals, organic solvents, methyl alcohol, ethylene glycol, insecti-
        cides, carbon monoxide.

Withdrawal syndromes
    Alcohol
    Sedatives and hypnotics

Metabolic
    Hypoxia
    Hypoglycemia
    Acid base imbalance: acidosis, alkalosis
    Electrolyte imbalance: elevated or decreased sodium, potassium, calcium, mag-
        nesium
    Water imbalance: inappropriate antidiuretic hormone, water intoxication, dehy-
        dration
    Failure of vital organs: liver, kidney, lung
    Inborn errors of metabolism: porphyria, Wilson's disease
    Remote effects of carcinoma, carcinoid syndrome
    Vitamin deficiency: thiamine (Wernicke's encephalopathy), nicotinic acid, folate,
        cyanocobalamin

Endocrine
    Thyroid: thyrotoxicosis, myxedema
    Parathyroid: hypo- and hyperparathyroidism
    Adrenal: Addison's disease, Cushing's syndrome
    Pancreas: hyperinsulinism, diabetes
    Pituitary hypofunction

CAUSES OF DELIRIUM

Organic causes of delirium have been reviewed by Lipowski (1980) and
Beresin (1988) and a partial list is found in Table 9–3.

Delirium must be distinguished from other organic mental syndromes and
functional psychiatric disorders. Dementia can be a confusing differential
diagnostic problem, especially because delirium is frequently superimposed
on a chronic dementing illness. As a general rule, any acute cognitive deterioration in a known demented patient is considered a delirium unless proven
otherwise and necessitates a thorough search for causes (Lipowski, 1980;
Beresin, 1985). Beresin (1988) outlined some comparative discriminators of
dementia from delirium (Table 9–4).

Table 9–3 *continued*
Organic Causes of Delirium

Cardiovascular
  Congestive heart failure
  Cardiac arrhythmia
  Myocardial infarction

Neurologic
  Head trauma
  Space occupying lesions: tumor, subdural hematoma, abscess, aneurysm
  Cerebrovascular diseases: thrombosis, embolism, arteritis, hemorrhage, hypertensive encephalopathy
  Degenerative disorders: Alzheimer's disease, multiple sclerosis
  Epilepsy

Infection
  Intracranial: encephalitis and meningitis (viral, bacterial, fungal, protozoal)
  Systemic: pneumonia, septicemia, subacute bacterial endocarditis, influenza, typhoid, typhus, infectious mononucleosis, infectious hepatitis, acute rheumatic fever, malaria, mumps, diphtheria, AIDS.

Hematologic
  Pernicious anemia
  Bleeding diatheses
  Polycythemia

Hypersensitivity
  Serum sickness
  Food allergy

Physical injury
  Heat: hyperthermia, hypothermia
  Electricity
  Burns

Reproduced with permission from Beresin EV: Delirium in the elderly. *J Geriatr Psychiatry Neurol* 1:132–133, 1988.

Usually, the demented patient's thoughts are impoverished; in contrast, the delirious patient typically has rich fantasies and perceptual disturbances (Lishman, 1978).

As noted in chapter 4, depression may present with cognitive disturbances and psychotically depressed patients may have delusions, paranoid ideation, poor attention and concentration, and restless sleep. Retarded depression can mimic hypoactive delirium or dementia with slowed thinking, decreased concentration, and memory impairments (Beresin, 1988). It is of utmost importance in sorting out the differential diagnosis to clarify how the patient had been recently. If the patient has had a dysphoric mood with sleep and appetite disturbances, a depressive syndrome would seem likely.

Table 9–4
Dementia versus Delirium

Features	Delirium	Dementia
Onset	Acute	Usually insidious
Duration	Brief	Chronic, unless reversible
Consciousness	Fluctuation	Static
Orientation	Abnormal, mistake familiar for unfamiliar	May be normal in mild cases
Memory	Recent defective (registration, retention, and recall)	Recent and later remote defective
Attention	Always impaired	May be intact
Perception	Frequently disturbed, contents vivid	Misperceptions may be absent, contents less florid
Thinking	Disorganized, contents rich	Impaired, contents empty and stereotyped
Judgment	Poor	Poor, occasional inappropriate social behavior
Sleep	Always disturbed	Usually normal
EEG	Invariably abnormal (slow, fast in withdrawal)	Normal or mild slowing

Reproduced with permission from Beresin EV: Delirium in the elderly. *J Geriatr Psychiatry Neurol* 1:138, 1988.

Depressed elderly patients frequently have a history of previous episodes, static mentation rather than fluctuations in consciousness, and predominance of depressive feelings.

Mania, on the other hand, can simulate hyperactive delirium with disorientation, agitation, rapid fluctuations in consciousness, diminished attention, and psychosis (Beresin, 1988; Carlson and Goodwin, 1973; Taylor and Abrams, 1973); in fact, one author used the term "acute delirious mania" (Bond, 1980). As with depressive disorders, there is usually a history of mania prior to old age (see chapter 4).

Because most elderly patients take a number of medications (Williamson, 1978), their propensity to drug-induced delirium is of major importance. Some of the major classes of medications that are associated with cognitive change in the elderly include the anticholinergic drugs, psychotropic agents, and cardiovascular medications (see Table 5–7).

Anticholinergic Delirium

Many of the drugs discussed in this book may be associated with anticholinergic side effects and delirium is frequently induced in elderly patients by such agents. It is well established that more than 600 commonly used drugs have anticholinergic actions that can produce serious neuropsychiatric toxic effects

(Granacher and Baldessarini, 1976). Diagnosis of delirium secondary to anti-cholinergic agents is tentatively established when there is a history of recent intake of one or more of these drugs, and when physical examination reveals the presence of peripheral muscarinic blockade. The latter may suggest the cause of delirium when a history of drug exposure is uncertain or absent (Lipowski, 1980).

Clinical Presentation
The signs and symptoms of peripheral muscarinic blockade include: dilated and poorly reactive pupils, tachycardia, facial flushing, dryness of skin and mucous membranes, blurred vision, urinary urgency, difficulty in initiating micturation, rise in blood pressure, and constipation. In some cases clinical manifestations such as fever, ataxia, dysarthria, muscle twitching, hyper-reflexia, convulsions, and overactivity are present.

Clinical Examples

Case 1: A 73-year-old man was brought to the emergency room from a local nursing home after he became confused and agitated. About one week prior to this incident, he had started to take amitriptyline because of withdrawn behavior and depression. In addition to confusion and agitation, the patient had a flushed face, dry skin, slight fever, and a pulse of 106. The physician diagnosed anticholinergic delirium and amitriptyline was discontinued.

Case 2: A 62-year-old woman had difficulty falling asleep for over a year. She treated herself with an over-the-counter medication which contained scopolamine. She gradually increased the dose to four capsules at bedtime. One night she awoke screaming. She was disoriented and convinced that her house was inhabited by strangers. Her husband took her to an emergency room where she was noted to have tachycardia and dilated pupils that were poorly responsive to light. She was treated with 1 mg of physostigmine intramuscularly and the symptoms resolved.

Commonly Implicated Medications
Nonprescription hypnotics   Many of these contain small quantities of scopolamine. Sominex is a typical offender.
Cycloplegics and mydriatics   Many elderly patients use eyedrops which contain atropine, scopolamine, and cyclopentolate. Even a small number of drops can induce delirium in the elderly. It is believed that such delirium may be due to swallowing of tears containing the drugs with subsequent absorption from the GI tract. Eyedrops appear to be particularly likely to precipitate severe toxic-confusional reactions in the elderly or brain-damaged individual and might lead to decompensation in mild dementia (Granacher and Baldessarini, 1976).

Antihistamines   Drugs such as diphenhydramine (Benadryl), hydroxyzine (Vistaril, Atarax), chlorpheniramine (Teldrin and others), and promethazine (Phenergan) are often prescribed as sedatives or antianxiety agents. These drugs have anticholinergic properties (Jenike, 1982).

Antiparkinsonian agents   Benztropine (Cogentin), trihexyphenidyl (Artane), and procyclidine (Kemadrin) are frequently used in the treatment of both disease-related and drug-induced extrapyramidal motor disorders. As little as 2 mg of benztropine can produce delirium in some patients (Ananth and Jain, 1979).

Antipsychotic drugs   Delirium with neuroleptics occurs most often in patients over the age of 50 and in brain-damaged patients (Angst and Hicklin, 1967; Helmchen, 1961). The delirium tends to follow rapid increases in dosage.

Low-potency neuroleptic drugs, such as chlorpromazine (Thorazine) and thioridazine (Mellaril), are much more likely to cause delirium than high-potency drugs such as haloperidol (Haldol), fluphenazine (Prolixin), and thiothixene (Navane).

Antidepressants   Tricyclic antidepressants are frequently associated with delirium in the elderly. Amitriptyline (Elavil and others) is the worst offender and has the highest antimuscarinic potency of the antidepressant drugs (see Table 9–5). Desipramine (Norpramin) has the least anticholinergic activity of the commonly used tricyclic antidepressants. Newer agents including maprotiline (Ludiomil) and trazodone (Desyrel) are said to have a low incidence of anticholinergic side effects (Gelenberg, 1981). Even in ordinary doses, antidepressants can produce a central delirium in the elderly without the striking peripheral parasympatholytic and pupillary signs seen with belladonna alkaloids (Baldessarini, 1978).

Other drugs   Antispasmotic medications such as Lomotil, commonly used for GI disorders, frequently contain atropine sulfate. Cimetidine (Tagamet) has been reported to cause delirium in elderly patients (Jenike, 1982a). It is unclear at present if a central anticholinergic mechanism is responsible, but three cases of patients in whom physostigmine rapidly reversed a presumed cimetidine-induced delirium have been reported (Mogelnicki et al, 1979; Jenike and Levy, 1983).

Management of Anticholinergic Delirium
If anticholinergic delirium is suspected, a trial of physostigmine (Antilirium) can be administered, typically by intramuscular or slow intravenous injection in doses of 1 to 2 mg. If the patient's mental status improves and symptoms of muscarinic blockade resolve after physostigmine injection, the diagnosis is confirmed. Physostigmine, the only anticholinesterase to freely cross the blood-brain barrier and reverse central anticholinergic effects, inhibits cholinesterase and thus promotes the action of acetylcholine.

The use of physostigmine is not without complications, including precipitation of asthmatic episodes and heart block resulting in myocardial infarction (Hall et al, 1981). The most serious consequences of excessive or too rapid administration of physostigmine are the provocation of acute respiratory embarrassment, heart block, or seizure (Granacher and Baldessarini, 1976). Because of these and other possible complications, some clinicians believe that it should be used conservatively (Baldessarini and Gelenberg, 1979). One report, however, contained 1,727 cases of successful treatment of central anticholinergic intoxication with no untoward effects (Holzgrafe et al, 1973). Toxicity resulting from physostigmine, manifested most commonly by nausea, vomiting, diarrhea, and bradycardia, can be reversed by the administration of 0.5 mg of atropine sulfate for each milligram of physostigmine administered.

Physostigmine has a relatively short half-life of 90 to 120 minutes. Thus, when anticholinergic toxicity is secondary to long-acting drugs, physostigmine may be needed at intervals of 30 minutes to two hours. For patients with a mild anticholinergic syndrome or elderly confused patients with uncertain cardiac status, one can manage the patient by withdrawal of the suspected toxin and the use of protective measures, reassurance, plus a benzodiazepine, such as lorazepam (Ativan) or oxazepam (Serax). Other central depressants, which themselves have anticholinergic properties, should not be used (Granacher and Baldessarini, 1976).

Psychotropic Drugs

A number of psychotropic agents can precipitate delirium in the elderly.

Antidepressants

As noted, antidepressants can produce delirium by an anticholinergic mechanism, but they can also cause sedation, postural hypotension, or cardiac toxicity (see chapter 4) and can produce delirium at even low dosages. Cardiac toxicity appears to increase when the ECG QRS complex is greater than 100 milliseconds (Spiker et al, 1975). Beresin (1988) pointed out that psychotic depressed elderly patients are at special risk when antidepressants are combined with antipsychotic medications. This often increases the anticholinergic load; high-potency agents, such as haloperidol, fluphenazine, or trifluoperazine, are less likely to produce anticholinergic effects than low-potency agents and should be used in combination with a low-anticholinergic antidepressant (see chapter 4). A similar problem of excessive anticholinergic burden might occur when the clinician is treating neuroleptic-induced parkinsonian side effects with an anticholinergic agent such as benztropine or diphenhydramine. Amantadine may be effective and less toxic in the elderly (see chapter 6).

Lithium
Lithium can cause toxicity at normal or even low levels. The signs and symptoms of toxicity (see chapter 4) include delirium, tremor, lethargy, dysarthria, neuromuscular irritability, diarrhea, seizures, stupor, and coma. When elderly patients taking lithium undergo ECT the risk for delirium may be even greater (Hoening and Chaulk, 1977; Mandel et al, 1980).

Benzodiazepines
These agents are unlikely causes of delirium in the young but are often implicated in the elderly. They are frequently prescribed medications in geriatric patients (Williamson, 1978) and can cause confusion and paradoxical excitement or rage reactions in the elderly. As outlined in chapter 7, long-acting agents are much more likely to be associated with drug-buildup and are more frequently implicated than the shorter-acting drugs, such as oxazepam and lorazepam.

Cardiovascular Medications

Many antihypertensive medications that have been associated with delirium include diuretics, clonidine, methyldopa, reserpine, propranolol, and metoprolol (Reus, 1979; Beresin, 1988). Diuretics, in fact, produce more adverse effects in the elderly than any other drugs (Morse and Litin, 1971) by producing dehydration, hypotension, hypokalemia, and hyponatremia (Beresin, 1985). Antiarrhythmic drugs such as quinidine, procainamide, and lidocaine can also produce delirium (Lipowski, 1980; Beresin, 1985).

Digitalis toxicity can produce delirium in as many as 20% of patients (Shear and Sacks, 1978 and 1978a; Portnoi, 1979) which can be manifested clinically by drowsiness, incoherence, fatigue, illusions, hallucinations, GI disturbances, and cardiac arrhythmias.

Cimetidine, currently a commonly prescribed drug, can cause delirium by at least two mechanisms (McMillen et al, 1978; Barnhart and Bowden, 1979): either directly by acting on the CNS or indirectly by decreasing hepatic blood flow and hence clearance of drugs or by reducing the efficacy of hepatic enzymes and thus the excretion of some drugs such as phenytoin, diazepan, chlordiazepoxide, warfarin, carbamazepine, theophylline, and lidocaine (McMillen et al, 1978; Barnhart and Bowden, 1979).

Some other drugs that can cause delirium are listed in Table 9–3.

Withdrawal Syndromes

When sedative-hypnotics or alcohol are stopped suddenly, a withdrawal delirium can result with autonomic arousal, irritability, tremor, positional nystagmus, and sleep disturbance (Gaitz and Baer, 1971). Mild abstinence syndromes can either abate or progress to seizures or delirium tremens (see chapter 10). The elderly alcoholic has many features that increase risk for delirium such as alcoholic cerebral damage, frequent pulmonary infections, head trauma, and vitamin deficiencies (Beresin, 1985 and 1988).

Metabolic Disturbances

Many metabolic aberations can produce delirium in the elderly and in many cases multiple disturbances occur in the same individual. For example, diuretic-induced dehydration can be complicated by electrolyte imbalance and alkalosis.

Hypoxia frequently presents as a delirium and can result from cardiovascular, pulmonary, and hematologic disorders (Beresin, 1988). Hypoglycemia is sometimes implicated and it appears that the rate of change more than the absolute level of glucose determines the amount of cognitive disturbance. Apparently the most common cause of hypoglycemia is improper insulin administration or inadequate food intake following insulin administration (Beresin, 1985 and 1988).

Hyponatremia secondary to ingestion of large amounts of water (psychogenic polydipsia) in some psychotic patients can produce delirium (Jose and Perez-Cruet, 1979). Also, inappropriate secretion of antidiuretic hormone can result from ingestion of a number of drugs, including antidepressants, antipsychotics, and carbamazepine (Moses and Miller, 1974).

Vitamin B_{12} and folate deficiencies commonly produce delirium and dementia in the elderly (Libow, 1973; Victor et al, 1971; Mitra, 1971; Strachan and Henderson, 1965). There is a report that almost a fourth of patients who have onset of Alzhiemer's disease after the age of 65 have low B_{12} levels (with normal red blood cell parameters) compared with those who have onset before the age of 65 who have normal levels (Gottfries, 1988). Vitamin B_{12} deficiency does not always produce the characteristic abnormal hematologic picture with a megaloblastic anemia prior to onset of cognitive symptoms. The significance of this finding is yet to be determined, but suggests that clinicians should pay close attention to vitamin levels in the elderly.

Thiamine deficiency, most common in elderly alcoholic patients, can produce Wernicke's encephalopathy (see chapter 10), with nystagmus, ataxia, ophthalmoplegia, and delirium (Victor et al, 1971).

Some medications, most notably the antipsychotic agents, can result in abnormal temperature regulation resulting in hypothermia in the winter or hyperthermia in the summer. Such patients can present with a delirium. When elderly patients have limited incomes, they might be forced to choose between food and heat or air conditioning and when they are given antipsychotic medications, alterations in body temperature can develop.

Cardiovascular Disorders

Cerebral hypoxia secondary to reduced blood flow with resultant delirium can result from a number of cardiac disorders including congestive heart failure,

Table 9–5
Antimuscarinic Potency of Commonly Used Drugs

Agent	Measure of Antimuscarinic Potency*
Scopolamine	0.3
Atropine	0.4
Trihexyphenidyl (Artane)	0.6
Benztropine (Cogentin)	1.5
Amitriptyline (Elavil)	10
Doxepin (Sinequan)	44
Imipramine (Tofranil)	78
Thioridazine (Mellaril)	150
Desipramine (Norpramin)	170
Chlorpromazine (Thorazine)	1000
Fluphenazine (Prolixin)	12,000
Thiothixene (Navane)	26,000
Haloperidol (Haldol)	48,000
Phenelzine (Nardil)	100,000

*The lower the number, the more likely the agent is to produce anticholinergic effects.
Adapted from Snyder S, Greenberg D, Yamamura H: Antimuscarinic potency of CNS agents. *Arch Gen Psychiatry* 31:173, 1974.

myocardial infarctions, arrhythmias, or postural hypotension (Beresin, 1986; Fine, 1978). Beresin (1988) noted that delirium may be the only symptom in paroxysmal tachyarrhythmias (Clark, 1970) and also in myocardial infarctions, which appear without pain in as many as 40% of geriatric patients (Varsamis, 1978).

Neurologic Disorders

In as many as 50% of elderly patients presenting with chronic subdural hematoma, there is no discernible history of head injury (Fogalholm et al, 1975). With age, the brain shrinks and bridging vessels from the skull to the cerebrum are stretched and as a result even minor trauma during sleep can produce a subdural hematoma. Such hematomas can imitate a number of disorders and affected patients may be delirious (Potter and Fruin, 1977).

Other mass lesions, such as primary or metastatic brain tumors, have their highest incidence in the elderly population and can present as a delirium or dementia.

Strokes and transient ischemic attacks can produce delirium even in the absence of focal neurologic signs (Mesulam, 1979).

Seizure disorders, such as petit mal status epilepticus, complex partial status epilepticus, postictal states, and interictal states associated with temporal lobe epilepsy can cause delirium (Beresin, 1988; Terzano et al, 1986). A recently described syndrome called periodic lateralized epileptiform discharges

(PLEDs) has been reported to cause a delirium which is sometimes responsive to carbamazepine treatment (Terzano et al, 1986).

Infection

In the elderly, infections are not universally associated with fever and should be considered in the evaluation of any delirious patient. Systemic, as well as CNS, infections can produce delirium, especially in the patient who has an already compromised brain (eg, Alzheimer's disease). Commonly implicated systemic infections include pulmonary, urinary tract, cholecystitis, and diverticulitis. In a dementing patient, even an uncomplicated urinary tract infection can dramatically worsen cognitive function by superimposing a delirious state. Such acute decompensations are almost universally reversible with appropriate treatment.

TREATMENT

Correct Organic Factors

In formulating a treatment plan for an individual patient, close attention must be paid to the correction of any organic or disease-related factors. Initially, life-threatening illnesses such as cerebral hypoxia, hypertensive encephalopathy, intracranial hemorrhage, meningitis, severe electrolyte and metabolic imbalances, hypoglycemia, and intoxications (Beresin, 1988) must be ruled out or corrected. If possible, all medications should be stopped and vital signs monitored at least every two hours. Transfer to an intensive care unit should be considered.

The patient must be protected from physical harm by using low beds, guard rails, and careful supervision.

Environmental Management

Attention to the immediate environment of the delirious patient is very important and even little manipulations can yield major improvements in clinical state. The underlying philosophy (Beresin, 1988) is to make the ward environment, including sensory input, personal contact, activities, and the physical plant, as consistent and familiar as possible (Table 9–6).

Beresin (1988) suggested supportive psychotherapy, which is particularly useful during lucid periods, to quell anxiety, provide comfort and reassurance, and promote reality testing by conveying instructions, explanations, and coping strategies (Hackett and Weisman, 1960 and 1960a). He believed that it is an error to interpret the meaning of unconscious fantasies that intrude into consciousness during delirious episodes. Family members should be told that delirious accusations, threats, and confessions are not related to reality.

Table 9–6
Ward Management of Delirium

Environment
  Sensory input: not excessive, inadequate, or ambiguous. Room should have adequate light and be quiet. Some patients prefer radio or television for familiar background stimulation
  Present one stimulus or task at a time
  Medication schedules should not interrupt sleep

Orientation
  Room should have a clock, calendar, and chart of the day's schedule
  Keep the patient in the same surroundings
  Verbal reminders of the time, day, and place should be used frequently
  Evaluate the need for eyeglasses, hearing aids, and foreign language interpreters

Familiarity
  Obtain familiar possessions from home to help orient the patient, particularly objects at the home bedside
  Request family members to stay with the patient. They provide the basis for orientation, effective communication, support, and aftercare planning
  Discuss familiar areas of interest, eg, hobbies, occupation
  Allow the same staff members to consistently care for the patient

Communication
  Instructions and explanations should be clear, slow-paced, simple, and repetitive
  Use face-to-face contact
  Convey an attitude of warmth and kind firmness
  Consistently address the patient as he/she prefers
  Begin each contact with orienting and identifying information
  Acknowledge the patient's emotions and encourage verbal expression

Activities
  Avoid physical restraint. Allow free movement, provided the patient is safe
  Encourage self-care and other personal activities to reinforce competence and enhance self-esteem

Reproduced with permission from Beresin EV: Delirium in the elderly. *J Geriatr Psychiatry Neurol* 1:140, 1988.

Beresin further recommended at least some discussions with the patient once the delirium has cleared since patients will have spotty recollections of the illness and not know with clarity what was fantasy and what was reality; some memories might be seriously disturbing and even posttraumatic stress syndrome has been reported (Mackenzie and Popkin, 1980).

Family Management

During a delirious episode, presence of close family members is of utmost help. They can provide support and orientation. Family members might instinctively interpret threats or confused statements as fact if not cautioned about the nature of delirious thinking. They may be traumatized when witnessing extreme confusion and agitation in a loved one and may require support and reassurance from clinicians associated with the care of their relative.

Drug Treatment of Delirium

Pharmacotherapy is required when the delirious elderly patient is excessively anxious, agitated, sleepless, or psychotic or when the patient is threatening to himself or others. If possible, medication should be avoided until specific organic causes are identified; this may not be possible, however. Short-acting benzodiazepines are helpful for treating anxiety and sleeplessness and are the drugs of choice for withdrawal syndromes. On the other hand, they may worsen agitation in demented patients with superimposed delirium and they are not helpful for psychotic symptoms.

Antipsychotic agents are often required to manage severely agitated or psychotic elderly patients. As outlined in chapter 6, high-potency agents, like haloperidol or thiothixene, are preferred over low-potency agents, such as chlorpromazine or thioridazine, because the low-potency drugs are more likely to produce anticholinergic effects that can further worsen cognition and can also precipitate cardiac arrhythmias and orthostatic hypotension. Haloperidol is the best studied and has been shown to be safe and effective over short periods of time (Beresin, 1988; Moore, 1977; Oldham and Bott, 1971; Ayd, 1978; Jenike, 1985; Tesar et al, 1985); it causes minimal sedation and has low anticholinergic potency and is safe in patients with cardiac and respiratory illness when given orally, intramuscularly, or intravenously. As in managing the disturbed demented patient, it is best to begin with modest doses such as 0.5 mg and increase the dose if there is no response. For milder behavioral disturbances, oral haloperidol is usually sufficient. For the very disturbed delirious patient, intravenous dosages of haloperidol of more than 200 mg/24 hours may be required (Tesar et al, 1985).

SUMMARY

The elderly are particularly likely to develop delirium, which is commonly underdiagnosed, and as many as 30% of delirious patients will progress to stupor, coma, and death. When optimally diagnosed and treated, delirium is often a compeletely reversible syndrome. The clinical presentations can be manifested in many ways and variability in symptoms is a hallmark of the disorder. Symptoms are often worse in the evening and at night.

Because of the potentially serious and sometimes life-threatening nature of delirium, rapid diagnosis and treatment are imperative. The clinician should do a complete mental status examination as outlined in chapter 2. Some delirious patients will be very embarrassed and secretive about cognitive deficits and one should proceed very gently after building some alliance with the patient. To establish a medical cause, a thorough history is required and should focus on medical history, medication (prescription and over-the-counter) use, and a complete review of systems. Physical and neurologic examinations as well as laboratory tests are required.

The early signs of delirium include feelings of uneasiness, malaise, headache, fatigue, decreased concentration, irritability, restlessness, anxiety, depression, or decreased interests. If delirium progresses, attention is reduced and distractibility and concentration problems follow. Language functions are always abnormal in patients with delirium and speech may be tangential, circumstantial, or slurred.

Delirium appears to be a common final pathway that can be reached by a number of ways. By definition, a biological stressor must be present for delirium to occur, but psychological or environmental factors are often involved. The pathologic mechanisms underlying delirium remain a mystery. Delirium must be distinguished from other organic mental syndromes and functional psychiatric disorders. Dementia can be a confusing differential diagnostic problem, especially because delirium is frequently superimposed on a chronic dementing illness.

Some of the commonly implicated drugs include: nonprescription hypnotics, cycloplegics and mydriatics, antihistamines, antiparkinsonian agents, antipsychotic drugs, and antidepressants. Alcohol and sedative-hypnotic withdrawal syndromes, infections, cardiovascular and neurologic disorders, and metabolic disturbances can produce delirium.

The management of delirious patients involves primarily withdrawal of the offending agent or correction of the organic illness. A number of environmental manipulations can help to minimize the seriousness of the delirium and facilitate improvement. Family members can provide invaluable assistance, but will likely need assistance in dealing with the trauma of seeing a delirious loved one. Short-term psychotherapeutic techniques may assist during the delirious episode, but should also be used in helping the recovered patient.

Physostigmine can be used for anticholinergic delirium but has some inherent dangers, such as induction of acute respiratory problems, heart block, or seizure. These can generally be avoided if the drug is given intramuscularly or slowly intravenously. For mild cases, reassurance plus a benzodiazepine may be adequate treatment. Haloperidol can be helpful for treating agitation or psychotic symptoms.

Above all, delirium must increasingly come to the awareness of clinicians who care for the aged, as early recognition and treatment can materially prolong survival of elderly patients.

REFERENCES

Ananth JV, Jain RC: Benztropine psychosis. *Can J Psychiatry* 18:409–414, 1979.
Angst J, Hicklin A: Delirose psychosen unter neuroleptica und antidepressiva. *Schweiz Med Wochenschr* 97:546–549, 1967.

Ayd FJ: Haloperidol: Twenty years' clinical experience. *J Clin Psychiatry* 39:807–814, 1978.

Baldessarini RJ, Gelenberg AJ: Using physostigmine safely. *Am J Psychiatry* 136:1609–1610, 1979.

Baldessarini RJ: *Chemotherapy in Psychiatry*. Cambridge, Mass, Harvard University Press, 1978.

Barnhart CC, Bowden CL: Toxic psychosis with cimetidine. *Am J Psychiatry* 136:725–726, 1979.

Bedford PD: General medical aspects of confusional states in elderly people. *Br Med J* 2:185–188, 1959.

Beresin E: Delirium in the elderly: Assessment and management. *Wyeth Monograph Series: Clinical Perspectives in Aging*, Wyeth Publications, 1985.

Beresin E: Delirium, in Sederer LI (ed): *Inpatient Psychiatry: Diagnosis and Treatment*, ed 2. Baltimore, Williams and Wilkins, 1986.

Beresin EV: Delirium in the elderly. *J Geriatr Psychiatry Neurol* 1:127–143, 1988.

Bond TC: Recognition of acute delirious mania. *Arch Gen Psychiatry* 37:553–554, 1980.

Carlson GA, Goodwin FK: The stages of mania. *Arch Gen Psychiatry* 28:221–228, 1973.

Chedru F, Geschwind N: Disorders of higher cortical functions in acute confusional states. *Cortex* 8:395–411, 1972.

Chedru F, Geschwind N: Writing disturbances in acute confusional states. *Neuropsychologia* 10:343–353, 1972a.

Clark ANG: Ectopic tachyarrhythmias in the elderly. *Gerontol Clin* 12:203–212, 1970.

DeVaul RA: Acute organic brain syndromes: Clinical considerations. *Tex Med* 72:51–54, 1976.

Engel GL: Delirium, in Freedman AM, Kaplan HI (eds): *Comprehensive Textbook of Psychiatry*. Baltimore, Williams and Wilkins, 1967.

Fine W: Postural hypotension. *Practitioner* 20:698–701, 1978.

Fogalholm R, Heiskanen O, Waltime O: Chronic subdural hematoma in adults. *J Neurosurg* 42:43–46, 1975.

Folstein MF, Folstein SE, McHugh PR: Mini-mental state: A practical method for grading the cognitive state of patients for the clinician. *J Psychiatr Res* 12:189–198, 1975.

Gaitz CM, Baer PE: Characteristics of elderly patients with alcoholism. *Arch Gen Psychiatry* 24:372–378, 1971.

Gelenberg AJ: New antidepressants. *Biol Ther Psychiatry* 4:5, 1981.

Gottfries CG: Alzheimer's disease. Presented at the International Workshop on Treatment and Diagnosis of Senile Dementia, Seefeld, Austria, Sep 24, 1988.

Granacher RP, Baldessarini RJ: The usefulness of physostigmine in neurology and psychiatry, in Klawans HL (ed): *Clinical Neuropharmacology*. New York, Raven Press, 1976, vol 1.

Hackett TP, Weisman AD: Psychiatric management of operative syndromes: I. The therapeutic consultation and the effect of non-interpretive intervention. *Psychosom Med* 22:267–282, 1960.

Hackett TP, Weisman AD: Psychiatric management of operative syndromes: II. Psychodynamic factors in formulation and management. *Psychosom Med* 22:356–372, 1960a.

Hall RCW, Feinsilver DL, Holt RE: Anticholinergic psychosis: Diagnosis and treatment. *Psychosomatics* 22:581–587, 1981.

Helmchen H: Delirante abliiufe unter psychiatrischer pharmakotherapie. *Arch Psychiatr Nervenkr* 202:395–411, 1961.

Hoening J, Chaulk R: Delirium associated with lithium and electroconvulsive therapy. *Can Med Assoc J* 116:837–838, 1977.

308

Holzgrafe RE, Vondrell JJ, Mintz SM: Reversal of postoperative reactions to scopolamine with physostigmine. *Anesth Analg (Cleve)* 52:921–925, 1973.

Jenike MA, Levy JC: Physostigmine reversal of cimetidine-induced delirium and agitation. *J Clin Psychopharmacol* 3:43–44, 1983.

Jenike MA: Cimetidine in elderly patients: Review of uses and risks. *J Am Geriatr Soc* 30:170–173, 1982a.

Jenike MA: *Handbook of Geriatric Psychopharmacology*. Littleton, Mass, PSG Publishing, 1985.

Jenike MA: Using sedative drugs in the elderly. *Drug Ther* 12:184–190, 1982.

Jose CJ, Perez-Cruet J: Incidence of morbidity of self-induced water intoxication in state mental hospital patients. *Am J Psychiatry* 136:221–222, 1979.

Kral MA: Confusional states: Description and management, in Howells JG (ed): *Modern Perspectives in the Psychiatry of Old Age*. New York, Bruner/Mazel, 1975.

Levin M: Varieties of disorientation. *J Ment Sci* 102:619–623, 1954.

Libow LS: Pseudosenility: Acute and reversible organic brain syndrome. *J Am Geriatr Soc* 21:112–120, 1973.

Lipowski ZJ: *Delirium*. Springfield, Ill, Charles C Thomas, 1980.

Lipowski ZJ: Organic mental disorders: Introduction and review of syndromes, in Kaplan HI, Freedman AM, Sadock BJ (eds): *Comprehensive Textbook of Psychiatry/III*. Baltimore, Williams and Wilkins, 1980a.

Lishman WA: *Organic Psychiatry: The Psychological Consequences of Cerebral Disorder*. Oxford, Blackwell Scientific Publications, 1978.

Liston EH: Delirium in the aged. *Psychiatr Clin North Am* 5:49–66, 1982.

Mackenzie TB, Popkin MK: Stress response syndrome occurring after delirium. *Am J Psychiatry* 137:1433–1435, 1980.

Mandel MR, Madsen J, Miller AL, et al: Intoxication associated with lithium and ECT. *Am J Psychiatry* 137:1107–1109, 1980.

McCartney JR, Palmateer LM: Assessment of cognitive deficits in geriatric patients: A study of physician behavior. *J Am Geriatr Soc* 33:467–471, 1985.

McMillen MA, Ambis D, Siegel JH: Cimetidine and mental confusion. *N Engl J Med* 298:283–285, 1978.

Mesulam M-M: Acute behavioral derangements without hemiplegia in cerebrovascular accidents. *Prim Care* 6:813–826, 1979.

Mitra ML: Confusional states in relation to vitamin deficiencies in the elderly. *J Am Geriatr Soc* 19:536–545, 1971.

Mogelnicki SR, Waller JL, Finlayson DC: Physostigmine reversal of cimetidine-induced mental confusion. *JAMA* 241:826–827, 1979.

Moore DP: Rapid treatment of delirium in critically ill patients. *Am J Psychiatry* 134:1431–1432, 1977.

Morse RM, Litin EM: The anatomy of a delirium. *Am J Psychiatry* 128:111–115, 1971.

Moses AM, Miller M: Drug-induced dilutional hyponatremia. *N Engl J Med* 191:1234–1239, 1974.

NIA Task Force: Senility reconsidered. *JAMA* 244:259–263, 1980.

Oldham AJ, Bott M: The management of excitement in a general hospital psychiatric ward by high dosage haloperidol. *Acta Psychiatr Scand* 47:369–376, 1971.

Portnoi MA: Digitalis delirium in elderly patients. *J Clin Pharmacol* 19:747–750, 1979.

Potter JF, Fruin AH: Chronic subdural hematoma—The great imitator. *Geriatrics* 32:61–66, 1977.

Purdie FR, Hareginan B, Rosen P: Acute organic brain syndrome: A review of 100 cases. *Ann Emerg Med* 10:455–461, 1981.

Reus VI: Behavioral side effects of medical drugs. *Prim Care* 6:283–294, 1979.

Shear MK, Sacks M: Digitalis delirium: Psychiatric considerations. *Int J Psychiatr Med* 8:371–381, 1978.

Shear MK, Sacks M: Digitalis delirium: Report of two cases. *Am J Psychiatry* 135:109–110, 1978a.

Simon A, Cahan RB: The acute brain syndrome in geriatric patients. *Psychiatr Res Rep* 16:8–21, 1963.

Snyder S, Greenberg D, Yamamura H: Antimuscarinic potency of CNS agents. *Arch Gen Psychiatry* 31:173, 1974.

Spiker DG, Weiss AN, Chang SS, et al: Tricyclic antidepressant overdose: Clinical presentation and plasma levels. *Clin Pharmacol Ther* 18:539–546, 1975.

Strachan RW, Henderson JG: Psychiatric syndromes due to avitaminosis B_{12} with normal blood and marrow. *Q J Med* 34:303–317, 1965.

Swigar ME, Benes FM, Rothman SLG, et al: Behavioral correlates of computerized tomographic (CT) scan changes in older psychiatric patients. *J Am Geriatr Soc* 33:96–103, 1985.

Taylor MA, Abrams R: The phenomenology of mania. *Arch Gen Psychiatry* 29:520–522, 1973.

Terzano MG, Parrino L, Mazzuchi A, et al: Confusional states with periodic lateralized epileptiform discharges (PLEDs): A peculiar epileptic syndrome in the elderly. *Epilepsia* 27:446–457, 1986.

Tesar GE, Murray GB, Cassem NH: Use of high-dose intravenous haloperidol in the treatment of agitated cardiac patients. *J Clin Psychopharmacol* 5:344–347, 1985.

Varsamis J: Clinical management of delirium. *Psychiatr Clin North Am* 1:71–80, 1978.

Victor M, Adams RD, Collins GH: *The Wernicke-Korsakoff Syndrome*. Philadelphia, FA Davis Co, 1971.

Williamson J: Prescribing problems in the elderly. *Practitioner* 220:749–755, 1978.

Wolff HG, Curran D: Nature of delirium and allied states. The dysergastic reaction. *AMA Arch Neurol Psychiatry* 33:1175–1215, 1935.

10

Alcohol and Drug Abuse in the Elderly

OVERVIEW

Alcohol and other substances are sometimes used as psychopharmacologic agents by elderly patients in an effort to treat undiagnosed or masked psychiatric illness. Blazer (1982) noted that alcoholic patients have a number of symptoms suggestive of a depressive disorder and that elderly alcoholics report a higher rate of suicide attempts and of social isolation.

A number of elderly patients, however, have primary alcoholism or drug abuse that requires treatment in its own right. In the past, alcohol and drug abuse were largely considered problems associated with youth and middle age, but more recent evidence suggests that this is not always the case (Atkinson, 1984); as many as 10% of adult alcoholics are over the age of 60 (Schuckit, 1977). One group found that alcohol and drug abuse together accounted for 10% of patients handled by a large geriatric mental health program (Reifler et al, 1982); in this study, only dementia and depression were more common. Alcoholism appears to be the most common substance abuse problem in the elderly (Atkinson, 1984).

CATEGORIES OF SUBSTANCE ABUSE

Types of Psychoactive Substances and Their Classification

According to DSM-III-R (1987), nine classes of psychoactive substances are associated with both abuse and dependence: alcohol; amphetamine or similarly acting sympathomimetics; cannabis; cocaine; hallucinogens; inhalants; opioids; phencyclidine (PCP) or similarly acting arylcyclohexylamines; and sedatives, hypnotics, or anxiolytics. Dependence, but not abuse, is seen with nicotine.

310

In DSM-III-R (1987) the category psychoactive substance use disorders (further categorized as either psychoactive substance dependence or psychoactive substance abuse) refers to the maladaptive behavior associated with more or less regular use of certain substances whereas the category psychoactive substance-induced organic mental disorders describes the direct acute or chronic effects of such substances on the CNS. Almost invariably, people who have a psychoactive substance use disorder will also have at least intermittent psychoactive substance-induced organic mental disorder, such as intoxication or withdrawal.

Psychoactive Substance Use Disorders

Psychoactive Substance Dependence
The dependent person generally continues to use the substance despite adverse consequences indicating impaired control of substance use. Dependence includes, but is not limited to, the physiologic symptoms of tolerance and withdrawal. At least three of the nine characteristic symptoms of dependence are necessary to make the diagnosis (see Table 10–1). In addition, the diagnosis of the dependence syndrome requires that some symptoms of the disturbance have persisted for at least one month, or have occurred repeatedly over a longer period of time, as in binge drinking. Dependence is further separated in terms of degree of severity (see Table 10–1).

Psychoactive Substance Abuse
This category is for noting maladaptive patterns of psychoactive substance use that have never met the criteria for dependence. Criteria for this disorder are listed in Table 10–2. An example of a situation when this category would apply is a student who binges on cocaine every few weekends and misses school for a few days because of "crashing."   Another would be a businessman who drives his car repeatedly when intoxicated with alcohol but has no other symptoms.

Psychoactive Substance-Induced Organic Mental Disorders

This category deals with the various organic mental syndromes, caused by direct effects of psychoactive substances on the nervous system, and is distinguished from the psychoactive substance use disorders that have been just discussed.

This category includes mental syndromes caused by the eleven classes of substances that most commonly are taken nonmedically to alter mood or behavior and include: alcohol; amphetamines or similarly acting sympathomimetics; caffeine; cannabis; cocaine; hallucinogens; inhalants; nicotine; opioids;

Table 10–1
Diagnostic Criteria for Psychoactive Substance Dependence

A. At least three of the following:
   (1) substance often taken in larger amounts or over a longer period than the person intended
   (2) persistent desire or one or more unsuccessful efforts to cut down or control substance use
   (3) a great deal of time spent in activities necessary to get the substance (eg, theft), taking the substance (eg, chain smoking), or recovering from its effects
   (4) frequent intoxication or withdrawal symptoms when expected to fulfill major role obligations at work, school, or home (eg, does not go to work because hung over, goes to school or work "high," intoxicated while taking care of his or her children), or when substance use is physically hazardous (eg, drives when intoxicated)
   (5) important social, occupational, or recreational activities given up or reduced because of substance use
   (6) continued substance use despite knowledge of having a persistent or recurrent social, psychological, or physical problem that is caused or exacerbated by use of the substance (eg, keeps using heroin despite family arguments about it, cocaine-induced depression, or having an ulcer made worse by drinking)
   (7) marked tolerance: need for markedly increased amounts of the substance (ie, at least a 50% increase) in order to achieve intoxication or desired effect, or markedly diminished effect with continued use of the same amount

   Note: The following items may not apply to cannabis, hallucinogens, or phencyclidine (PCP):

   (8) characteristic withdrawal symptoms
   (9) substance often taken to relieve or avoid withdrawal symptoms
B. Some symptoms of the disturbance have persisted for at least one month, or have occurred repeatedly over a longer period of time.

Criteria for severity of psychoactive substance dependence:
   Mild: Few, if any, symptoms in excess of those required to make the diagnosis, and the symptoms result in no more than mild impairment in occupational functioning or in usual social activities or relationships with others.
   Moderate: Symptoms or functional impairment between "mild" and "severe."
   Severe: Many symptoms in excess of those required to make the diagnosis, and the symptoms markedly interfere with occupational functioning or with usual social activities or relationships with others.
   In Partial Remission: During the past six months, some use of the substance and some symptoms of dependence.
   In Full Remission: During the past six months, either no use of the substance, or use of the substance and no symptoms of dependence.

Reprinted with permission from the *Diagnostic and Statistical Manual of Mental Disorders, third edition, revised.* Copyright 1987. American Psychiatric Association.

phencyclidine; and sedatives, hypnotics, or anxiolytics. Each drug can cause a number of mental syndromes (eg, alcohol) or only one (eg, caffeine). Table 10–3 lists some of the organic mental syndromes associated with each substance.

Table 10–2
Diagnostic Criteria for Psychoactive Substance
Abuse

A. A maladaptive pattern of psychoactive substance use indicated by at least one of the following:
  (1) continued use despite knowledge of having a persistent or recurrent social, occupational, psychological, or physical problem that is caused or exacerbated by use of the psychoactive substance
  (2) recurrent use in situations in which use is physically hazardous (eg, driving while intoxicated)
B. Some symptoms of the disturbance have persisted for at least one month, or have occurred repeatedly over a longer period of time.
C. Never met the criteria for psychoactive substance dependence for this substance.

Reprinted with permission from the *Diagnostic and Statistical Manual of Mental Disorders, third edition, revised*. Copyright 1987. American Pyschiatric Association.

Since the majority of the psychoactive substance-induced organic mental disorders are quite rare in the elderly we only review in detail alcohol-induced organic mental disorders and sedative-, hypnotic-, or anxiolytic-induced organic mental disorders. For diagnostic criteria for other substance-induced organic mental disorders, DSM-III-R (1987) should be consulted.

Alcohol-Induced Organic Mental Disorders
A number of organic mental syndromes occur with some regularity in elderly patients who are abusing alcohol:

Alcohol intoxication   The essential feature of this disorder is maladaptive behavioral changes as a result of recent ingestion of alcohol (Table 10–4).

Most people become intoxicated at blood alcohol levels between 100 and 200 mg/dL and death, usually by direct CNS depression or by aspiration of vomitus, has been reported at levels ranging from 400 to 700 mg/dL. Alcoholics are often abusing other drugs concomitantly and multiple complicated syndromes are not uncommon.

Alcohol idiosyncratic intoxication   This disorder is characterized by many of the same behavioral changes as noted in the previous paragraph but results from the ingestion of relatively small amounts of alcohol that would not be enough to induce intoxication in most people (Table 10–5). This has been called "pathological intoxication."

Uncomplicated alcohol withdrawal   This disorder is characterized by the symptoms outlined in Table 10–6 and typically follow within several hours after cessation of or reduction in alcohol ingestion by a person who has been drinking alcohol for several days or longer. This diagnosis is not made if the patient meets criteria for alcohol withdrawal delirium.

Symptoms almost always disappear within five to seven days unless delirium sets in. Seizures develop in occasional patients, especially those with

Table 10-3
Organic Mental Syndromes Associated with Psychoactive Substances

	Intoxication	Withdrawal	Delirium	Withdrawal Delirium	Delusional Disorder	Mood Disorder	Other Syndromes
Alcohol	x	x		x			[1]
Amphetamine and related substances	x	x	x		x		
Caffeine	x						
Cannabis	x				x		
Cocaine	x	x	x		x		
Hallucinogen	x (hallucinosis)				x	x	[2]
Inhalant	x						
Nicotine		x					
Opioid	x	x					
Phencyclidine (PCP) and related substances	x		x		x	x	[3]
Sedative, hypnotic, or anxiolytic	x	x		x			[4]

[1] Alcohol idiosyncratic intoxication, Alcohol hallucinosis, alcohol amnestic disorder, dementia associated with alcoholism.
[2] Posthallucinogen perception disorder.
[3] Phencyclidine (PCP) or similarly acting arylcyclohexylamine organic mental disorder NOS.
[4] Sedative, hypnotic or anxiolytic amnestic disorder.
Reprinted with permission from the *Diagnostic and Statistical Manual of Mental Disorders, third edition, revised.* Copyright 1987. American Psychiatric Association.

Table 10–4
Diagnostic Criteria for 303.00 Alcohol
Intoxication

A. Recent ingestion of alcohol (with no evidence suggesting that the amount was insufficient to cause intoxication in most people).
B. Maladaptive behavioral changes, eg, disinhibition of sexual or aggressive impulses, mood lability, impaired judgment, impaired social or occupational functioning.
C. At least one of the following signs:
    (1) slurred speech
    (2) incoordination
    (3) unsteady gait
    (4) nystagmus
    (5) flushed face
D. Not due to any physical or other mental disorder.

Reprinted with permission from the *Diagnostic and Statistical Manual of Mental Disorders, third edition, revised.* Copyright 1987. American Psychiatric Association.

preexisting history of epilepsy. Malnutrition, fatigue, affective illness, and concomitant physical illness can worsen this syndrome.

Alcohol withdrawal delirium Occurring much less commonly than uncomplicated alcohol withdrawal, this syndrome, whose essential feature is delirium (see chapter 9), develops, usually within one week, after recent cessation of or reduction in alcohol intake (Table 10–7). Besides delirium, marked autonomic activity is noted with tachycardia and sweating. This has often been referred to as delirium tremens. Concomitant physical illness appears to predispose to delirium and in a physically healthy person delerium rarely develops during withdrawal from alcohol (DSM-III-R).

Alcohol hallucinosis Vivid and persistent hallucinations of either an auditory or a visual nature sometimes (usually within 48 hours) develop after cessation of or reduction in alcohol ingestion (Table 10–8). The hallucinations are generally upsetting to the patient and usually consist of voices discussing the patient in the third person. Some patients complain of hissing or buzzing sounds. Delirium is not present.

This syndrome usually follows 10 years or more of heavy drinking (DSM-III-R). A chronic form of this disorder has been described for the patient

Table 10–5
Diagnostic Criteria for 291.40 Alcohol
Idiosyncratic Intoxication

A. Maladaptive behavioral changes, eg, aggressive or assaultive behavior, occurring within minutes of ingesting an amount of alcohol insufficient to induce intoxication in most people.
B. The behavior is atypical of the person when not drinking.
C. Not due to any physical or other mental disorder.

Reprinted with permission from the *Diagnostic and Statistical Manual of Mental Disorders, third edition, revised.* Copyright 1987. American Psychiatric Association.

Table 10–6
Diagnostic Criteria for 291.80 Uncomplicated
Alcohol Withdrawal

A. Cessation of prolonged (several days or longer), heavy ingestion of alcohol or reduction in the amount of alcohol ingested, followed within several hours by coarse tremor of hands, tongue, or eyelids, and at least one of the following:
  (1) nausea or vomiting
  (2) malaise or weakness
  (3) autonomic hyperactivity, eg, tachycardia, sweating, elevated blood pressure
  (4) anxiety
  (5) depressed mood or irritability
  (6) transient hallucinations or illusions
  (7) headache
  (8) insomnia
B. Not due to any physical or other mental disorder, such as alcohol withdrawal delirium.

Reprinted with permission from the *Diagnostic and Statistical Manual of Mental Disorders, third edition, revised.* Copyright 1987. American Psychiatric Association.

who develops ideas of reference and other poorly systematized persecutory delusions and the clinical situation may be indistinguishable from schizophrenia, with vague and illogical thinking, tangential associations, and inappropriate affect (see chapter 6). There is some evidence that the chronic form is more likely to develop from repeated episodes of the disorder (DSM-III-R).

Alcohol amnestic disorder   Rarely chronic alcoholics, not meeting criteria for either delirium (see chapter 9) or dementia (see chapter 5), develop profound memory problems (Table 10–9). This syndrome, when caused by thiamine deficiency is also known as Korsakoff's syndrome.

Associated features often include peripheral neuropathy, cerebellar ataxia, and myopathy. This disorder often follows an acute episode of Wernicke's encephalopathy, manifested by confusion, ataxia, eye-movement abnormalities (gaze palsies, nystagmus), and other neurologic signs. As these manifestations subside, memory impairment can remain. As noted later, if Wernicke's disease is treated early with thiamine, alcohol amnestic disorder can be averted. Once developed, however, alcohol amnestic disorder generally

Table 10–7
Diagnostic Criteria for 291.00 Alcohol
Withdrawal Delirium

A. Delirium developing after cessation of heavy alcohol ingestion or a reduction in the amount of alcohol ingested (usually within one week).
B. Marked autonomic hyperactivity, eg, tachycardia, sweating.
C. Not due to any physical or other mental disorder.

Reprinted with permission from the *Diagnostic and Statistical Manual of Mental Disorders, third edition, revised.* Copyright 1987. American Psychiatric Association.

Table 10–8
Diagnostic Criteria for 291.30 Alcohol
Hallucinosis

A. Organic hallucinosis with vivid and persistent hallucinations (auditory or visual) developing shortly (usually within 48 hours) after cessation of or reduction in heavy ingestion of alcohol in a person who apparently has alcohol dependence.
B. No delirium as in alcohol withdrawal delirium.
C. Not due to any physical or other mental disorder.

Reprinted with permission from the *Diagnostic and Statistical Manual of Mental Disorders, third edition, revised.* Copyright 1987. American Psychiatric Association.

persists, although a little improvement has been noted in some patients over time.

Dementia associated with alcoholism Rarely dementia (see chapter 5) follows prolonged and heavy ingestion of alcohol (Table 10–10). In order to make this diagnosis, all other causes of dementia must be excluded and at least three weeks must have elapsed since cesssation of alcohol ingestion.

Sedative-, Hypnotic-, or Anxiolytic-Induced Organic Mental Disorders
Drugs in this category include many of the drugs discussed in this book including hypnotics such as the benzodiazepines, ethchlorvynol, glutethimide, chloral hydrate, methaqualone, and barbiturates.

Sedative, hypnotic, or anxiolytic intoxication The essential features of this syndrome are outlined in Table 10–11 and include behavioral changes associated with certain physical signs such as slurred speech, incoordination, gait problems, and impaired attention or memory. Patients may appear as if they were intoxicated with alcohol; there is, however, no known syndrome corresponding to alcohol idiosyncratic reaction. Patients are also less likely to become hostile or violent while intoxicated from sedatives. Respiratory depression and hypotension are dangers as patients increase dosages to maintain an effect or overdose.

Uncomplicated sedative, hypnotic, or anxiolytic withdrawal Typical features include nausea or vomiting; malaise or weakness; autonomic hyperactivity; anxiety or irritability; orthostatic hypotension; coarse tremor of the hands, tongue, and eyelids; insomnia; and grand mal seizures (Table 10–12).

Table 10–9
Diagnostic Criteria for 291.10 Alcohol Amnestic
Disorder

A. Amnestic Syndrome following prolonged, heavy ingestion of alcohol.
B. Not due to any physical or other mental disorder.

Reprinted with permission from the *Diagnostic and Statistical Manual of Mental Disorders, third edition, revised.* Copyright 1987. American Psychiatric Association.

Table 10–10
Diagnostic Criteria for 291.20 Dementia
Associated with Alcoholism

A. Dementia following prolonged, heavy ingestion of alcohol and persisting at least three weeks after cessation of alcohol ingestion.
B. Exclusion, by history, physical examination, and laboratory tests, of all causes of dementia other than prolonged heavy use of alcohol.

Reprinted with permission from the *Diagnostic and Statistical Manual of Mental Disorders, third edition, revised.* Copyright 1987. American Psychiatric Association.

These symptoms develop following cessation of several weeks or more of sedative, hypnotic, or anxiolytic use or a reduction in the amount of the substance that was regularly used (Jenike, 1987). Withdrawal has been reported in people receiving as little as 15 mg of diazepam daily for eight months or more, but is more likely to be found with cessation of doses in the range of 40 mg daily of diazepam or its equivalent.

Sedative, hypnotic, or anxiolytic withdrawal delirium Delirium associated with marked autonomic activity, such as tachycardia and sweating, can develop after cessation of or reduction in heavy use of drugs in this category (Table 10–13). Visual, auditory, or tactile hallucinations are common; tremor and fever can occur. The onset is usually on the second or third day after cessation of or reduction in dosage of the drug and rarely appears more than a week after abstinence.

Sedative, hypnotic, or anxiolytic amnestic syndrome Following prolonged heavy use, the amnestic syndrome can occur (Table 10–14). Unlike alcohol amnestic disorder, full recovery may occur.

Table 10–11
Diagnostic Criteria for 305.40 Sedative,
Hypnotic, or Anxiolytic Intoxication

A. Recent use of a sedative, hypnotic, or anxiolytic.
B. Maladaptive behavioral changes, eg, disinhibition of sexual or aggressive impulses, mood lability, impaired judgment, impaired social or occupational functioning.
C. At least one of the following signs:
   (1) slurred speech
   (2) incoordination
   (3) unsteady gait
   (4) impairment in attention or memory
D. Not due to any physical or other mental disorder.
Note: When the differential diagnosis must be made without a clear-cut history or toxicologic analysis of body fluids, it may be qualified as "Provisional."

Reprinted with permission from the *Diagnostic and Statistical Manual of Mental Disorders, third edition, revised.* Copyright 1987. American Psychiatric Association.

Table 10–12
Diagnostic Criteria for 292.00 Uncomplicated
Sedative, Hypnotic, or Anxiolytic Withdrawal

A. Cessation of prolonged (several weeks or more) moderate or heavy use of a sedative, hypnotic, or anxiolytic, or reduction in the amount of substance used, followed by at least three of the following:
(1) nausea or vomiting
(2) malaise or weakness
(3) autonomic hyperactivity, eg, tachycardia, sweating
(4) anxiety or irritability
(5) orthostatic hypotension
(6) coarse tremor of hands, tongue, and eyelids
(7) marked insomnia
(8) grand mal seizures
B. Not due to any physical or other mental disorder, such as sedative, hypnotic, or anxiolytic withdrawal delirium.
Note: When the differential diagnosis must be made without a clear-cut history or toxicologic analysis of body fluids, it may be qualified as "Provisional."

Reprinted with permission from the *Diagnostic and Statistical Manual of Mental Disorders, third edition, revised.* Copyright 1987. American Psychiatric Association.

SUBSTANCE USE AND ABUSE IN THE ELDERLY

Alcohol Abuse

Prevalence
Heavy alcohol drinking drops sharply in people older than 75 years (Atkinson and Kofoed, 1982) and the prevalence in women is lower than that in men. In addition, women start to drink less in their 50s and 60s. Atkinson (1984) reported that about 5% to 12% of men and 1% to 2% of women in their 60s are problem drinkers, as ascertained by household survey methods.

Depending on the type of institution, from 5% to 60% of elderly men admitted to acute medical wards are active alcoholics. Of elderly patients in psychiatric clinics, 3% to 17% are alcoholics and from 23% to 44% of elderly patients admitted to acute psychiatric wards are drinking excessively at admission.

Some factors that contribute to a reduced prevalence of alcoholism in the very elderly include the following: (1) many severe alcoholics die young, (2) lower income in old age might limit consumption, (3) some alcoholics recover, and (4) underdiagnosis of elderly alcoholics can be an important contributing factor. Underreporting can result from: (1) the fact that elderly abusers tend to be middle class and do not fit the stereotypes that society has come to recognize; (2) clinicians have a low index of suspicion for abuse in the elderly; (3) clinical presentation of alcoholism in the elderly may be nonspecific and

320

Table 10–13
Diagnostic Criteria for 292.00 Sedative,
Hypnotic, or Anxiolytic Withdrawal Delirium

A. Delirium developing after the cessation of heavy use of a sedative, hypnotic, or anxiolytic, or a reduction in the amount of substance used (usually within one week).
B. Autonomic hyperactivity, eg, tachycardia, sweating.
C. Not due to any physical or other mental disorder.
Note: When the differential diagnosis must be made without a clear-cut history or toxicologic analysis of body fluids, it may be qualified as "Provisional."

Reprinted with permission from the *Diagnostic and Statistical Manual of Mental Disorders, third edition, revised.* Copyright 1987. American Psychiatric Association.

the patients may appear to have chronic medical illnesses, cognitive decline, or a mood disorder; and (4) the elderly are generally observed less closely in their daily life; that is, they may no longer be working or may not have a spouse or close relatives. In addition, certain biological alterations may be operative as people age; there is an increased tendency for alcohol to induce cognitive impairment, unpleasant mood, or physical symptoms that can reduce positive feedback or induce negative feelings about the effects of alcohol with age (Atkinson, 1984).

Predictive Factors and Patterns of Drinking Habits
With age, nonalcoholics tend to drink less alcohol. Also, many problem drinkers eventually quit alcohol intake entirely even without treatment. One report of a 35-year follow-up of nearly 400 boys reported that of 102 who later became alcoholics, 21 became abstinent (ie, no alcohol in last three years) by the age of 47 (Vaillant and Milofsky, 1982; Vaillant, 1983). Factors associated with increased likelihood of abstinence included reliance on other dependencies such as food, drugs, work, religion, and gambling; medical problems that were perceived as secondary to alcohol intake; participation in Alcoholics Anonymous; and new love relationships. Of the 21 abstainers, only four were in active treatment during the first year of sobriety.

The majority of elderly alcoholics used alcohol heavily as young adults

Table 10–14
Diagnostic Criteria for 292.83 Sedative,
Hypnotic, or Anxiolytic Amnestic Disorder

A. Amnestic syndrome following prolonged heavy use of a sedative, hypnotic, or anxiolytic.
B. Not due to any physical or other mental disorder.
Note: When the differential diagnosis must be made without a clear-cut history or toxicologic analysis of body fluids, it may be qualified as "Provisional."

Reprinted with permission from the *Diagnostic and Statistical Manual of Mental Disorders, third edition, revised.* Copyright 1987. American Psychiatric Association.

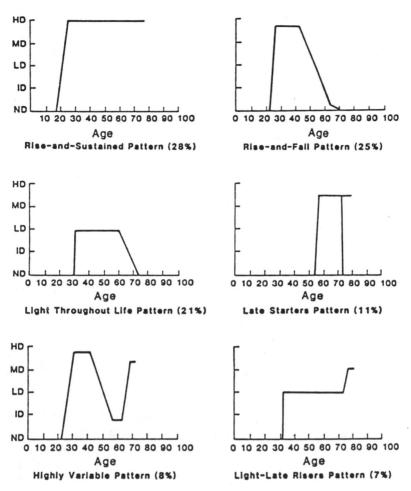

Figure 10–1 Lifetime drinking patterns reported by 85 persons aged 60 years and older who had used alcohol. HD = heavy drinking; MD = moderate drinking; LD = light drinking; ID = intermittent drinking; ND = no drinking. Reproduced with permission from Dunham RG: Aging and changing patterns of alcohol use. *J Psychoactive Drugs* 13:4, 1981.

and can be viewed as having a lifelong problem that persisted into old age. However, some patients who are referred to as late-onset alcoholics do not in fact begin to have a problem with alcohol until late in life. Dunham (1981) reviewed the lifetime drinking patterns of 85 persons who were at least 60 years old and who had used alcohol. The patterns of drinking that he encountered as well as the percentage of each type are outlined in Figure 10–1.

Compared to older heavy drinkers, younger alcoholics report higher rates of family alcoholism (Jones, 1972; Penick et al, 1978). Confirming the above,

Atkinson (1984) reported stratifying elderly patients in their program according to age of onset of alcoholism and found a significant inverse relationship between reported family alcoholism and age of onset of problem drinking in the patients; a positive family history of alcoholism, however, was identified in 41% of patients who had onset after the age of 40, suggesting that genetic influences may be operant in at least some of the patients with the late-onset alcoholism. Supporting the hypothesis that genetic influences can be less of a factor in elderly compared with young alcoholics is the finding that 86% of patients with early-onset alcoholism reported a positive family history for alcoholism.

Biological Changes in Alcohol Metabolism
Associated with Age

As noted in chapter 3, as people age, total body water decreases, lean body mass is reduced, and body fat increases (Bruce et al, 1980; Novak, 1972; Forbes and Reina, 1970). From the age of 20 to 60 years, body water levels can decrease from 25% to 18%. Therefore, ethanol, which is distributed primarily in body water, will have higher levels for a given dose in a typical elderly person because of an apparent decrease in the size of the reservoir (Vestal et al, 1977). Thus, at a fixed dose of alcohol, effects can be greater in the elderly than in younger people. Vestal and colleagues (1977) reported that a fixed intravenously administered alcohol load produced a peak blood alcohol level that was 20% higher in men over the age of 60 than in men under the age of 45 (Atkinson, 1984).

Alcohol's association with cognitive alterations is well documented (Hartford and Samorajski, 1982). Atkinson (1984) noted that an association between chronic heavy alcohol consumption and findings of dementia has been demonstrated in clinical surveys, in CT brain scan studies, and in neuropsychological testing. Apart from dementia, other more subtle deficits of abstract reasoning, cognitive adaptation to novel stimuli, and memory in alcohol abusers and even more moderate drinkers have been reported. Older social drinkers (Parker and Noble, 1980; Parker et al, 1982) and alcohol abusers (Parsons and Leber, 1981) seem to have greater cognitive loss than younger drinkers and the reversibility of the cognitive deficits with abstinence is not clear.

When an elderly person is acutely intoxicated, the metabolism of many drugs is reduced; chronic alcohol abuse, however, can increase drug metabolism by inducing liver enzyme activity. When alcohol and psychoactive drugs are simultaneously ingested, delirium, confusion, or heavy sedation may result. Unexpected responses to prescribed medication may be the clinician's first clue to undisclosed substance abuse (Atkinson, 1984). Cognitive loss from alcohol may further impair coping ability, and alcohol use is probably often a contributing factor in suicide among the elderly (Martin and Streissguth, 1982).

Table 10–15
Clinical Presentation of Elderly Alcohol Abuse

Nonspecific presentation is most common; any of the following symptoms may be prominent:

Self neglect	Injuries
Falls	Diarrhea
Confusion	Malnutrition
Lability	Myopathy
Depression	Incontinence
Unusual behavior	Hypothermia

Classical findings of intoxication, dependence, or withdrawal are less common
Dementia from all causes coexists in 25% to 60% of cases

Reproduced with permission from Atkinson RM: *Alcohol and Drug Abuse in Old Age*. Copyright 1984. American Psychiatric Association.

Factors Predisposing to Alcoholism in the Elderly

Losses are commonly associated with aging; loss of job and self-esteem (retirement), death of spouse or close friends, declining health, lowered energy level, and loss or lowering of income. Studies yielded conflicting data on the relationship of life stress to alcoholism (Atkinson, 1984); some showed that life stress and alcoholism in elderly are directly associated (Bailey et al, 1965), others indicated that elderly persons under the least stress are most at risk for alcoholism (Barnes, 1979), while still others showed no relationship between life stress and alcoholism (Borgatta et al, 1982). Thus it is not at all clear that life stress does indeed lead to alcoholism. Besides this body of conflicting evidence, it is clear that most elderly persons are subjected to many of these same stresses and the majority of them do not become alcohol abusers.

As many as one-fourth to one-third of patients with major depression increase their alcohol intake during depressive episodes (Schuckit, 1979).

Recognizing the Elderly Alcoholic

The clinician dealing with elderly patients must overcome stereotypes and inquire about alcohol use routinely. Because denial is common, family members should also be questioned in reference to the elderly patient's drinking patterns. Many elderly alcoholics present with nonspecific medical or psychiatric findings (Table 10–15). Schuckit and Miller (1976) reported that physicians miss the diagnosis of alcoholism initially in 20% or more of elderly patients evaluated on acute medical wards and misdiagnosis of dementia in these patients is especially problematic (Kafetz, 1982).

Acute Treatment of Alcoholism in the Elderly

Overall treatment for older alcoholics is similar to that for younger patients and consists of initial hospital management of severe or medically complicated patients followed by prolonged outpatient rehabilitation. Compliant, medically stable patients can begin outpatient treatment without hospitalization.

324

Table 10–16
The Brief Michigan Alcoholism Screening Test (MAST)*

Questions	Check One	
1. Do you feel you are a normal drinker?	Yes (0)	No (2)
2. Do friends or relatives think you are a normal drinker?	Yes (0)	No (2)
3. Have you ever attended a meeting of Alcoholics Anonymous (AA)?	Yes (5)	No (0)
4. Have you ever lost friends or girlfriends or boyfriends because of drinking?	Yes (2)	No (0)
5. Have you ever gotten into trouble at work because of drinking?	Yes (2)	No (0)
6. Have you ever neglected your obligations, your family, or your work for two or more days in a row because you were drinking?	Yes (2)	No (0)
7. Have you ever had delirium tremens (DTs), severe shaking, heard voices, or seen things that weren't there after heavy drinking?	Yes (2)	No (0)
8. Have you ever gone to anyone for help about your drinking?	Yes (5)	No (0)
9. Have you ever been in a hospital because of drinking?	Yes (5)	No (0)
10. Have you ever been arrested for drunk driving or driving after drinking?	Yes (2)	No (0)

*Note: Alcoholism is indicated by a score of greater than five. Test scores are determined by tallying values for answers, which are on a progressive scale of zero, two, and five.
Reproduced with permission from Pokorny AD, Miller BA, Kaplan HB: The brief MAST: a shortened version of the Michigan Alcoholism Screening Test. *Am J Psychiatry* 129:342, 1972.

Cassem (1984) noted that it is easier to make the diagnosis than to get the patient to accept it and that total honesty with the patient is the rule. The possibility that severe alcoholism can be fatal, as well as some of the present and future medical consequences, must be discussed with each patient. He recommended giving the patient a copy of the Michigan Alcoholism Screening Test (MAST) (Pokorny et al, 1972). Even if the patient does not complete the form, knowing that a score of greater than 5 defines an alcoholic can help the patient to take treatment considerations more seriously (Table 10–16). This can also help to cut through denial evidenced by family members.

To better understand the concept of an addiction, the patient needs to know that feeling the need for alcohol and the dread of going without it are part of what addiction means (Cassem, 1984). The patient must be made to understand that he does not have a character flaw, but a complicated disease produced by a drug that causes tolerance and psychologic and physical dependence. The fact that alcoholism can be treated and that abstinence rates approach 80% for some groups (Seixas, 1970; Kerr, 1977; Bateman and Peterson, 1971; Blaney et al, 1975) must be communicated.

If the patient is presently drinking heavily, a period of inpatient detoxification might be required in order to avert potentially life-threatening consequences of alcohol withdrawal. When alcohol is abruptly discontinued after prolonged periods of ingestion, neuronal excitability and catecholamine release occur with the production of muscle tension and tremor, hyperacuity of sensory modalities, hyperreflexia, overalertness, anxiety, sleeplessness, and a reduction of seizure threshold (Cassem, 1984; Sellers and Kalant, 1976). In about 5% of such patients these symptoms progress to full-blown delirium tremens.

In addition to the problems of withdrawal, other medical hurdles such as infection or head injury can present concomitant challenges. Patients undergoing withdrawal may also be combative and uncooperative.

Symptoms of mild withdrawal include tremulousness, sleeplessness, and irritability and are usually present within six hours after alcohol intake has stopped. They typically resolve within 48 hours. Cassem (1984) recommended the following as treatment for mild withdrawal:

1. administer thiamine, 50 mg intramuscularly
2. sedate, eg, with chlordiazepoxide, 50 to 100 mg orally
3. observe for two hours
4. discharge with four-day supply of chlordiazepoxide, 25 mg orally, to be taken four times a day.
5. enlist help of relatives
6. arrange for rehabilitation follow-up

With the older patient, attention must be directed to the potential for overprescribing chlordiazepoxide, thus leading to increased memory problems, which may increase agitation, or frank stupor (Blazer, 1982). Benzodiazepines like chlordiazepoxide and their active metabolites may have greatly increased half-lives in the elderly (see chapter 7). Even if the drugs are prescribed at a progressively lower dose each succeeding day, the highest blood levels can occur three to four days after initial prescription (Blazer, 1982). If an elderly patient has increased memory problems, dysarthria, and ataxia at this point in withdrawal, the clinician must, among other things, suspect potential drug intoxication. If drug intoxication occurs, administration should be discontinued for a 24- to 36-hour period, and the patient should be observed carefully with the drug readministered at a much lower dose, and the withdrawal procedure should be continued.

During the examination and observation period, any of the following is an indication for hospitalization (Cassem, 1984):

1. symptoms of severe withdrawal (see next paragraph)
2. fever over 38.3° C (101° F)
3. Wernicke's encephalopathy (ataxia, nystagmus, gaze palsy)
4. head trauma with an episode of unconsciousness
5. presence of major complication such as severe malnutrition, alcoholic hepatitis, respiratory failure or infection, GI bleeding, pancreatitis
6. seizure

Severe withdrawal, also called delirium tremens, rarely occurs in patients less than 30 years old. Severe symptoms are most likely to occur 48 to 60 hours after drinking is stopped and consist of severe tremulousness, seizures (9% of patients), auditory or visual hallucinations (or both), tachycardia, confusional state, diaphoresis, and agitation. Once this condition has developed, mortality is estimated to be as high as 15% overall and may be higher in the elderly alcoholic.

Because this situation is a potentially fatal emergency, close observation in a medical setting is essential. Cassem (1984) defined the goals of therapy as prompt sedation with relief of physical symptoms, prevention of complications, management of associated conditions, and preparation for long-term rehabilitation. Thiamine is given immediately, 50 mg intramuscularly. Benzodiazepines are the drugs of first choice in sedating the alcoholic and heavy smokers might need higher doses of these agents.

Ideally, a calm state should be produced as swiftly as possible, with the patient still awake. If possible, the oral or intravenous route should be used since intramuscularly administered benzodiazepines (with exception of lorazepam) are inconsistently absorbed. Average daily dosage of chlordiazepoxide ranges from 100 to 400 mg the first day, although some patients may require 2,000 mg (Cassem, 1984; Sellers and Kalant, 1976). Doses are generally tapered by about 20% to 25% each day thereafter. The mean duration of delirium tremens in one study was 56 hours (Thompson et al, 1975).

Patients are particularly vulnerable to complications if they have a fever higher than 40° C (104° F), are malnourished, or have fluid and electrolyte disturbances. Potassium and magnesium typically need to be replaced to decrease likelihood of cardiac arrhythmias (Fisher and Abrams, 1977). Intramuscularly administered magnesium is an important adjunct to the initial therapeutic treatment of the acute alcoholic (Beard and Knott, 1968).

Complaints of thirst and dry mucous membranes frequently lead the clinician to believe that dehydration is a severe problem in the alcoholic and iatrogenic overhydration then results. After establishing intravenous therapy, the clinician can give the severe alcoholic 500 to 1,000 mg of 5% normal saline solution while awaiting the results of blood chemistry tests (Blazer, 1982). With high fever, infection must be ruled out. During withdrawal, grand mal seizures can occur; they are most common within 31 to 48 hours after drinking is discontinued. Unless the patient has a prior history of seizures, the administration of phenytoin is usually unnecessary.

Giving glucose to a withdrawing alcoholic who has not received prior treatment with thiamine can deplete the patient's last stores of available thiamine and precipitate acute Wernicke's encephalopathy which is diagnosed on the basis of gaze palsies, nystagmus, and ataxia.

Korsakoff's psychosis is a disorder of cognitive function in which memory is impaired and confabulation frequently occurs. Two features are essential to the diagnosis of Korsakoff's psychosis: impaired ability to recall past events and impaired ability to learn new information. It appears that some patients have a genetic defect that makes them particularly vulnerable to thiamine deficiency (Blass and Gibson, 1977). The early signs of Wernicke's encephalopathy herald the onset of a grave medical emergency. When treated immediately with intravenously administered thiamine, the acute encephalopathy is reversible and ocular palsies reverse within hours, with improvement of horizontal nystagmus following slowly thereafter. Mild ocular palsies and nystagmus persist in about half of the patients who are treated. Cassem (1984) noted that even if Korsakoff's psychosis has developed, recovery is complete in almost a quarter of the patients and significant improvment occurs in 50% of patients within several months.

Chronic Treatment of the Elderly Alcoholic

The long-term or rehabilitative treatment of the alcoholic requires considerable expertise and is best left in the hands of experts. Unless the clinician is heavily involved in the treatment of alcoholic patients, referral to a specialized clinic or to Alcoholics Anonymous (AA) is recommended.

Every effort should be made by the clinician to ensure that the elderly alcoholic patient actually presents himself or herself for treatment. This will involve coordinating with family members and asking the unit or clinician accepting the referral to contact you if the patient does not follow through (Cassem, 1984).

A number of poor prognostic indicators for treatment that have been identified include: antisocial personality traits, dementia, skid row or socially isolated life-style, and family drinking partners (Atkinson, 1984). Involvement in a group, a sense of helping others, and interaction with individuals at other stages of the life cycle provide a reintegration of such individuals into society. Unfortunately, many older persons refuse to participate in self-help groups (Blazer, 1982), often secondary to denial of the severity of the problem coupled with the inhibition to increase social participation that is frequently noted in alcoholics of all ages.

The elderly are overrepresented in the group referred to as "skid row alcoholics" compared with the general population (Bahr and Caplow, 1973; Bouge, 1963; Blazer, 1982). In a review of the literature on this topic, Schuckit and Pastor (1979) noted that the residents of skid row often demonstrate physical and psychologic disabilities coupled with downward economic mobility. In contrast with young skid row residents, older residents show the highest rates of degenerative physical diseases such as cardiovascular disease, genitourinary disease, and perceptual problems. The older residents frequently cite inadequate pensions, unemployment, or specific physical disabilities as patterns for arrival on skid row.

Wiseman (1970) noted that obtaining and consuming alcohol and recovering from the effects of alcohol are the central characteristics of the lifestyle on skid row (Blazer, 1982). However, Bouge (1963) suggested that the alcoholic image may be inappropriate for the older skid row residents, who are less likely to be heavy drinkers than are those at other stages of the life cycle. Affective disorders are more common in older skid row residents than in the younger ones (Goldfarb, 1970). In general, little improvement is reported with the elderly skid row population although occasional success stories make the effort worthwhile (Blazer, 1982).

The treatment of the depressed patient with an alcohol use disorder must include pharmacologic therapy, psychotherapy, and therapeutic intervention with the family (Blazer, 1982). Themes of loneliness, dependency, uselessness, and physical health are frequent in discussions with older alcoholics. Antidepressant therapy is an important adjunct to the treatment of the depressed alcoholic, but it should not be started before the patient is withdrawn from alcohol and before a baseline assessment of affect is made following withdrawal. Sometimes, depressive symptoms are the results of the depressive effect of alcohol itself and these will resolve shortly after abstinence begins. If after a few weeks depressive symptoms return, antidepressant therapy can be started.

Older patients comprise 2% to 25% of patients in alcoholism treatment programs (Atkinson, 1984) and outpatient follow-up data from at least nine studies indicate that elderly alcoholics have outcomes equal or superior to that of younger patients (Atkinson and Kofoed, 1982; Rix, 1982; Janik and Dunham, 1983; Wiens et al, 1983; Kofoed et al, 1984; Atkinson, 1984). There is some controversy around whether or not special elderly-oriented treatment programs are required or whether the elderly alcoholic can do just as well in traditional programs (Janik and Dunham, 1983). Despite the fact that no careful study of comparative approaches has been done, some data on which clinicians can base treatment plans are available. Atkinson (1984) reported that elderly-oriented outpatient treatment for alcoholism has been conducted effectively in both general geriatric programs (Zimberg, 1978) and alcoholism programs (Dunlop et al, 1982). There is general consensus that group treatment is desirable (Blazer, 1982) and there are anecdotal reports of several elderly-oriented Alcoholics Anonymous chapters (Atkinson, 1984).

There is some evidence that treatment of elderly alcoholics should be different from that in younger patients. Linn (1978) noted that the elderly experience greater social bonding and fewer conflicts with authority, that they interact differently with staff, and that they are less psychologically minded in general. Dunlop and colleagues (1982) suggested that elderly alcoholics have stronger guilt feelings, exhibit more denial, and resist change more than younger alcoholics. On the other hand, older patients tend to be more stable and less likely to regress after progress has been made.

At least one group (Kofoed et al, 1984) reported that many older Veterans Administration patients feel uncomfortable when outnumbered by younger patients and they suggested the use of peer group treatment programs for older alcoholic veterans (Zimburg, 1978). Their groups meet once weekly for 1½ hours and during the daytime because access to public transportation is better and because patients with poor vision are reluctant to drive or even go out at night. In addition to the standard groups, occasional potluck social gatherings are held. Kofoed and associates (1984) noted that, as opposed to groups of younger alcoholics, elderly patients rapidly develop a strong attachment among group members. Many of their older patients entered treatment denying a serious alcoholism problem, but stayed in the group because of social attachment and maintained sobriety without candid acknowledgment of the alcohol problems.

As with all age groups, therapeutic intevention with the family is essential if return to alcohol abuse is to be avoided. Family members should be warned of the severe and potentially irreversible memory problems that can result from chronic alcohol abuse over time. Blazer (1982) noted that most families express great concern about the immediate effects of acute alcohol intoxication; older persons who drink themselves into delirium or stupor are great burdens on their families, yet families demonstrate a remarkable tolerance of this behavior, often waiting weeks or months before referring patients for appropriate help.

Once families recognize that help is available and after the clinician has shown care and attention to the patients and families, they are frequently more willing to contact the clinician early if a deterioration is noted. However, older patients, especially individuals who have maintained dominant roles in their families in the past, can intimidate or threaten family members who contact the clinician. To avoid these potential conflicts, Blazer (1982) recommended meeting with patient and family early in the course of treatment and establishing a strong and positive alliance with the patient for the purpose of defeating the alcoholism, which is recognized as dangerous. The clinician can emphasize to the patient and his or her family that, by the nature of the condition, weakening of resolve is to be expected; therefore, the clinician encourages, in front of the patient, that family members make contact when they suspect problems are imminent.

Although controversy has surrounded the question of whether or not alcoholics can ever drink socially without risk of relapse (Armor et al, 1976; Block, 1976; Pattison, 1976; Cohen, 1976), it appears that abstinence is the only safe approach (Cassem, 1984; Fox, 1976). Thus the goal of long-term rehabilitation must include the establishment of strict control of drinking, preferably by total abstinence. The goals of any rehabilitation program must include the replacement of the alcohol addiction with other addictions that are nonchemical, time-consuming, and heavily supported by a network of human relationships and that increase the alcoholics self-esteem (Cassem, 1984). Alcoholics Anonymous (Bean, 1975) has the essential elements of an outstanding program: education about the effects of alcohol; network of supporting persons (meetings seven nights a week, a buddy system); group support; group pressure not to drink; group forgiveness when relapse occurs; involvement of spouse and family; multiple methods for restoring shattered self-esteem; provision of a sense of belonging and of being understood; alleviation of loneliness; opportunities for self-expression, confession, and catharsis; reassurance by hearing that individuals whom the patient might admire, such as successful professionals or business people, have similar problems; and the satisfaction of being able to help other alcoholics recover (Cassem, 1984).

Drug Abuse

Prevalence

Although less is known about drug abuse than alcoholism in the elderly, it appears that for every four of five alcoholics there is one elderly person who abuses drugs of some sort (Redich, 1980; Reifler et al, 1982). While abuse of stimulants, hallucinogens, and marijuana is very uncommon in the elderly and abuse is generally limited to chronic opioid abusers, prescription drug abuse is not unusual among the aged, with women presumably at greater risk than men because they are prescribed psychoactive agents twice as often as men (Atkinson and Kofoed, 1982). Commonly abused over-the-counter (OTC) medications include laxatives, sedatives, analgesics, and cold preparations. The fact that these drugs are easily obtained, generally inexpensive, and are perceived as completely safe by many elderly people leads to frequent abuse.

The most commonly prescribed drugs are analgesics, antianxiety agents, and sedative-hypnotics. In one community survey (Stephens et al, 1982) about 18% of older patients were receiving psychoactive prescription drugs; of these, one-third were not taking the drugs as prescribed. Interestingly, most consumed less than prescribed. In institutions, elderly patients receive psychotropics more frequently, often for control of agitated or violent behaviors (see chapters 5 and 6).

Often the elderly drug abuser originally obtained a psychoactive substance by prescription from a physician for treatment of anxiety or insomnia, but has gradually increased the dose and frequency of use on his or her own (DSM-III-R). The person continues to justify the use on the basis of treating symptoms, but substance-seeking behavior becomes prominent, and the person might go to several doctors in order to obtain sufficient supplies of the substance. Tolerance can be remarkable, with doses of more than 100 mg of diazepam daily producing little sedation. Older people are apparently less likely to rely on illegal sources of medication and the initial reason for using the medications is rarely to obtain a high from the substance.

Late onset addiction to opioids is virtually nonexistent (Atkinson, 1984); opioid addicts do, however, live to old age and form a small group. As with alcoholics, early mortality of opioid addicts may contribute to declining prevalence of opioid addiction with age (Duvall et al, 1963; O'Donnell, 1964; Vaillant, 1973; Harrington and Cox, 1979; Atkinson, 1984). Some elderly addicts stop drug use secondary to decreased drive and physical illness, but this occurs less frequently than for alcoholics (Atkinson, 1984). Surviving addicts may remain free of street drugs by receiving close parole supervision, by being in a methadone program, or by becoming alcoholic (Vaillant, 1973; Harrington and Cox, 1979).

Over-the-Counter Drug Abuse

Some elderly persons medicate themselves in an effort to relieve chronic arthritic pain or other medical problems, insomnia (see chapter 8), or feelings of anxiety and/or depression. It is reported that the elderly are seven times more likely to use OTC medication as the general population and that at least half of these medications are analgesics (Thompson et al, 1983). Although considered safe by most elderly patients, OTC medications are potentially dangerous and these dangers increase with age. Guttman (1978) found that 69% of those over the age of 60 use OTC drugs; strikingly, 40% reported taking these agents on a daily basis (Kofoed, 1984) and 80% of these patients also used alcohol, prescribed drugs, or both. Some explanations for increased OTC use include the facts that problems such as arthritis, constipation, and pain become more common with age (Gillies and Skyring, 1972; Jarvik and Perl, 1981; Kofoed, 1984) and that some manufacturers of OTC drugs target the elderly with their advertising. Ten percent of older men and as many as 20% of older women use aspirin compounds daily, and as many as 5% use acetaminophen regularly (Stewart et al, 1982). For elderly people on fixed incomes, OTC medications may seem a more reasonable way to manage chronic problems than frequent visits to doctors or clinics (Guttman, 1978); also, older persons are less likely than younger persons to have a regular personal physician (Kofoed and Bloom, 1982).

Specific dangers of drug use   Chronic OTC medication users are prone to have a number of difficulties including analgesic nephropathy, colon changes from laxative abuse, chronic salicylism, emphysema, and cancer associated with tobacco use (Kofoed, 1984). Rebound symptoms from anticholinergic agents, sedatives, nasal decongestants, and laxatives can tend to promote chronic use. As the elderly are very likely to be taking prescription drugs in combination with OTC medication, they are at increased risk for clinically significant drug interactions (Caranasos et al, 1974; Chien et al, 1978; Guttman, 1978; Salzman, 1979; Sangiorgi, 1979; Pascarelli, 1981).

Analgesics   Aspirin is reportedly the most frequently used drug that leads to hospitalization (Caranasos et al, 1974), with GI bleeding the leading complaint. Chronic use of aspirin (salicylism) can mimic neurologic disorders and is most common in the elderly (Greer et al, 1965; Gardner and Hall, 1982). Aspirin potentiates the effects of oral hypoglycemics (Kofoed, 1984). Acetaminophen can elevate serum alkaline phosphatase levels, and fatal liver damage can occur with overdose (Stewart et al, 1982). Analgesic nephropathy reportedly occurs with both chronic aspirin and acetaminophen use (Gillies and Skyring, 1972; Gardner and Hall, 1982). Kofoed (1984) reported that analgesic overuse and abuse is seldom considered prior to serious illness or organ damage.

Laxatives   Almost a third of the US population over the age of 60 regularly uses laxatives and about 10% of these overuse or abuse these agents (Cummings et al, 1974; Chien et al, 1978). Patients who have been abusing laxatives may present with hypokalemia, chronic diarrhea, or malabsorption syndromes. Osteomalacia or abdominal pain develop in occasional patients (Frame et al, 1971; Cummings, 1974). Laxative abusers tend to deny or lie about use of these agents. Stool tests for phenolphthalein can assist in the diagnosis. Although young laxative abusers are usually female, older abusers may be of either sex (Kofoed, 1984).

Anticholinergic agents　These agents are commonly used in both OTC and prescription drugs and their side effects, which are additive when more than one drug is used, are frequently encountered in clinical practice. Common OTC preparations include cold and allergy agents, sleep preparations (eg, Sominex), and antidiarrhea compounds. Antihistamines, which are prominent anticholinergic agents (Jenike, 1982), such as diphenhydramine (Benadryl), hydroxyzine (Vistaril, Atarax), chlorpheniramine (Teldrin and others), and promethazine (Phenergan), are often prescribed as sedatives or antianxiety agents. Many of the drugs discussed in this book may be associated with anticholinergic side effects that are additive with OTC anticholinergic medications. Delirium is frequently induced in elderly patients by such agents. It is also well established that more than 600 commonly used drugs have anticholinergic actions that can produce serious neuropsychiatric toxic effects (Granacher and Baldessarini, 1976). Diagnosis of delirium, to which the elderly are particularly vulnerable, secondary to anticholinergic agents is tentatively established when there is a history of recent intake of one or more of these drugs, and when physical examination reveals the presence of peripheral muscarinic blockade. The latter may suggest the cause of delirium when a history of drug exposure is uncertain or absent (Lipowski, 1980). Management of toxic anticholinergic states is covered in detail in chapter 9.

Sympathomimetics　Many OTC decongestant preparations contain sympathomimetics like ephedrine and phenylpropanolamine which can be dangerous when combined with MAOIs or antihypertensive agents. Also, nasal decongestants produce rebound symptoms that can lead to chronic abuse.

Others　Some cough syrups contain alcohol and are occasionally abused by elderly alcoholic patients. Antacids have been reported to produce psychiatric and physical symptoms related to their calcium, aluminum, or magnesium content (Hall et al, 1978). Caffeine is found in many OTC medications and is easily available in coffee, tea, and soft drinks. Of men older than 60 years, 85% continue to drink coffee or tea daily and almost 35% consume four or more cups daily (Vestal et al, 1976; Chien et al, 1978). Overuse of these agents contributes to anxiety, panic disorders, cardiac arrhythmias, gastric disorders, and osteoporosis (Heaney, 1981; Kofoed, 1984). Cigarette smoking appears to decline in old age but large surveys show that 17% to 25% of men older than 60 smoke versus 48% of those between 40 and 59 years old (Vestal et al, 1976; Chien et al, 1978). The dangers of oral and lung cancers and heart disease are now well documented, but lesser known problems include osteoporosis, weight loss, decreased muscular strength, and decreased exertion tolerance (Daniell, 1976; Mellstrom et al, 1982).

Management of the OTC drug abuser In many cases, elderly patients are abusing OTC medications because they are not aware of the potential dangers and view their use as completely harmless. The alert physician can increase the likelihood of identifying potential problems by taking a careful drug history. When questioned, many elderly patients only report use of prescription drugs and do not consider OTC medications worthy of report. They also often forget to mention eye medications which are often prescribed by a separate physician. Specific questions aimed at identifying OTC drug use include: Are you taking any medications that you get yourself from the store without a prescription? Do you borrow medications from a friend? How do you manage problems like insomnia, constipation, or nasal congestion? Just asking these questions will identify the majority of the OTC drug users; some, however, will be reluctant to be honest about such use because of various fears.

Kofoed (1984) reported that the diagnosis of OTC drug abuse is rarely made until psychiatric symptoms or organ damage occurs. This trend can only be reversed by patient and physician education aimed at heightening awareness of these dangers for the elderly person. OTC drug use should be considered routinely in the diagnostic evaluation of all older patients (Atkinson and Kofoed, 1982).

Prescription Drug Abuse in the Elderly

Demographics Even though the elderly comprise only 11% of the US population, they use about 25% of the prescription drugs (Basen, 1977). The majority of these agents are used to treat medical or psychological symptoms and identification of abusing patients is difficult (Finlayson, 1984). Pascarelli (1981) found that the most widely prescribed drugs to elderly patients are the cardiovascular, sedative-hypnotic, and analgesic agents. Analgesics are the drugs most frequently used by the elderly and chronic pain syndromes are a major source of substance abuse, with the abuse being responsible for much of the illness behavior observed and reported (Finlayson, 1984).

Even though there is some evidence that late-onset alcoholism is often a reaction to losses and stresses associated with increasing age (Zimberg, 1974), this does not seem to be the case with prescription drug abuse in the elderly (Finlayson, 1984). In a series of 225 patients who were hospitalized for prescription drug abuse, Swanson and colleagues (1973) found that the patients were generally high achievers who had complicated medical histories and that superimposed alcohol abuse was often present. These patients had a fairly even distribution from adolescence through old age. Finlayson (1984) confirmed this lack of clustering by age.

Finlayson (1984), reporting on a group of 248 patients older than 65 who were treated at an Alcohol and Drug Dependency Unit over an eight-year period, found that 214 (86%) were dependent on alcohol alone; 19 (8%) were dependent on prescription drugs alone; and 15 (6%) were dependent on a combination of prescription drugs and alcohol. Examining demographic characteristics of the 34 drug abusing subjects, Finlayson found that they were mainly socially and economically stable and that they were equally divided among men and women. Slightly more than 82% were married and only 15% were living alone. They and others (Swanson et al, 1973) found that the elderly were not interested in stimulants. Eighteen of the 34 patients were abusing analgesics and reported that pain was the reason for drug use. The duration of abuse ranged from 2 to 40 years, with a mean duration of 16 years. Seven patients began abuse before they were 45 and only eight when they were 65 or older.

Finlayson (1984) noted that prescription drug abuse may be more difficult to detect than alcoholism in the elderly because of the multiple legitimate reasons older persons can muster for taking medication. In addition, clinicians and family members may be reluctant to refer the older drug-dependent person, even more reluctant than they are to refer the older alcoholic.

Some of the conditions, and therefore warning signs, associated with prescription drug abuse by the elderly include pain disorders, depression, organic mental disorders, low levels of psychosocial functioning, change in tolerance to drugs, accident proneness, and defensiveness (Finlayson, 1984). One useful sign of analgesic dependence is continued analgesic use in the face of an admitted lack of pain relief by the drug (Finlayson, 1984).

Treatment   If the elderly patient is abusing drugs, but is not dependent, outpatient treatment is generally indicated. Often education and correction of associated psychological problems, such as anxiety, loneliness, grief, or depression, will improve the situation. Finlayson (1984) noted that the elderly respond quite well to emotional support, encouragement, and strengthening of their social system; family involvement enhances treatment outcome. Total abstinence might not be possible in some elderly patients who have multiple or severe medical problems and physicians and family members will have to judiciously monitor drug intake.

Once dependence is recognized, hospitalization will likely be required for management of withdrawal symptoms and observation. Optimal management of medical problems should precede attempts at withdrawal. When major affective illness is present, pharmacologic management may have to go hand in hand with withdrawal. Just getting the elderly patient to accept hospitalization may be a major obstacle and once accomplished both patient and family members may be relieved to have the problem in the open where solutions at least seem possible. Although independent living should be the goal after treatment, this may not always be possible. Consultation with caring family members is essential in determining posthospitalization disposition. Alcoholics Anonymous can be helpful for alcoholic drug abusing elderly patients.

Prevention of prescription drug abuse Primary physicians must maintain a high index of suspicion and must keep a conspicuous inventory of both prescription and OTC medications in each patient's chart (Salzman, 1982). Monitoring frequency and dosages of prescribed medications will help to detect the patient who is increasing dosages as well as noncompliant patients who are taking less medication than prescribed.

SUMMARY

Even though substance abuse problems are relatively uncommon in the elderly, when they occur they can be difficult to manage. Clinicians tend to underestimate the serious consequences of substance use in the elderly. Questions about alcohol and drug usage (including OTC medications) should be asked of each elderly patient regardless of presenting symptoms. Diagnostic and management issues have been reviewed.

REFERENCES

Armor DJ, Polich JM, Stambul HB: *Alcoholism and Treatment*. Santa Monica, Cal, Rand Corporation, 1976, p vi.

Atkinson RM, Kofoed LL: Alcohol and drug abuse in old age: a clinical perspective. *Subst Alcohol Actions Misuse* 3:353–368, 1982.

Atkinson RM: *Alcohol and Drug Abuse in Old Age*. Washington, DC, American Psychiatric Association Press, 1984.

Bahr HM, Caplow T: *Old Men Drunk and Sober*. New York, Oxford University Press, 1973.

Bailey MB, Haberman PW, Alksne H: The epidemiology of alcoholism in an urban residential area. *J Stud Alcohol* 26:19–40, 1965.

Barnes GM: Alcohol use among older persons: findings from a western New York State general population survey. *J Am Geriatr Soc* 27:244–250, 1979.

Basen AB: The elderly and drugs: problem, overview and program strategy. *Public Health Rep* 92:43–48, 1977.

Bateman NI, Petersen DM: Variables related to outcome of treatment for hospitalized alcoholics. *Int J Addict* 6:215–224, 1971.

Bean M: Alcoholics Anonymous (pts 1 and 2). *Psychiatr Ann* 3:7, 5:2, 1975.

Beard JD, Knott DH: Fluid and electrolyte balance during acute withdrawal in chronic alcoholic patients. *JAMA* 204:133, 1968.

Blaney R, Radford IS, MacKenzie G: A Belfast study of outcome in the treatment of alcoholism. *Br J Addict* 70:41–50, 1975.

Blass JP, Gibson GE: Abnormality of a thiamine-requiring enzyme in patients with Wernicke-Korsakoff syndrome. *N Engl J Med* 297:1367, 1977.

Blazer DG: *Depression in Late Life*. St Louis, CV Mosby, 1982.

Block MA: Don't place alcohol on a pedestal (editorial). *JAMA* 235:2103, 1976.

Borgatta EF, Mongomery RJV, Borgatta ML: Alcohol use and abuse, life crisis events, and the elderly. *Res Aging* 4:378–408, 1982.

Bouge DJ: *Skid Row in American Cities*. Chicago, Community and Family Study Center, University of Chicago, 1963.

Bruce A, Anderson M, Arvidsson B, et al: Body composition. Prediction of normal body potassium, body water and body fat in adults on the basis of body height, body weight and age. *Scand J Clin Lab Invest* 40:461–473, 1980.

Caranasos GJ, Stewart GB, Cluff LE: Drug-induced illness leading to hospitalization. *JAMA* 228:713–717, 1974.

Cassem NH: Alcoholism. *Sci Am Med* Sect VI:131–14, 1984.

Chien CP, Townsend EJ, Ross-Townsen A: Substance use and abuse among the community elderly: the medical aspect. *Addict Dis* 3:357–372, 1978.

Cohen S: Alcoholics: can they become social drinkers? *Drug Abuse Alcoholism Newsletter* 5:no 8, Oct 1976.

Cummings JH: Progress report: laxative abuse. *Gut* 15:758–765, 1974.

Daniell HW: Osteoporosis and the slender smoker. *Arch Intern Med* 136:298–304, 1976.

Diagnostic and Statistical Manual of Mental Disorders, ed 3, revised. Washington DC, American Psychiatric Association Press, 1987.

Dunham RG: Aging and changing patterns of alcohol use. *J Psychoactive Drugs* 13:143–151, 1981.

Dunlop J, Skorney B, Hamilton J: Group treatment for elderly alcoholics and their families. *Soc Work Groups* 5:78–92, 1982.

Duvall HJ, Locke BZ, Brill L: Follow-up study of narcotic drug addicts five years after hospitalization. *Public Health Rep* 78:185–193, 1963.

Finlayson RE: Prescription drug abuse in older persons, in Atkinson RM (ed): *Alcohol and Drug Abuse in Old Age*. Washington DC, American Psychiatric Association Press, 1984, pp 62–70.

Fisher J, Abrams J: Life-threatening ventricular tachyarrhythmias in delirium tremens. *Arch Intern Med* 137:1238, 1977.

Forbes GB, Reina JC: Adult lean body mass declines with age: Some longitudinal observations. *Metabolism* 19:653–663, 1970.

Fox V: The controlled drinking controversy (editorial). *JAMA* 236:863, 1976.

Frame B, Guiang H, Frost H, et al: Osteomalacia induced by laxative (phenolphthalein) ingestion. *Arch Intern Med* 128:794–796, 1971.

Gardner ER, Hall RCW: Psychiatric symptoms produced by over-the-counter drugs. *Psychosomatics* 23:186–190, 1982.

Gillies MA, Skyring AP: The pattern and prevalence of aspirin ingestion as determined by interview of 2,921 inhabitants of Sydney. *Med J Aust* 1:974–979, 1972.

Goldfarb C: Patients nobody wants: skid row alcoholics. *Dis Nerv System* 31:274, 1970.

Granacher RP, Baldessarini RJ: The usefulness of physostigmine in neurology and psychiatry, in Klawans HL (ed): *Clinical Neuropharmacology*. New York, Raven Press, 1976, vol 1.

Greer JK, Ward HP, Corbin KB: Chronic salicylate intoxication in adults. *JAMA* 193:85–88, 1965.

Guttman D: Patterns of legal drug use by older Americans. *Addict Dis* 3:337–356, 1978.

Hall RCW, Gardner ER, Perl M, et al: Psychiatric and physiological reactions produced by over-the-counter medications. *J Psychedelic Drugs* 10:2432–2498, 1978.

Harrington P, Cox TJ: A twenty-year follow-up of narcotic addicts in Tucson, Arizona. *Am J Drug Alcohol Abuse* 6:25–37, 1979.

Hartford JT, Samorajski T: Alcoholism in the geriatric population. *J Am Geriatr Soc* 30:18–24, 1982.

Heaney RP: Nutritional factors in post-menopausal osteoporosis. *Roche Semin Aging* 5:8, 1981.

Janik SW, Dunham RG: A nationwide examination of the need for specific alcoholism treatment programs for the elderly. *J Stud Alcohol* 44:307–317, 1983.

Jarvik LF, Perl M: Overview of physiologic dysfunctions related to psychiatric problems in the elderly, in Levenson AJ, Hall RCW (eds): *Neuropsychiatric Manifestations of Physical Disease in the Elderly*. New York, Raven Press, 1981, pp 1–15.

Jenike MA: Drug abuse. *Sci Am Med* Sect VI:1–8, 1987.

Jenike MA: Using sedative drugs in the elderly. *Drug Ther* 12:184–190, 1982.

Jones RW: Alcoholism among relatives of alcoholic patients. *Q J Stud Alcohol* 33:810, 1972.

Kafetz K: Alcohol excess and the senile squalor syndrome. *J Am Geriatr Soc* 30:706, 1982.

Kerr A: Fighting alcoholism at its weakest links. *McLean Rev* 7(3):1, 1977.

Kofoed L, Bloom JD: Geriatric sexual dysfunction: a case survey. *J Am Geriatr Soc* 30:437–440, 1982.

Kofoed LL, Tolson RL, Atkinson RL, et al: Elderly groups in an alcoholism clinic, in Atkinson RM (ed): *Alcohol and Drug Abuse in Old Age*. Washington DC, American Psychiatric Association Press, 1984.

Kofoed LL: Abuse and misuse of over-the-counter drugs by the elderly, in Atkinson RM (ed): *Alcohol and Drug Abuse in Old Age*. Washington DC, American Psychiatric Association Press, 1984, pp 50–59.

Linn MW: Attrition of older alcoholics from treatment. *Addict Dis* 3:437–447, 1978.

Lipowski ZJ: *Delirium*. Springfield, Ill, Charles C Thomas, 1980.

Martin JC, Streissguth AP: Alcoholism and the aged, in Oattison EM, Kaufman E (eds): *Encyclopedic Handbook of Alcoholism*. New York, Gardner Press, 1983, pp 779–791.

Mellstrom D, Rundgren A, Jagenburg R, et al: Tobacco smoking, aging and health among the elderly: a longitudinal population study of 70-year-old men and an age cohort comparison. *Age Ageing* 11:45–58, 1982.

Novak LP: Aging, total body potassium, fat-free mass, and cell mass in males and females between ages 18 and 35 years. *J Gerontol* 27:438–443, 1972.

O'Donnell J: A follow-up of narcotic addicts. *Am J Orthopsychiatry* 34:948–954, 1964.

Parker ES, Noble EP: Alcohol consumption and the aging process in social drinkers. *J Stud Alcohol* 41:170–178, 1980.

Parker ES, Parker DA, Brody JA, et al: Cognitive patterns resembling premature aging in male social drinkers. *Alcoholism (NY)* 6:46–52, 1982.

Parsons OA, Leber WR: The relationship between cognitive dysfunction and brain damage in alcoholics: causal, interactive, or epiphenomenal? *Alcoholism (NY)* 5:326–343, 1981.

Pascarelli EF: Drug abuse and the elderly, in Lowinson JH, Ruiz P (eds): *Substance Abuse: Clinical Problems and Perspectives*. Baltimore, Williams and Wilkins, 1981, pp 752–757.

Pattison EM: Nonabstinent drinking goals in the treatment of alcoholism: a clinical typology. *Arch Gen Psychiatry* 33:923, 1976.

Penick EC, Read MR, Crowley PA, et al: Differentiation of alcoholics by family history. *J Stud Alcohol* 39:1944–1948, 1978.

Pokorny AD, Miller BA, Kaplan HB: The brief MAST: a shortened version of the Michigan Alcoholism Screening Test. *Am J Psychiatry* 129:342, 1972.

Redich KRW, cited by Blazer D: The epidemiology of mental illness in late life, in Busse EW, Blazer DG (eds): *Handbook of Geriatric Psychiatry*. New York, Van Nostrand Reinhold, 1980, p 256.

Reifler B, Raskind M, Kethley A: Psychiatric diagnoses among geriatric patients seen in an outreach program. *J Am Geriatr Soc* 30:530–533, 1982.

Rix KJB: Elderly alcoholics in the Edinburgh psychiatric services. *J Roy Soc Med* 75:177–180, 1982.

338

Salzman C: Basic principles of psychotropic drug prescription for the elderly. *Hosp Community Psychiatry* 33:133–136, 1982.

Salzman C: Polypharmacy and drug-drug interactions in the elderly, in Nandy K (ed): *Geriatric Psychopharmacology*. New York, Elsevier-North Holland, 1979, pp 117–126.

Sangiorgi GB: Alcohol and drugs: interactions and iatrogenic injuries, in Orimo H, Shimada K, Ikiri M, et al (eds): *Recent Advances in Gerontology*. Amsterdam, Exerpta Medica, 1979, pp 626–628.

Schuckit MA, Miller PL: Alcoholism in elderly men: a survey of a general medical ward. *Ann NY Acad Sci* 273:558–571, 1976.

Schuckit MA, Pastor PA: Alcohol-related psychopathology in the aged, in Kaplan HI (ed): *Psychopathology of Aging*. New York, Academic Press, 1979, pp 211–227.

Schuckit MA: Alcoholism and affective disorder: diagnostic confusion, in Goodwin DW, Erickson CK (eds): *Alcoholism and Affective Disorder*. New York, Spectrum Publications, 1979, pp 9–19.

Schuckit MA: Geriatric alcoholism and drug abuse. *Gerontologist* 17:168–174, 1977.

Seixas JA: Alcoholism, a practical synthesis for physicians. South Plainfield, NJ, Ayerst Laboratories, 1970 (available from National Council on Alcoholism, NY).

Sellers EM, Kalant H: Alcohol intoxication and withdrawal. *N Engl J Med* 294:757, 1976.

Stephens RC, Haney CA, Underwood S: *Drug Taking Among the Elderly*. National Institute on Drug Abuse Treatment Research Report. DHHS Publication No. ADM83–1229. Washington DC, US Government Printing Office, 1982.

Stewart RB, Hale WE, Marks RG: Analgesic drug use in an ambulatory elderly population. *Drug Intell Clin Pharm* 16:833–836, 1982.

Stewart RB, Hale WE, Marks RG: Analgesic drug use in the elderly. *N Engl J Med* 308:134–138, 1983.

Swanson DW, Weddige RL, Morse RM: Abuse of prescription drugs. *Mayo Clin Proc* 48:359–367, 1973.

Thompson TL II, Moran MG, Nies AS: Psychotropic drug use in the elderly. *N Engl J Med* 308:134–138, 1983.

Thompson WL, Johnson AD, Maddrey WL, et al: Diazepam and paraldehyde for treatment of severe delirium tremens: a controlled trial. *Ann Intern Med* 82:175, 1975.

Vaillant GE, Milofsky ES: Natural history of male alcoholism. IV. Paths to recovery. *Arch Gen Psychiatry* 39:127–133, 1982.

Vaillant GE: A 20-year follow-up of New York narcotic addicts. *Arch Gen Psychiatry* 29:237–241, 1973.

Vaillant GE: *The Natural History of Alcoholism*. Cambridge, Harvard University Press, 1983.

Vestal RE, McGuire EA, Tobin JD, et al: Aging and ethanol metabolism. *Clin Pharmacol Ther* 21:343–354, 1977.

Vestal RE, Norris AH, Tobin JD, et al: Antipyrine metabolism in man: influence of age, alcohol, caffeine and smoking. *Clin Pharmacol Ther* 18:425–432, 1976.

Wiens AN, Menustik CE, Miller SI, et al: Medical-behavioral treatment of the older alcoholic patient. *Am J Drug Alcohol Abuse* 9:461–475, 1983.

Wiseman JP: *Stations of the Lost: the Treatment of Skid Row Alcoholics*. Englewood Cliffs, NJ, Prentice Hall, 1970.

Zimberg S: Psychosocial treatment of elderly alcoholics, in Zimberg S, Wallace J, Blums SB (eds): *Practical Approaches to Alcoholism Psychotherapy*. New York, Plenum, 1978, pp 237–251.

Zimberg S: Two types of problem drinkers: both can be managed. *Geriatrics* 29:135–139, 1974.

11

Obsessive-Compulsive Disorders in the Elderly

The onset of obsessive-compulsive disorder (OCD) is quite rare after the age of 50; in reviewing data at the Massachusetts General Hospital OCD Clinic and Research Unit, only 1 (1%) of 100 consecutively evaluated outpatients had the onset of the disorder after the age of 50. However, review of the data from a later group of consecutively evaluated patients revealed that 22 (12%)of 183 patients were older than 50 when they first presented to the clinic, and 8 (4%) of the 183 were 60 years or older. Thus, even though the onset of the disorder is rare in older people, the percentage of elderly patients with OCD is significant. Many of these elderly patients had never been treated and of those who had been treated (some for decades), most never received appropriate therapeutic modalities. The majority of these elderly patients with OCD were markedly improved after a few months of appropriate treatment.

It is now known that if patients receive proper therapy, usually consisting of behavior therapy and psychotropic medication, the majority will improve substantially, and occasionally completely, within a few months (Jenike et al, 1986).

DIAGNOSTIC CRITERIA

The currently accepted definition of obsessive-compulsive disorder (OCD) is given in the DSM-III-R (1987), and requires that a patient have either obsessions or compulsions that are a significant source of distress or that interfere with social or role functioning (Table 11–1).

Obsessions are defined in DSM-III-R as:

"Recurrent, persistent ideas, thoughts, images, or impulses that are ego-dystonic; that is, they are not experienced as voluntarily produced, but rather as thoughts

Table 11–1
Diagnostic Criteria for 300.30 Obsessive-
Compulsive Disorder

A. Either obsessions or compulsions:
   Obsessions: (1), (2), (3), and (4):
   (1) recurrent and persistent ideas, thoughts, impulses, or images that are experienced, at least initially, as intrusive and senseless, eg, a parent's having repeated impulses to kill a loved child, a religious person's having recurrent blasphemous thoughts
   (2) the person attempts to ignore or suppress such thoughts or impulses or to neutralize them with some other thought or action
   (3) the person recognizes that the obsessions are the product of his or her own mind, not imposed from without (as in thought insertion)
   (4) if another Axis I disorder is present, the content of the obsession is unrelated to it, eg, the ideas, thoughts, impulses, or images are not about food in the presence of an eating disorder, about drugs in the presence of a psychoactive substance use disorder, or guilty thoughts in the presence of a major depression

   Compulsions: (1), (2), and (3):
   (1) repetitive, purposeful, and intentional behaviors that are performed in response to an obsession, or according to certain rules or in a stereotyped fashion
   (2) the behavior is designed to neutralize or to prevent discomfort or some dreaded event or situation; however, either the activity is not connected in a realistic way with what it is designed to neutralize or prevent, or it is clearly excessive
   (3) the person recognizes that his or her behavior is excessive or unreasonable (this may not be true for young children; it may no longer be true for people whose obsessions have evolved into overvalued ideas)

B. The obsessions or compulsions cause marked distress, are time-consuming (take more than an hour a day), or significantly interfere with the person's normal routine, occupational functioning, or usual social activities or relationships with others.

that invade consciousness and are felt to be senseless or repugnant. Attempts are made to ignore or suppress them."

Compulsions are defined in DSM-III-R as:

"Repetitive and seemingly purposeful behaviors that are performed according to certain rules or in a stereotyped fashion. The behavior is not an end in itself, but is designed to produce or prevent some future event or situation. However, either the activity is not connected in a realistic way with what it is designed to produce or prevent or it may be clearly excessive. The act is performed with a sense of subjective compulsion coupled with desire to resist the compulsion (as least initially). The individual generally recognizes the senselessness of the behavior (this may not be true for young children) and does not derive pleasure from carrying out the activity, although it provides a release of tension."

Table 11–2
Diagnostic Criteria for 301.40 Obsessive-
Compulsive Personality Disorder

A pervasive pattern of perfectionism and inflexibility, beginning by early adulthood and present in a variety of contexts, as indicated by at least *five* of the following:
(1) perfectionism that interferes with task completion, eg, inability to complete a project because own overly strict standards are not met
(2) preoccupation with details, rules, lists, order, organization, or schedules to the extent that the major point of the activity is lost
(3) unreasonable insistence that others submit to exactly his or her way of doing things, **or** unreasonable reluctance to allow others to do things because of the conviction that they will not do them correctly
(4) excessive devotion to work and productivity to the exclusion of leisure activities and friendships (not accounted for by obvious economic necessity)
(5) indecisiveness: decision making is either avoided, postponed, or protracted, eg, the person cannot get assignments done on time because of ruminating about priorities (do not include if indecisiveness is due to excessive need for advice or reassurance from others)
(6) overconscientiousness, scrupulousness, and inflexibility about matters of morality, ethics, or values (not accounted for by cultural or religious identification)
(7) restricted expression of affection
(8) lack of generosity in giving time, money, or gifts when no personal gain is likely to result
(9) inability to discard worn-out or worthless objects even when they have no sentimental value

Reprinted with permission from the *Diagnostic and Statistical Manual of Mental Disorders, third edition, revised.* Copyright 1987. American Psychiatric Association.

DISTINCTION FROM OBSESSIVE-COMPULSIVE PERSONALITY DISORDER

OCD is frequently confused with obsessive-compulsive personality disorder. OCD is an Axis I disorder in DSM-III-R, while obsessive-compulsive personality disorder is an Axis II disorder. Although patients who are diagnosed as having obsessive-compulsive personality disorder (Table 11–2) may have some obsessions and minor compulsions associated with their perfectionism, indecisiveness, or procrastination, these rituals do not interfere with the patient's life to the extent that OCD does. However, some patients with OCD also have obsessive-compulsive personality traits, and some do meet DSM III-R criteria for obsessive-compulsive personality disorder (Rasmussen and Tsuang, 1986).

The differential diagnosis of these two disorders has important implications for treatment. For example, although traditional psychotherapy produces little change in OCD obsessions and compulsions, it may be of some value in the treatment of patients with obsessive-compulsive personality disorder (Jenike, 1986c). Conversely, although controlled trials of behavior therapy and psychopharmacologic treatments have been found to be very effective for

OCD symptoms, there has been little research in using these approaches for obsessive-compulsive personality disorder.

PREVALENCE AND SIGNIFICANCE

Although traditional estimates of the prevalence of OCD in the general population were approximately 0.05%, results of recent studies suggested a much higher lifetime prevalence of 2% to 3% of the entire population (Myers et al, 1984; Robins et al, 1984); thus OCD is not the rare psychiatric disorder it was once thought to be.

Obsessions and compulsions of OCD can be severely incapacitating; not only is depression a frequent concomitant problem, but also the symptoms often spread to interfere with social and occupational functioning and often involve the person's family. We have seen several patients in the Massachusetts General Hospital OCD clinic whose entire families were moved to a new house in an attempt to escape the patient's contamination fears and cleaning rituals.

SUBTYPES OF OBSESSIVE-COMPULSIVE DISORDER

Obsessive-compulsive symptoms tend to fall into one of several major categories: checking rituals, cleaning rituals, obsessive thoughts, obsessional slowness, or mixed rituals. Checking and cleaning rituals form the overwhelming majority of compulsive rituals (53% and 48%, respectively) (Rachman and Hodgson, 1980). The elderly probably have the same types of symptoms as younger patients; of the elderly patients followed in the Massachusetts General Hospital OCD Clinic and Research Unit, all types of OCD symptoms were represented and there was not a predominance of one particular symptom. Some vignettes are presented to illustrate typical symptoms.

Cleaning Compulsions

A 70-year-old man presented with fears of being contaminated by touching various objects he considered dirty. He had to cover various "dirty objects" with paper towels before he was able to touch them. If, however, he did happen to touch his laundry, his bed, door handles in public restrooms, his shoes, the gas cap on his car, or other "dirty" objects, he experienced vague feelings of dirtiness and discomfort, and he would engage in extensive washing of his hands, along with any clothing he believed had come into contact with the object. The patient kept one hand "clean" at all times and refused to place this hand in his trouser pocket or to use it to shake hands.

As a result of these OCD symptoms, the patient was unable to work full time and his social life dwindled.

(Note: Rachman and Hodgson [1980] noted similarities between patients with cleaning rituals and those with simple phobias. In both types of patients a specific environmental situation triggers the fear and the person engages in passive avoidance of the situation or the contaminant, resulting in a rapid decrease in anxiety.)

Checking Compulsions

A 66-year-old woman who engaged in repetitive checking behaviors when she was not sure whether she had performed an action correctly presented to the clinic. She would plug and unplug electric appliances 20 times or more to be sure that she actually took the plug out of the socket. She would do the same with light switches, turning them on and off repeatedly to ensure that she in fact had turned them off.

She stared at the addresses on envelopes for as long as several minutes to ensure that she had actually seen her name on the envelope. She repetitively counted money, and her arithmetic required so many recalculations that she totally avoided financial paperwork and could no longer work in her previous job as a bookkeeper. The patient was no longer able to read because she continually returned to sentences she had already read to be sure she had actually seen them.

Primary Obsessional Disorder

Virtually all patients with compulsive rituals also have frequent obsessive thoughts. However, there is a subgroup of patients with OCD whose primary problem is obsessive thoughts, with few or no rituals (Jenike et al, 1987). These obsessive thoughts are typically of an aggressive, sexual, or religious nature, and are repulsive to the sufferer.

As an example, a 53-year-old man could no longer enter public places because of obsessive thoughts and impulses to shout obscenities or to accuse "unsavory" characters of having committed some illegal act. Similarly, a 62-year-old woman no longer entered public places because she would experience intolerable sexual thoughts about individuals she saw in these places.

Other Types

Less common subtypes of OCD symptoms are (a) patients who engage in rituals that involve placing objects in a certain order, and (b) patients with primary obsessional slowness, who become "stuck" for hours while performing everyday tasks such as dressing.

As clinicians see larger numbers of patients with OCD, relatively rare subtypes being identified include patients with obsessions and compulsions primarily aimed at controlling an overwhelming fear of having a bowel movement or being incontinent of urine in public (Jenike et al, 1987a) or young women who have extensive face picking rituals that can last for hours each day. We have not as yet seen any elderly patients with these disorders. Other disorders closely related to OCD are monosymptomatic hypochondriasis

(Brotman and Jenike, 1984), dysmorphophobia (Jenike, 1984), and obsessive fear of AIDS (Jenike and Pato, 1986; Jenike, 1987b), cancer, or some other illness (Jenike, 1986a). Obsessive fear of illness does present in elderly patients.

SOMATIC THERAPIES FOR OBSESSIVE-COMPULSIVE DISORDERS

Drugs

Much has been learned about somatic treatments for OCD in just the last few years. There are now medications that predictably help more than half of the patients with OCD. The number of controlled trials is growing rapidly as staff at a number of OCD clinics are seeing large numbers of patients. The typical randomized prospective placebo-controlled trial, which proved so useful in depression research, had until recently been almost impossible because of the small numbers of patients with OCD available to any one researcher. We will review the anecdotal evidence and the few controlled trials that underscore the effectiveness of pharmacotherapy in some patients.

Heterocyclic Antidepressants
Numerous antidepressants that have been reported to be useful in treating patients with OCD include imipramine (Geissman and Kammerer, 1964; Angst and Theobald, 1980; Hussain and Ahad, 1970; Turner et al, 1980), amitriptyline (Hussain and Ahad, 1970; Snyder, 1980), doxepin (Ananth et al, 1975; Bauer and Nowak, 1969), desipramine (Gross et al, 1969), zimeldine (Kahn et al, 1984), fluoxetine (Fontaine and Chouinard, 1985), trazodone (Prasad, 1984; Lydiard, 1986), and fluvoxamine (Price et al, 1987; Perse et al, 1987). Most of these reports, however, involved a small number of patients and no control subjects. Responses were unpredictable and not clearly related to depression; there was, however, dramatic improvement in some patients.

Clomipramine (Anafranil), a tricyclic antidepressant, has been available in Europe and Canada for over a decade and studies indicate that it has specific antiobsessional properties apart from its antidepressant qualities (Lopez-Ibor, 1969; DeVorvrie, 1968; Jiminez, 1968; Grabowski, 1968; Fernandez and Lopez-Ibor, 1967; Rack, 1977; Marshall and Micev, 1973; Yaryura-Tobias et al, 1976, Yaryura-Tobias and Neziroglu, 1975; Waxman, 1977; Coombe, 1982; Wyndowe et al, 1975; Capstick, 1977; Ananth et al, 1981; Stroebel et al, 1984). A few carefully controlled studies have confirmed preliminary results that clomipramine is indeed superior to placebo in the treatment of OCD (Thoren et al, 1980a and 1980b; Marks et al, 1980; Montgomery, 1980; Ananth et al, 1979; Insel et al, 1983; Jenike et al, 1989).

A large multicenter trial of clomipramine, funded by Ciba-Geigy Pharmaceutical Company, was recently completed in the United States and if preliminary positive findings hold up, one would expect that clomipramine will be on the market sometime in 1990. The main drawback to clomipramine is that it has occasional troublesome side effects that are primarily of an anticholinergic nature. Sexual difficulties are common and there is a small incidence of seizures when taken at higher doses.

A recent report of an open trial of a large number of OCD patients indicated that fluoxetine (Prozac) may be particularly helpful for these patients (Jenike et al, 1989a). Smaller samples of patients with OCD have also been reported to respond to this medication (Turner et al, 1985; Fontaine and Chouinard, 1986; Bremner, 1984). Fluoxetine is relatively free of toxic side effects, but is quite expensive at this time (eg, $1.50/20-mg pill).

Monoamine Oxidase Inhibitors

There are still no controlled studies of MAOI in OCD. A number of case reports (Joel, 1959; Annesley, 1969; Jain et al, 1970; Jenike, 1981 and 1982; Swinson, 1984; Rimher et al, 1982; Jenike et al, 1983) and anecdotal evidence suggest that they may be particularly helpful for patients who concomitantly have OCD and panic attacks or severe anxiety. Affective illness in patients or their families did not appear to be a good predictor of responsiveness to MAOI (Jenike et al, 1983).

Lithium Carbonate

A link between manic-depressive illness and OCD has been suggested (Black, 1974; Stern and Jenike, 1983; Joseph Lipinski, personal communication, 1985). Cycling obsessive-compulsive symptoms have been described, but there are very few reports on the successful use of lithium carbonate in treating OCD. One double-blind crossover trial of six OCD patients carried out in Denmark reported that lithium was as ineffective as placebo in symptom resolution (Geisler and Schou, 1970). On the other hand, there are a few case reports of patients with classic OCD who improved with lithium carbonate (Forssman and Walinder, 1969; Van Putten and Sander, 1975; Stern and Jenike, 1983) .

Obsessive-compulsive behaviors are sometimes found in patients who have bipolar affective disorder (Black, 1974; Baer et al, 1985). Although behavior therapy using in vivo exposure and response prevention is highly effective in treating these behaviors (see next section), until recently there were no reports of their use in patients who had bipolar disorder and concomitant OCD. A recent report of two patients who met criteria for both disorders and who were treated with a combination of therapist-aided and self-administered exposure and response prevention demonstrated that behavior therapy was effective only after the affective disorder was effectively controlled with lithium and neuroleptics (Baer et al, 1985).

Rasmussen (1984) reported the case of a 22-year-old woman with classic OCD who did not respond to clomipramine alone, but who improved greatly a few days after lithium carbonate was added with a stabilized lithium blood level of 0.9 mEq/L. Whether or not lithium augmentation of other tricyclic antidepressants or MAOIs for obsessive-compulsive symptoms is helpful remains to be tested. As noted in chapter 4, improvement in depressives has been demonstrated in tricyclic nonresponders after lithium was added to the antidepressant (DeMontigny et al, 1981).

Antipsychotic Agents

Under stress, the severe obsessional patient may appear psychotic, an observation that prompted clinicians to attempt amelioration with neuroleptic drugs. Commonly patients receive neuroleptics for many years even though there is no evidence that they have been of any help.

There are only a few case reports of patients in whom treatment with these agents was successful (Altschuler, 1962; O'Regan, 1970 and 1970a; Hussain and Ahad, 1970; Rivers-Buckeley and Hollender, 1982) and most of these patients were atypical and some resembled the clinical picture of schizophrenia rather than classic OCD. It may be that the schizophrenic features were partly, or even substantially, responsible for the improvement with neuroleptic agents.

In view of the absence of data on the efficacy of these drugs and the frequency of toxic side effects, especially in the elderly (see chapter 6), their use can only be recommended for the more acutely disturbed obsessional patient. When these agents are tried, patients should be evaluated at regular intervals of not more than one month and the neuroleptic discontinued if there is no definite improvement.

Anxiolytic Agents

There are also no good studies that address the use of anxiolytics in patients with OCD. Most clinicians believe that these agents are of little use in the treatment of obsessions or compulsions but that they do help with the anxiety that many OCD patients have. If antidepressants improve OCD symptoms, usually anxiety decreases without the use of anxiolytics.

The literature contains a few anecdotal reports of success (Breitner, 1960; Hussain and Ahad, 1970; Bethume, 1964; Tesar and Jenike, 1984; Tollefson, 1985) and a couple of controlled trials (Venkoba Rao, 1964; Orvin, 1967) in which the inclusion and outcome criteria were unclear.

Results of a recent small (n=14) open trial of buspirone (Buspar) in younger OCD patients indicated that it was not helpful in improving symptoms (Jenike and Baer, 1988).

In view of the occasional spontaneous remission and often fluctuating course of OCD, it is difficult to make a strong case for the use of anxiolytic drugs on the basis of available data.

Other Agents

Since a deficit in the serotonergic brain system is sometimes hypothesized as the cause of OCD, the use of the serotonin precursor, tryptophan, is of interest. Most of the work on tryptophan has been done by one group and results have not been replicated by others; Yaryura-Tobias and colleagues (1977, 1979, and 1981) reported the cases of a number of patients who improved with tryptophan.

Rasmussen (1984) reported the case of a male patient with OCD who had a partial response to clomipramine which was dramatically boosted when 6 g/day of L-tryptophan was added. This patient relapsed when tryptophan was stopped and improved again when it was restarted. Whether tryptophan would boost the antiobsessional effects of other tricyclic antidepressants or MAOIs remains to be determined. Walinder and associates (1976), however, demonstrated that L-tryptophan potentiated tricyclic antidepressant effects in endogenously depressed patients who did not have OCD.

Because the administration of tryptophan stimulates the enzyme that causes the breakdown of tryptophan, to be maximally effective, nicotinamide and probably vitamins B_6 and C should also be administered. It is likely that the administration of other large neutral amino acids should also be controlled in the diet and not taken in close proximity to doses of tryptophan (Cole et al, 1980; Jenike et al, 1986d).

Electroconvulsive Therapy

As patients with OCD have been refractory to usual treatments, many receive courses of ECT. Many of the severe patients with OCD who have been referred by clinicians to Massachusetts General Hospital OCD Clinic over the past few years have had at least one course of ECT. Most did not have a major affective disorder and the main reason for administering ECT was for treatment of OCD. Overall, ECT was an extremely ineffective treatment modality in these patients.

ECT is generally regarded as not useful in the OCD patient who is not endogenously depressed (Gruber, 1971; APA Task Force Report No. 14, 1978), although scant literature exists concerning the effects of ECT alone on OCD symptoms. In a review of this subject, Mellman and Gorman (1984) found a few studies reporting that ECT in combination with other treatment modalities was associated with clinical improvement in some OCD patients. They also reported the case of one atypical patient (obsessions only, which developed after wife's death) who had a good response to ECT after he did not respond to a number of treatments including a 12-week trial of clomipramine.

Walter and colleagues (1972) assessed the combined effects of ECT, modified narcosis, and antidepressants on obsessional neurotics (unclear diagnostic criteria) and found that 40% of the patients improved. The relative effect of each form of treatment separately was obscure. Grimshaw (1965) studied

100 patients who had obsessional symptoms, which were also poorly defined, and concluded that ECT had little effect on obsessional states.

Psychosurgery

Most OCD patients who undergo psychosurgery have very severe illness that has not responded to multiple therapeutic approaches, and thus the results of surgical intervention are impressive (LeBeau, 1952; Whitty and Duffield, 1952; Birley, 1964; Sykes and Tredgold, 1964; Strom-Olsen and Carlisle, 1971; Tan et al, 1971; Kelly et al, 1972; Bridges et al, 1974; Bailey et al, 1975; Bernstein et al, 1975; Mitchell-Heggs et al, 1976; Smith et al, 1976; Tippen and Henn, 1982; Jenike et al, 1986; Ballantine et al, 1987).

Tippen and Henn (1982) reviewed the results of six studies of modified leukotomy that included 110 patients who had obsessional disease. Eighty-nine patients (81%) were at least "improved," while more than half of those improved were in complete remission. The long-term outcome of these patients remained undetermined.

Side effects of modern site-specific lesion techniques are rare. The data on the efficacy of surgical treatment for OCD should be interpreted with some caution, however, as negative results are rarely reported and inclusion criteria and outcome measures for surgical patients were not well described. Hopefully, over the next few years, research efforts will clarify the indications for and optimal type of psychosurgery in the treatment of refractory OCD patients. At present, the role of surgical procedures is unclear.

BEHAVIOR THERAPY FOR OBSESSIVE-COMPULSIVE DISORDER

Description

Behavior therapy is a directive psychotherapeutic approach, based on proven learning principles, which teaches the patient how to directly alter his or her compulsive rituals. The techniques most consistently effective in reducing compulsive behaviors (and along with them obsessive thoughts) are exposure to the feared situation or object, and response prevention, in which the patient is helped to resist the urge to perform the compulsion after this exposure.

Behavior therapy produces the largest changes in rituals, such as compulsive cleaning or checking, whereas changes in obsessive thoughts are less predictable (Marks, 1981). This is in contrast to traditional psychotherapy, where any changes that might be produced are mainly in obsessional thoughts, while little effect is seen in rituals (Sturgis and Meyer, 1980). This difference reflects the specific effects of behavioral treatment, where the behaviors themselves are the targets of treatment. Consequently behavior therapy is now regarded as the treatment of choice (usually in combination with medications) when behavioral rituals predominate (Marks, 1981).

History of Behavioral Treatments for Obsessive-Compulsive Disorder

The use of behavioral techniques to treat obsessions and compulsions is not new. Decades ago Janet (1908, as cited by Marks, 1981) gave a remarkably accurate description of what is now termed exposure therapy, including the name itself:

> The guide, the therapist, will specify to the patient the action as precisely as possible. He will analyze it into its elements if it should be necessary to give the patient's mind an immediate and proximate aim. By continually repeating the order to perform the action, that is, exposure, he will help the patient greatly by words of encouragement at every sign of success, however insignificant, for encouragement will make the patient realize these little successes and will stimulate him with the hopes aroused by glimpses of greater successes in the future. Other patients need strictures and even threats and one patient told [Janet], 'Unless I am continually being forced to do things that need a great deal of effort I shall never get better. You must keep a strict hand over me.'

This outline of the behavioral treatment of OCD remains concise and accurate today, and exposure therapy as described by Janet remains the major behavioral treatment of OCD almost a century later. Yet despite the fact that behavioral techniques were successfully employed a century or more ago, it was not until the late 1960s that these techniques were widely and effectively employed in the treatment of this disorder. The reason can be found in the impact of psychoanalytic theory at the turn of this century. Soon after Janet gave his description of exposure therapy, Freud published his analysis of semantic conditioning in the formation of obsessions and compulsions in the patient known as the Rat Man (Freud, 1983), and interest turned toward the meaning of obsessions and compulsions and away from considering the compulsive behaviors as treatment targets in and of themselves.

A behavior therapist who has seen a large number of patients with OCD would agree that the presentation of many of these cases appears to coincide with psychodynamic themes. However, although psychodynamic formulations have descriptive value, they have not yielded effective techniques for modifying obsessions and compulsions. The need for direct behavioral treatment, even when behavior can also be explained in psychodynamic terms, finds support in an unexpected observation by Freud (1924) when he discussed the psychoanalytic treatment of a related anxiety disorder, agoraphobia:

> Our technique grew up in the treatment of hysteria and is still directed principally to the cure of this affliction. But the phobias have made it necessary for us to go beyond our former limits. One can hardly master a phobia if one waits till the patient lets the analysis influence him to give it up . . . take the example of agoraphobia. It succeeds only when one can induce them through

the influence of the analysis to behave like the first class, that is, to go out alone and to struggle with their anxiety while they are making the attempt. One first achieves therefore, a considerable moderation of the phobia and it is only when this has been attained by the physician's recommendation that the associations and memories come into the patient's mind, enabling the phobia to be solved.

Common Misconceptions about Behavior Therapy

We have found that in some cases patients are not given behavior therapy because of long-standing misconceptions about this form of treatment. Corrections of the most common misconceptions are as follows: (a) Behavior therapy will not lead to the formation of substitute symptoms, (b) interrupting compulsive rituals is not dangerous in any way to the patient, (c) the patient's thoughts and feelings are not ignored in behavior therapy, (d) behavior therapy no longer assumes that all maladaptive behavior is learned through simple conditioning processes, (e) the use of medication is not incompatible with behavior therapy, and (f) behavior therapists recognize that their methods are not equally effective for all patients (Baer and Minichiello, 1986).

Outcome Studies

Controlled outcome studies of exposure and response prevention for OCD over the past 15 years, involving more than 200 patients in various countries, have found that 60% to 70% of patients with ritualistic behaviors were much improved after behavioral treatment. Approximately 20% to 30% of the patients were resistant to the treatment, and the dropout rate averaged 20% (Marks, 1981; Rasmussen and Tsuang, 1984; Rachman and Hodgson, 1980). Treatment was carried out over a relatively short period averaging 3 to 7 weeks, with a 10-session treatment program most common. At follow-up of two years or more, improvements in rituals were maintained in almost all of the patients (Marks, 1981). Patients who had obsessive thoughts without ritualistic activity have been studied separately, with unpredictable results (Marks, 1981).

Foa and associates (1980) found that exposure and response prevention components of behavior therapy can produce differential effects in the treatment of compulsive washers. Exposure therapy was found to help mainly in reducing the anxiety component, while response prevention had its greatest effect in reducing the ritualistic washing. The combined treatment was more effective than either component alone. These authors also found that in treating checking rituals, a combination of imaginal exposure (ie, having the patient vividly imagine the most feared consequences of not ritualizing) plus response prevention is superior to response prevention alone. This may occur because the catastrophic consequences that many patients with checking rituals fear will never actually occur in real life, so habituation must be carried out in imagination (Foa et al, 1980).

The use of cognitive techniques in the treatment of obsessions and compulsions has been less predictable than the treatment package of exposure plus response prevention (Marks, 1981). Although the technique of thought-stopping is widely used to treat obsessive thoughts, clear empirical support for its usefulness remains lacking. Because OCD patients engage in obvious cognitive errors in inference and assessing the probability of danger, the application of cognitive therapy techniques to directly change these cognitive processes would seem to be useful. However, the only controlled study in this area found that the cognitive therapy technique did not add significantly to therapeutic effects of exposure in vivo (Emmelkamp et al, 1980). This negative finding is consistent with results of studies of other disorders treated with behavioral techniques: cognitive techniques do not add significantly to the results obtained with behavioral techniques aimed at the targeted behaviors (Latimer and Sweet, 1984).

Although obsessive and compulsive symptoms are usually greatly reduced with behavioral treatment, and interference with occupational and social functioning is reduced, the ritualistic behavior is rarely totally eliminated. Marks (1981) observed:

> Although most patients who are cooperative (and those are the great majority) improve with exposure in vivo, few of them are totally cured. Patients are generally told that they need to acquire a coping set to deal with tendencies to ritualize that might recur after discharge. Occasionally brief booster treatment is needed, but this is minimal apart from explicit advice about regular homework, which may be needed for many months after discharge.

PREDICTORS OF TREATMENT FAILURE

Predictors of treatment failure in behavior therapy for OCD are noncompliance with treatment, concomitant severe depression (Foa, 1979), absence of rituals, fixed beliefs in rituals, presence of concomitant personality disorder (Jenike et al, 1986a and 1986b; Minichiello et al, 1987), and type of compulsive ritual. Patients with schizotypal and possibly other severe personality disorders (Axis II in DSM-III-R) also do poorly with pharmacotherapy (Jenike, 1986b).

Findings from outcome studies and anecdotal evidence indicated that poor compliance is the most common reason for treatment failure with behavioral therapy for OCD (Marks, 1981). Behavior therapy is more demanding of the patient than many other forms of psychotherapy, and the patient must comply with behavioral instructions both during treatment sessions and during "homework" assignments. If the patient is inconsistent in doing this, treatment is unlikely to be successful.

The aid of a family member or friend in carrying out homework assignments is often critical to ensure compliance. In addition, the use of antidepressants concomitantly with behavior therapy often increases patients' compliance with exposure treatments (Marks et al, 1980). New methods of improving compliance with behavioral treatment that are under investigation include the use of portable computers that assist the patient in carrying out homework assignments (Baer et al, 1987).

Severe depression has also been found to be a negative predictor for improvement with behavior therapy of OCD (Foa, 1979). In patients with severe depression (eg, neurovegetative signs), the behavioral processes of physiological habituation to the feared stimuli do not occur, regardless of the length of exposure (Lader and Wing, 1969). Patients with severe depression often respond well to behavior therapy after depression is controlled with medication, however (Baer and Minichiello, 1986).

If a patient has only obsessive thoughts without rituals, behavior therapy is unlikely to succeed. In these cases pharmacotherapy is the treatment of choice (Jenike et al, 1987).

Patients who strongly hold the belief that their compulsive rituals are necessary to forestall future catastrophes (ie, overvalued ideas) appear to have a poorer outcome with behavioral treatments (Foa, 1979). For example, the patient who really believes that someone in his family will die if he does not wash his entire house every day is unlikely to give up rituals with behavior therapy alone. In some cases, treatment with antidepressant medication will produce changes in a patient's fixed beliefs, and behavior therapy might then be successful in eliminating rituals.

As noted, patients meeting DSM-III-R criteria for both OCD and schizotypal personality disorder do not respond well to either behavior therapy or pharmacotherapy. The idea of concomitant schizotypal personality disorder as a poor prognostic indicator in OCD appears to have validity in light of the literature on treatment failure. This personality disorder encompasses several of the poor predictive factors just reviewed. Most noticeably these patients have strongly held beliefs that their rituals are necessary to prevent some terrible event. Also, these patients have a difficult time complying with prescribed treatment and assigned record-keeping. Rachman and Hodgson (1980) similarly found that an abnormal personality is a negative predictor of outcome in behavior therapy for OCD; and more recently, Solyom and colleagues (1985) reported on a subcategory of patients with obsessional psychosis similar to the subgroup of patients with OCD and schizotypal personality, who also respond poorly to both behavior therapy and pharmacotherapy.

If a patient is found to meet the criteria for schizotypal personality disorder, we attempt to arrange for placement in a structured environment such as a day treatment center or half-way house during and after behavioral treatment. This intervention often produces small decreases in the patient's obsessive and compulsive symptoms, along with moderate improvements in overall functioning.

Patients with contamination fears and cleaning rituals appear to respond best to behavioral treatment (Rachman and Hodgson, 1980), while patients with checking compulsions might not respond as well. Even when responsive to behavioral techniques, patients with checking rituals appear to improve more slowly than those with cleaning rituals (Foa and Goldstein, 1978). A possible explanation for this difference is that many patients with checking rituals are unable to engage in the prescribed response prevention, especially those who check excessively at home (Rachman and Hodgson, 1980). In addition, patients with primary obsessional slowness respond more slowly to behavior therapy than do patients with either cleaning or checking rituals (Baer and Minichiello, 1986).

CONCLUSIONS

Initial Evaluation

The majority of patients with OCD who are seen as resistant to treatment have, in fact, not received appropriate treatments for the disorder. The majority of clinician-referred OCD patients presenting to the Massachusetts General Hospital clinic have never had trials of behavior therapy and almost half have not undergone antidepressant trials.

In order to outline a treatment plan for an OCD patient, it is necessary to have a clear idea of exactly what the problem is, what exacerbates and what improves it, how it has evolved over the life of the patient, and what other symptoms and difficulties exist concomitantly. This optimally requires history taking which combines behavioral, psychodynamic, and family principles. To determine the appropriate treatment and understand the individual's potential for noncompliance, a thorough mental status examination will be required. A depressed, manic, cognitively impaired, or psychotic patient will require a special treatment strategy. It is very unlikely that behavioral treatments will be effective until associated functional illnesses are well controlled. Also, elderly alcoholic patients usually need treatment for alcoholism (see chapter 10) before they can comply with treatment aimed specifically at their obsessive-compulsive symptoms.

Medical Evaluation

It is extremely unusual for a medical or neurologic illness to be associated with classic OCD. If onset of the illness is after the age of 50, the likelihood of associated disease probably increases. Possible neurologic causes are reviewed elsewhere (Jenike, 1984a and 1986e).

Treatment

Patients with Only Obsessive Thoughts
In patients who have obsessive thoughts only and do not have rituals, a trial of antidepressant medication is a reasonable first choice. Since fluoxetine is

now available by prescription in the United States, it may be best to begin with this drug. The optimal dose is unknown, but the staff at the Massachusetts General Hospital OCD clinic is increasing the drug dose to 80 mg/day as tolerated. Drug trials take three months and many patients will appear not to have responded during one or two months of medication, only to make significant strides in the third month.

If fluoxetine is not helpful, at this time clomipramine is probably the next drug to try. It can now be obtained directly from Ciba-Geigy Pharmaceutical Company. Adequate trials can require administration of as much as 250 mg/day for as long as 12 weeks. Troublesome anticholinergic side effects may limit dosage increases in the elderly. Other standard antidepressants might work, but they seem to be effective in a smaller percentage of patients. Newer agents, such as fluvoxamine and sertraline, may also turn out to be effective, but they are only available through experimental protocols at the time of this writing. A number of studies are underway to evaluate the effectiveness of the newer agents.

Rarely obsessions improve within a few days. Anecdotal experience indicates that the onset of effect of MAOIs may be particularly rapid.

Behavior therapy has little to offer the patient who does not have rituals. In those patients who are drug nonresponders, thought stopping, assertiveness training, systematic desensitization, imaginal flooding, and cognitive restructuring might assist in lowering symptoms.

Patients with Rituals
A few patients who have compulsive rituals will respond completely to either drugs or behavior therapy alone, but the majority require a combination of the two approaches for optimal clinical improvement. The techniques of exposure plus response prevention as outlined earlier are the mainstay of behavioral treatment. In patients who have concomitant major depression, psychosis, or mania, it is unlikely that behavior therapy will be of help until these symptoms are well controlled pharmacologically. In such patients, initial treatment should be drug oriented and behavior therapy should begin only after these affective or psychotic symptoms are optimally controlled.

In patients who only perform rituals at home, behavioral treatments will have to take place in the home. Family members will need to function as surrogate therapists and supervise the exposure plus response prevention. Many patients can be treated in an office setting with homework given to the patient at the end of each session.

Patients with Personality Disorders
Assessment of personality disorders in OCD patients is important in predicting outcome and the preferred treatment approach. As noted earlier, patients with severe personality disorders are largely refractory to usual therapeutic

strategies. These patients respond differently to previously validated behavioral techniques of exposure plus response prevention and also are usually not responsive to drug therapy. In particular, schizotypal personality disorder significantly impairs treatment outcome and should be considered along with other predictors of poor outcome such as severe depression, overvalued ideation, and noncompliance. This effect appears to be so strong that investigators should analyze data separately for patients meeting criteria for this disorder and those who do not. These patients are now often excluded from experimental drug protocols.

Until further data are available on management of OCD patients with concomitant severe personality disorder, clinicians can focus on reducing stress and conflict in their environments which is best done with behavioral family or couples counseling. In addition, attempt to arrange for day treatment, placement in a halfway house, or other alternative living arrangements away from the usually stressful environment where obsessive-compulsive symptoms often are exacerbated and reinforced. Once the patient is removed from the stressful environment, supportive therapy, with encouragement in exposure and response prevention and strong verbal reinforcement of the slightest gains, has been helpful to date in producing modest improvements in obsessions and compulsions. The long-term fate of these patients remains to be determined.

Medication Trials
Probably the initial drug of choice for OCD at this time is fluoxetine (Prozac). The Massachusetts General Hospital OCD clinic has more than 130 patients who are taking this drug at the time of this writing and results have been striking in more than half of the patients. At present treatment is begun with 20 mg taken each morning (it may cause insomnia) and gradually (over a few weeks) increased to 80 mg. A reasonable trial takes 10 to 12 weeks and it is relatively unusual for patients who are eventually going to respond well to show much improvement before 4 to 8 weeks on the drug. Occasionally patients respond early, but this will be the exception. Patients should be advised at the onset of treatment that drug trials in this disorder are fairly lengthy endeavors. If patients have a good response at a dose of 80 mg, we gradually decrease the dose to the minimum that is consistent with symptom reduction.

Clomipramine can be obtained from Canada, Mexico, or Europe. In addition, it is now much easier to obtain clomipramine directly from Ciba-Geigy Pharmaceutical Company. Because the elderly are likely to be sensitive to clomipramine's prominent anticholinergic side effects, it is best avoided in the elderly until other potentially less toxic agents have been tried.

Research centers may have access to experimental agents. If none of these drugs are available in a particular community for refractory patients, any of the standard heterocyclic agents can be tried. Dosages should be in the antidepressant range and blood levels may be helpful for imipramine, nortriptyline, and desipramine (Task Force, 1985).

If two antidepressant trials fail or if the patient also has panic attacks, a MAOI trial is a reasonable next step. Tranylcypromine, as much as 60 mg daily, or phenelzine, to 90 mg daily, are the two most commonly used drugs. Dietary and drug precautions are mandatory (see chapter 4).

Prior to changing antidepressant medication, it is probably worth trying to augment the response by adding lithium carbonate or tryptophan for a four-week period. Based on case reports with clomipramine, this strategy will occasionally yield positive results.

Anxiolytic agents are often used as adjuncts to other medications and may be helpful in facilitating behavior therapy in patients who are unable to tolerate the anxiety produced by exposure and response prevention techniques. It is unlikely that anxiolytic agents will have significant effect on OCD symptoms when used alone.

Electroconvulsive Therapy or Psychosurgery
ECT is generally not helpful in patients with OCD. However, in OCD patients who have clear-cut depression that precedes obsessive-compulsive symptoms, it may be worth trying.

From the collective data on psychosurgery, it appears that more than half of the severe OCD patients improve. Postoperative personality changes are not evident with modern restricted operations and surgical complications are few. A patient who for years has had disabling OCD that has responded poorly to more conventional therapies may have a reasonable chance of favorable outcome with relatively few risks. Despite the lack of reliable data, it appears that when more conservative treatments fail, psychosurgery is a viable option. Whether or not it will improve the clinical situation of the very severe OCD patients with concomitant personality disorder is unknown.

OBSESSIVE-COMPULSIVE DISORDERS FOUNDATION

This group has been formed within the last two years. They have a newsletter which updates current areas of interest to OCD patients and their families. Patients can join the foundation by writing to them at the OCD Foundation, Inc, P.O. Box 9573, New Haven, CT 06535.

REFERENCES

Altschuler M: Massive doses of trifluoperazine in the treatment of compulsive rituals. *Am J Psychiatry* 119:367, 1962.
Ananth J, Pecknold JC, van den Steen N, et al: Double-blind study of clomipramine

and amitriptyline in obsessive neurosis. *Prog Neuropsychopharmacol* 5:257–262, 1981.

Ananth J, Solyom L, Bryntwick S, et al: Clomipramine therapy for obsessive compulsive neurosis. *Am J Psychiatry* 136:700–720, 1979.

Ananth J, Solyom L, Solyom C, et al: Doxepin in the treatment of obsessive compulsive neurosis. *Psychosomatics* 16:185–187, 1975.

Angst J, Theobald W: *Tofranil*. Berne, Switzerland, Verlag Stampl, 1980, pp 11–32.

Annesley PT: Nardil response in a chronic obsessive compulsive. *Br J Psychiatry* 115:748, 1969.

APA Task Force Report No. 14 on Electroconvulsive Therapy. Washington DC, American Psychiatric Association, 1978.

Baer L, Minichiello WE, Jenike MA: Behavioral treatment of obsessive-compulsive disorder with concomitant bipolar affective disorder. *Am J Psychiatry* 142:358–360, 1985.

Baer L, Minichiello WE, Jenike MA: Use of a portable-computer program in behavioral treatment of obsessive-compulsive disorder. *Am J Psychiatry* 144:1101, 1987.

Baer L, Minichiello WE: Behavior therapy for obsessive-compulsive disorder. In Jenike MA, Baer L, Minichiello WE (eds): *Obsessive-Compulsive Disorders: Theory and Management*. Littleton, Mass, PSG Publishing, 1986.

Bailey HR, Dowling JL, Davies E: Cingulotomy and related procedures for severe depressive illness: studies in depression, IV, in Sweet WH, Obrador S, Martin-Rodriguez JG (eds): *Neurosurgical Treatment in Pain and Epilepsy*. Baltimore, University Park Press, 1975.

Ballantine HT, Bouckoms AJ, Thomas EK, et al: Treatment of psychiatric illness by stereotactic cingulotomy. *Biol Psychiatry* 22:807–819, 1987.

Bauer G, Nowak H: Doxepine: ein neues Antidepressivum Wirkungs-Verleich mit Amitriptyline. *Arzneimittelforsch* 19:1642–1646, 1969.

Bernstein IC, Callahan WA, Jaranson JM: Lobotomy in private practice. *Arch Gen Psychiatry* 32:1041–1047, 1975.

Bethume HC: A new compound in the treatment of severe anxiety states: Report on the use of diazepam. *N Engl J Med* 63:153–156, 1964.

Birley JLT: Modified frontal leucotomy: A review of 106 cases. *Br J Psychiatry* 110:211–221, 1964.

Black A: The natural history of obsessional neurosis, in Beech HR (ed): *Obsessional States*. London, Methuen, 1974, pp 16–54.

Breitner C: Drug therapy in obsessional states and other psychiatric problems. *Dis Nerv Syst* 21(suppl):31–35, 1960.

Bremner JD: Fluoxetine in depressed patients: A comparison with imipramine. *J Clin Psychiatry* 45:414–419, 1984.

Bridges PK, Goktepe EO, Moratos J: A comparative review of patients with obsessional neurosis and depression treated by psychosurgery. *Br J Psychiatry* 123:663–674, 1974.

Brotman AW, Jenike MA: Monosymptomatic hypochondriasis treated with tricyclic antidepressants. *Am J Psychiatry* 141:1608–1609, 1984.

Capstick N: Clinical experience in the treatment of obsessional states. *J Int Med Res* 5(suppl 5):71, 1977.

Cole JO, Hartmann E, Brigham P: L-Tryptophan: Clinical studies. *McLean Hosp J* 5:37–71, 1980.

Coombe PD: Clomipramine and severe obsessive-compulsive neurosis. *Aust NZ J Psychiatry* 16:293–297, 1982.

DeMontigny C, Grunberg F, Mayer A, et al: Lithium induces rapid relief of depression in tricyclic antidepressant drug non-responders. *Br J Psychiatry* 138:252–256, 1981.

DeVorvrie GV: Anafranil (G34586) in obsessive neurosis. *Acta Neurol Belg* 68:787–792, 1968.

Diagnostic and Statistical Manual of Mental Disorders, ed 3, revised. Washington DC, American Psychiatric Association Press, 1987.

Emmelkamp PMG, van der Helm M, van Zanten BL, et al: Treatment of obsessive-compulsive patients: The contribution of self-instructional training to the effectiveness of exposure. *Behav Res Ther* 18:61–66, 1980.

Fernandez CE, Lopez-Ibor JJ: Monochlorimipramine in the treatment of psychiatric patients resistant to other therapies. *Actas Luso Esp Neurol Psiquiatr* 26:119–147, 1967.

Foa EB, Goldstein A: Continuous exposure and strict response prevention in the treatment of obsessive-compulsive neurosis. *Behav Ther* 17:169–176, 1978.

Foa EB, Steketee G, Milby JR: Differential effects of exposure and response prevention in obsessive-compulsive washers. *J Consult Clin Psychol* 48:71–79, 1980.

Foa EB: Failure in treating obsessive-compulsives. *Behav Res Ther* 17:169–176, 1979.

Fontaine R, Chouinard G: An open clinical trial of fluoxetine in the treatment of obsessive-compulsive disorder. *J Clin Psychopharmacol* 6:98–101, 1986.

Fontaine R, Chouinard G: Antiobsessive effect of fluoxetine. *Am J Psychiatry* 142:989, 1985.

Forssman H, Walinder J: Lithium treatment of atypical indication. *Acta Psychiatr Scand Suppl* 207:34–40, 1969.

Freud S: Turnings in the ways of psychoanalytic therapy, in *Collected Papers*. London, Hogarth Press, 1924, vol 2, pp 399–400.

Freud S: Strachey J, trans: The Complete Psychological Works of Sigmund Freud. London, Hogarth Press, 1983, vols 1–24.

Geisler A, Schou M: Lithium ved tvangsneuroser. *Nord Psychiatr Tidsskr* 23:493–495, 1970.

Geissman P, Kammerer T: L'imipramine dans la neurose obsessionelle: Etude de 39 cas. *Encephale* 53:369–382, 1964.

Grabowski JR: Treatment of severe depression and obsessive depression with G3486. *Folia Med* 57:265–270, 1968.

Grimshaw L: The outcome of obsessional disorder: a follow-up study of 100 cases. *Br J Psychiatry* 111:1051–1056, 1965.

Gross M, Slater E, Roth M (eds): *Clinical Psychiatry*. Paris, Bailliere Tindall and Casel, 1969.

Gruber RP: ECT for obsessive-compulsive symptoms. *Dis Nerv Syst* 32:180–182, 1971.

Hussain MZ, Ahad A: Treatment of obsessive compulsive neurosis. *Can Med Assoc J* 103:648–650, 1970.

Insel TR, Murphy DL, Cohen RM, et al: Obsessive-compulsive disorder. A double-blind trial of clomipramine and clorgyline. *Arch Gen Psychiatry* 40:605–612, 1983.

Jain VK, Swinson RP, Thomas JE: Phenelzine in obsessional neurosis. *Br J Psychiatry* 117:237–238, 1970.

Janet P: *Les obsessions et la psychasthenie,* ed 2. Paris, Bailliere, 1908.

Jenike MA, Armentano M, Baer L: Disabling obsessive thoughts responsive to antidepressants. *J Clin Psychopharmacol* 7:33–35, 1987.

Jenike MA, Baer L, Minichiello WE, et al: Concomitant obsessive-compulsive disorder and schizotypal personality disorder. *Am J Psychiatry* 143:530–533, 1986b.

Jenike MA, Baer L, Minichiello WE, et al: Concomitant obsessive-compulsive disorder and schizotypal personality disorder: A poor prognostic indicator. *Arch Gen Psychiatry* 43:296, 1986a.

Jenike MA, Baer L, Minichiello WE: *Obsessive-Compulsive Disorders: Theory and Management*, Littleton, Mass, PSG Publishing, 1986.

Jenike MA, Baer L: An open trial of buspirone in obsessive-compulsive disorder. *Am J Psychiatry* 145:1285–1286, 1988.

Jenike MA, Buttolph L, Baer L: Fluoxetine in obsessive-compulsive disorder: an open trial. *Am J Psychiatry*, in press, 1989a.

Jenike MA, Pato C: Disabling fear of AIDS responsive to imipramine. *Psychosomatics* 27:143–144, 1986.

Jenike MA, Summergrad P, Baer L, et al: Clomipramine for obsessive-compulsive disorder: A double-blind placebo controlled trial. Submitted for publication, 1989.

Jenike MA, Surman OS, Cassem NH, et al: Monoamine oxidase inhibitors in obsessive-compulsive disorder. *J Clin Psychiatry* 44:131–132, 1983.

Jenike MA, Vitigliano HL, Rabinovitz J, et al: Bowel obsessions: A variant of obsessive-compulsive disorder responsive to antidepressants. *Am J Psychiatry* 144:1347–1348, 1987a.

Jenike MA: Illnesses related to obsessive-compulsive disorder, in Jenike MA, Baer L, Minichiello WE (eds): *Obsessive-Compulsive Disorders: Theory and Management*. Littleton, Mass, PSG Publishing, 1986a.

Jenike MA: Predictors of treatment failure, in Jenike MA, Baer L, Minichiello WE (eds): *Obsessive-Compulsive Disorders: Theory and Management*. Littleton, Mass, PSG Publishing, 1986b.

Jenike MA: Psychotherapy of the Obsessional, in Jenike MA, Baer L, Minichiello WE (eds): *Obsessive-Compulsive Disorders: Theory and Management*. Littleton, Mass, PSG Publishing, 1986c.

Jenike MA: Somatic treatments, in Jenike MA, Baer L, Minichiello WE (eds): *Obsessive-Compulsive Disorders: Theory and Management*. Littleton, Mass, PSG Publishing, 1986d.

Jenike MA: A case report of successful treatment of dysmorphophobia with tranylcypromine. *Am J Psychiatry* 141:1463–1464, 1984.

Jenike MA: Coping with fear responses to AIDS. *Hum Sexuality* 21:22–28, 1987b.

Jenike MA: Obsessive compulsive disorder: A question of a neurologic lesion. *Compr Psychiatry* 25:298–304, 1984a.

Jenike MA: Rapid response of severe obsessive-compulsive disorder to tranylcypromine. *Am J Psychiatry* 138:1249–1250, 1981.

Jenike MA: Use of monoamine oxidase inhibitors in obsessive-compulsive disorder. *Br J Psychiatry* 140:159, 1982.

Jenike MA:.Theories of etiology, in Jenike MA, Baer L, Minichiello WE (eds): *Obsessive-Compulsive Disorders: Theory and Management*. Littleton, Mass, PSG Publishing, 1986e.

Jiminez F: A clinical study of Anafranil in depressive, obsessional and schizophrenic patients. *Folia Neuropsiquat Sur Este Esp* 3:189, 1968.

Joel SW: Twenty month study of iproniazid therapy. *Dis Nerv Syst* 20:1–4, 1959.

Kahn RS, Westenberg HGM, Jolles J: Zimeledine treatment of obsessive-compulsive disorder. *Acta Psychiatr Scand* 69:259–261, 1984.

Kelly DHW, Walter C, Mitchell-Heggs N, et al: Modified leucotomy assessed clinically, physiologically and psychologically at six weeks and eighteen months. *Br J Psychiatry* 120:19–29, 1972.

Lader M, Wing L: Physiological measures in agitated and retarded depressed patients. *J Psychiatr Res* 7:89–100, 1969.

Latimer PR, Sweet AA: Cognitive versus behavioral procedures in cognitive-behavior therapy: A critical review of the evidence. *J Behav Ther Exp Psychiatry* 15:9–22, 1984.

Le Beau J: The cingular and precingular areas in psychosurgery (agitated behavior, obsessive compulsive states, epilepsy. *Acta Psychiatr Neurol Scand* 27:305–316, 1952.

Lopez-Ibor JJ: Intravenous infusions of monochlorimipramine. Technique and results, in *Proceedings of the Sixth International Congress of the CINP, Taragona, Spain, April 1968.* Amsterdam, Exerpta Medica, 1969, pp 519–521. Foundation International Congress Series No. 180.

Lydiard RB: Obsessive-compulsive disorder successfully treated with trazodone. *Psychosomatics* 27:858–859, 1986.

Marks IM, Stern RS, Mawson D, et al: Clomipramine and exposure for obsessive compulsive rituals. *Br J Psychiatry* 136:1–25, 1980.

Marks IM: Review of behavioral psychotherapy, I: Obsessive-compulsive disorders. *Am J Psychiatry* 138:584–592, 1981.

Marshall WK, Micev V: Clomipramine in the treatment of obsessional illness and phobic anxiety states. *J Int Med Res* 1:403–412, 1973.

Mellman LA, Gorman JM: Successful treatment of obsessive-compulsive disorder with ECT. *Am J Psychiatry* 141:596–597, 1984.

Minichiello WE, Baer L, Jenike MA: Schizotypal personality disorder: A poor prognostic indicator for behavior therapy in the treatment of obsessive-compulsive disorder. *J Anxiety Dis* 1:273–276, 1987.

Mitchell-Heggs N, Kelly D, Richardson A: Stereotactic limbic leucotomy: A follow-up at 16 months. *Br J Psychiatry* 128:226–240, 1976.

Montgomery SA: Clomipramine in obsessional neurosis: A placebo controlled trial. *Pharmacol Med* 1:189–192, 1980.

Myers JK, Weissman MM, Tischler GL, et al: Six month prevalence of psychiatric disorders in three commitments. *Arch Gen Psychiatry* 41:949–958, 1984.

O'Regan B: Treatment of obsessive compulsive disorder (letter). *Can Med Assoc J* 103:648–650, 1970.

O'Regan B: Treatment of obsessive compulsive neurosis with haloperidol. *Can Med Assoc J* 103:167–168, 1970a.

Orvin GH: Treatment of the phobic obsessive compulsive patient with oxazepam, an improved benzodiazepine compound. *Psychosomatics* 8:278–280, 1967.

Perse TL, Griest JH, Jefferson JW, et al: Fluvoxamine treatment of obsessive-compulsive disorder. *Am J Psychiatry* 144:1543–1548, 1987.

Prasad AJ: Obsessive-compulsive disorder and trazodone. *Am J Psychiatry* 141:612–613, 1984.

Price LH, Goodman WK, Charney DS, et al: Treatment of severe obsessive-compulsive disorder with fluvoxamine. *Am J Psychiatry* 144:1059–1061, 1987.

Rachman SJ, Hodgson RJ: *Obsessions and Compulsions.* Englewood Cliffs, NJ, Prentice-Hall, 1980.

Rachman SJ: *Fear and Courage.* San Francisco, WH Freeman, 1978.

Rack PH: Clinical experience in the treatment of obsessed states. *J Int Med Res* 5(suppl 5):81–96, 1977.

Rasmussen SA, Tsuang MT: Epidemiology and clinical features of obsessive-compulsive disorder, in Jenike MA, Baer L, Minichiello WE (eds): *Obsessive-Compulsive Disorders: Theory and Management.* Littleton, Mass, PSG Publishing, 1986.

Rasmussen SA, Tsuang MT: The epidemiology of obsessive compulsive disorder. *J Clin Psychiatry* 45:450–457, 1984.

Rasmussen SA: Lithium and tryptophan augmentation in clomipramine-resistant obsessive-compulsive disorder. *Am J Psychiatry* 141:1283–1285, 1984.

Rimher Z, Szantok, Arato M, et al: Response of phobic disorders with obsessive symptoms to MAO inhibitors. *Am J Psychiatry* 139:1374, 1982.

Rivers-Buckeley N, Hollender MH: Successful treatment of obsessive-compulsive disorder with loxapine. *Am J Psychiatry* 139:1345–1346, 1982.

Robins LN, Helzer JE, Weissman MM, et al: Lifetime prevalence of specific psychiatric disorders in three sites. *Arch Gen Psychiatry* 41:958–967, 1984.

Smith B, Kilom LF, Cochrane N, et al: A prospective evaluation of open prefrontal leucotomy. *Med J Aust* 1:731–735, 1976.

Snyder S: Amitriptyline therapy of obsessive-compulsive neurosis. *J Clin Psychiatry* 41:286–289, 1980.

Solyom L, DiNicola VF, Phil M, et al: Is there an obsessive psychosis? Aetiological and prognostic factors of an atypical form of obsessive-compulsive neurosis. *Can J Psychiatry* 30:372–380, 1985.

Stern TA, Jenike MA: Treatment of obsessive-compulsive disorder with lithium carbonate. *Psychosomatics* 24:671–673, 1983.

Stroebel CF, Szarek BL, Glueck BC: Use of clomipramine in treatment of obsessive-compulsive symptomatology. *J Clin Psychopharmacol* 4:98–100, 1984.

Strom-Olsen R, Carlisle S: Bifrontal stereotactic tractotomy: A follow-up study of its effects in 210 patients. *Br J Psychiatry* 118:141–154, 1971.

Sturgis ET, Meyer V: Obsessive compulsive disorders, in Turner SM, Calhoun KC, Adams HE (eds): *Handbook of Clinical Behavior Therapy*. New York, John Wiley and Sons, 1980, pp 68–102.

Swinson RP: Response to tranylcypromine and thought stopping in obsessional disorder. *Br J Psychiatry* 144:425–427, 1984.

Sykes M, Tredgold R: Restricted orbital undercutting: A study of its effects on 350 patients over the ten years 1951–1960. *Br J Psychiatry* 110:609–640, 1964.

Tan E, Marks I, Marset P: Bimedial leucotomy in obsessive-compulsive neurosis: A controlled serial enquiry. *Br J Psychiatry* 118:155–164, 1971.

Task Force on the use of laboratory tests in psychiatry: tricyclic antidepressants—blood level measurements and clinical outcome. *Am J Psychiatry* 142:142–149, 1985.

Tesar GE, Jenike MA: Alprazolam as treatment for a case of obsessive-compulsive disorder. *Am J Psychiatry* 141:689–690, 1984.

Thoren P, Asberg M, Cronholm B, et al: Clomipramine treatment of obsessive compulsive disorder. I. A controlled clinical trial. *Arch Gen Psychiatry* 37:1281–1285, 1980a.

Thoren P, Asberg M, Cronholm B, et al: Clomipramine treatment of obsessive compulsive disorder. II. *Arch Gen Psychiatry* 37:1286–1294, 1980b.

Tippin J, Henn FA: Modified leukotomy in the treatment of intractable obsessional neurosis. *Am J Psychiatry* 139:1601–1603, 1982.

Tollefson G: Alprazolam in the treatment of obsessive symptoms. *J Clin Psychopharmacol* 5:39–42, 1985.

Turner SM, Hersen M, Bellack AS, et al: Behavioral and pharmacological treatment of obsessive-compulsive disorders. *J Nerv Ment Dis* 168:651–657, 1980.

Turner SM, Jacob RG, Beidel DC, et al: Fluoxetine treatment of obsessive-compulsive disorder. *J Clin Psychopharmacol* 5:207–212, 1985.

Van Putten T, Sander DG: Lithium in treatment failures. *J Nerv Ment Dis* 161:255–264, 1975.

Venkoba Rao A: A controlled trial with Valium in obsessive compulsive states. *J Indian Med Assoc* 42:564–567, 1964.

Walinder J, Skott A, Carlsson A, et al: Potentiation of the antidepressant action of clomipramine by tryptophan. *Arch Gen Psychiatry* 33:1384–1389, 1976.

Walter CJ, Mitchell-Heggs N, Sargant W: Modified narcosis, ECT, and antidepressant drugs: a review of technique and immediate outcome. *Br J Psychiatry* 120:651–652, 1972.

Waxman D: A clinical trial of clomipramine and diazepam in the treatment of phobic and obsessional illness. *J Int Med Res* 5(suppl 5):99–110, 1977.

Whitty CWM, Duffield JE: Anterior cingulectomy in the treatment of mental disease. *Lancet* 262:475–481, 1952.

Wyndowe J, Solyom L, Ananth J: Anafranil in obsessive compulsive neurosis. *Curr Ther Res* 18:611–617, 1975.

Yaryura-Tobias JA, Bhagavan HN: L-Tryptophan in obsessive-compulsive disorders. *Am J Psychiatry* 134:1298–1299, 1977.

Yaryura-Tobias JA, Neziroglu MS, Bergman L: Clomipramine for obsessive compulsive neurosis: An organic approach. *Curr Ther Res* 20:541–548, 1976.

Yaryura-Tobias JA, Neziroglu MS, Bhagavan H: Obsessive-compulsive disorders: A serotonergic hypothesis, in Saletu B, Berner P, Hollister L (eds): *Neuropsychopharmacology: Proceedings of the 11th Congress of the CINP*. Oxford, England, Pergamon Press, 1979, pp 117–125.

Yaryura-Tobias JA, Neziroglu MS: The action of clorimipramine in obsessive compulsive neurosis: A pilot study. *Curr Ther Res* 17:1, 1975.

Yaryura-Tobias JA: Tryptophan may be adjuvant to obsessive-compulsive therapy. *Clin Psychiatr News* September 1981, p 16.

12

Therapy and Management of Older Persons

OVERVIEW

A discussion of the hundreds of types of psychotherapies that are available is clearly beyond the scope of this book. Therapeutic issues as they pertain to particular psychiatric (eg, depression, anxiety, insomnia) or neurologic (eg, dementia, Parkinson's disease) disorders have been reviewed in individual chapters. This chapter reviews some of the general matters that arise in non-pharmacologic treatments of the elderly. Practical management issues that confront the clinician treating elderly patients who have personality disorders or styles that impede treatment are included.

The elderly are underrepresented in the population using outpatient psychiatric services (Steuer, 1982). In 1968, for example, only 2% of patients who attended outpatient psychiatric facilities or were treated by psychiatrists in private practice were older than 65. This situation appears to have changed only slightly over the last two decades; a more recent estimate is that only 2.7% of all clinical services provided by psychologists go to older adults (Vandenbos et al, 1981) and that the portion of community mental health center services rendered to this group has remained relatively stable at around 4% over the last decade (General Accounting Office, 1982).

This underutilization of services may be the result of many factors. It may reflect a cultural bias where professionals might believe that resources should go to younger patients who have more years of life ahead of them and who are more economically productive. Some clinicians may view the elderly as inflexible or consider decline inevitable, while others may think that special knowledge is required to help the aged.

Countertransference issues may surface. Some elderly patients may view therapists as their children (Grotjahn, 1955) and unresolved conflicts with the

363

therapist's own parents may interfere with objective observation and therapy. It has also been argued, however, that mental health system factors—reimbursement system inequities, lack of cooperation among community mental health centers and physicians, discrepant perceptions of the help that is needed, and the lack of referrals from other physicians who have contact with older patients who need mental health services—are the most important explanations of why so few older adults are seen by mental health professionals (Kahn, 1975).

THERAPEUTIC APPROACHES

On the one hand, there are many types of psychotherapeutic approaches that can be used with the elderly, but on the other hand, no good studies address the outcome of psychotherapy which the clinician can use as a guide.

Based on few data, it has been suggested that four common principles underlie the process of all psychotherapeutic approaches in the elderly: (1) fostering a sense of control, self-efficacy, and hope; (2) establishing a relationship with the caregiver; (3) providing or elucidating a sense of meaning; and (4) establishing constructive contingencies in the environment (Butler, 1975).

Butler (1960, 1968, 1975, and 1975a) pointed out themes common in old age, such as dysfunctioning of one's body, independence and dependence, concerns with time, and stereotypes of the young. Questions concerning meaningfulness and feelings of uselessness are also common, and therapists may help the older patient to resolve existential crises through reminiscence and self-evaluation.

Busse and Pfeiffer (1977) recommended that the therapist be active in mapping and clarifying the patient's problems and suggested the establishment of limited goals such as symptom relief, support for adaptation to changing life circumstances, acceptance of greater dependency as a normal aspect of aging, and renewed or continued involvement in useful activity. They also encouraged social conversation during part of each session to enhance the patient's thoughts of being part of a meaningful relationship.

A number of practical tips for dealing effectively with elderly patients have surfaced. Blume and Tross (1980) pointed out the importance of regularly scheduled sessions as a source of constancy in what may be a life filled with change. As a means of increasing a patient's sense of self-worth, Burnside (1978) recommended that the therapist consider touching geriatric patients to express caring and to gain the patient's attention. Linden (1957) stressed the importance of optimism in the therapist and emphasized that the personality of the therapist is a main consideration in psychotherapy outcome.

When depressed elderly patients are being treated with medication, the drug will likely be more effective when used in combination with some type of psychotherapy (Goff and Jenike, 1986).

PSYCHOSOCIAL INTERVENTIONS

Because the problems of old people are likely to be social as well as intrapsy-chic, practical interventions are important, and the therapist should have a knowledge of community social agencies and referral sources. A number of agencies and groups are particularly useful in the management of particular types of patients and their families. Support groups and programs involving home visits to frail elderly with the purpose of reducing social isolation have been demonstrated to reduce psychiatric symptoms (Mulligan and Bennett, 1977–1978). Programs that enlist elderly persons as teachers, advisors, and consultants benefit both helpers and the helped (Sherman, 1981). Foster grand-parent programs place older adults in positions to help children in various school or hospital settings (Saltz, 1977; Hirschowitz, 1973). Pet therapy is reported to improve feelings of isolation, loneliness, and uselessness (Lago et al, 1983). Pets may afford companionship, demand responsibility in terms of caring for them, and provide physical contact.

Encouraging family members of dementing patients to join local and national chapters of the Alzheimer's Disease and Related Disorders Association (ADRDA) often greatly facilitates adjustment to these overwhelmingly stressful disorders (see chapter 5).

PERSONALITY TYPES AND IMPACT OF PSYCHIATRIC OR MEDICAL ILLNESS

Overview

When people become ill, certain aspects of their individual personalities may become accentuated and they may behave in puzzling, if not destructive, ways. Geringer and Stern (1986) expanded on earlier work of Kahana and Bibring (1965) and outlined specific psychological conflicts that may arise when pa-tients with various character types become physically ill. The effects of charac-ter type on coping ability and particular strategies that the clinician can use to maximize coping are worth reviewing as these issues arise daily in psychiatric and medical practice with elderly patients.

Medical and psychiatric illnesses are often associated with psychological regression that generates problems with dependency, trust, and self-control. Three common tasks that should be completed to successfully cope with medical illness are: acknowledging the illness, allowing oneself to be depen-dent on others, and restoring normal functioning, if possible.

Each patient's habitual personality style will influence how successfully that person works through the psychological tasks created by being ill. Kahana and Bibring (1965) outlined seven personality types that can be utilized to illustrate patient's reactions to illness. They delineated personality characteris-tics and conflicts that can occur in the context of the physician-patient relation-ship, and provided a useful bridge between dynamic and descriptive psychiatry that is of practical use to the clinician. These personality types are briefly reviewed and practical tips for managing each type, based on the information provided by Kahaha and Bibring (1965) and Gehringer and Stern (1986), are presented.

Oral Personality

The person with the classic oral personality is dependent, demanding, and usually impulsive. A decreased tolerance of frustration can lead to anger and depression, fear of being alone, and addictive tendencies. The clinician may note increased demands and the expectation that he or she has unlimited time and resources in caring for such a patient. Depression, anger, and blaming the clinician are common when unrealistic expectations are invariably not met.

Patients are best managed through gentle and firm limit-setting, particularly on the amount of time spent with the patient and the amount of medication prescribed. They may do well with frequent, short visits, rather than infrequent, long appointments. It may be best for a physician to see such patients not just when they are ill, as this reinforces their desire to remain dependent, but also briefly at regular intervals when they are well. Patients then will not have to remain ill to keep up the relationship with the caregiver.

Compulsive Personality

Patients with a compulsive personality are very controlled, orderly, rational, and emotionally reserved. They tend to focus on minute details and often "miss the forest for the trees." They tend to be conscientious and preoccupied with moral issues, and they are self-disciplined and frugal. It has been suggested that they are trying to control aggressive impulses by their style, and illness may be viewed as a potential loss of self-control.

Their characteristic response to being ill is to become more rigid and to seek more information from the physician. They may have the most difficulty with illnesses that involve compromised control over themselves and their environment, such as being on an intraaortic balloon pump or respirator, having a delirium or dementing process that compromises cognitive function, or losing bowel or bladder control.

They may have trouble making decisions and these patients are best managed by giving careful, methodical instructions and information, and by allowing them as much participation and control over care as possible. If there are a number of possible options to treatment or management, allow them to help make decisions. They can do such things as take their own pulse, help with dressing changes, or even decide medication dose if there is a range allowable.

Hysterical Personality

Patients with a hysterical personality are characteristically charming, imaginative, seductive, dramatizing, and strive to form intense personal relationships. They may desire a close and often flirtatious clinician-patient relationship. These patients have an excessive need for admiration and reassurance of their attractiveness. Illness evokes a threat to their masculinity or feminity. Men fear bodily damage and loss of physical prowess while women typically fear loss of attractiveness.

They are best managed by reassurance, support for their attractiveness or physical prowess, and affective ventilation. As opposed to the compulsive person, these patients often want the "big picture" and, in fact, may be overwhelmed by details of their illness. Such patients would be expected to have difficulty with illnesses that compromise physical prowess or attractiveness, such as burns, congestive heart failure, Parkinson's disease, and coronary artery disease.

Masochistic Personality

Patients with a masochistic personality have a history of repeated suffering and a strong tendency to incur misfortune, coupled with an exhibitionistic display of suffering. They tend to have self-sacrificing relationships and may believe that they are a burden to others. These patients often have childhood histories of being loved and attended to only when they were sick or suffering. They may see illness both as a deserved punishment and as a permissible way of being cared for. Thus, efforts to reassure patients and reduce symptoms may fail, because the wish for care often supersedes the wish for reduction of symptoms.

It is best to acknowledge their suffering and ask them to help themselves so that they can effectively continue their self-sacrifice for others. If such a patient has a chronic disease, it may be best not to emphasize improvement but to focus on the disability that remains.

Schizoid Personality

Patients with a schizoid personality are typically remote, reclusive, and reserved, and exhibits a paucity of involvement with others; they are classic loners. Illness forces them to interact with others and threatens to intrude on their solitude. Often this fear of involvement will result in denial of illness as a way to defend against the fear of intrusion.

Once under medical care, they are apt to remain reclusive, make little eye contact, and ask few questions. Well-intentioned caregivers may try to draw a schizoid person out with the opposite result. Management that preserves and respects the schizoid person's intense need and love of privacy is indicated.

Paranoid Personality

The paranoid personality has a fearful, guarded, and suspicious nature, along with oversensitivity to criticism or slights and fear of being hurt. Patients with this personality type expect the worst in others and may hasten to attack in a manner out of proportion to any actual insult. Such patients often engender anger in those whom they encounter, anger which is then taken as evidence to support their initial point of view. Illness may be viewed as another potential attack and this intensifies their mistrust and anger toward caregivers.

They are optimally managed by keeping some interpersonal distance, acknowledging the paranoid person's viewpoint, and being as firm and consistent as possible about necessary procedures and routines.

Narcissistic Personality

The narcissistic patients view themselves as all-important and are smug, grandiose, vain, and arrogant, or, when seemingly humble, patronizing. Grandiosity may be a cover-up for fragile self-esteem. Such patients may alternatively idealize and devalue the treating physician, because there is a need to be cared for by the most outstanding physician and a simultaneous need for the patient to surpass everyone encountered. Illness is experienced as a threat to autonomy and the image of perfection.

Clinicians need to enhance the patient's self-esteem and sense of autonomy while caring for their psychiatric or medical needs.

Management Plan

During psychiatric or medical illnesses, some of these features may surface to the detriment of the patient's care. For the personality types just described, illness usually results in an intensification of the characteristic personality style. Patients may become more dependent, controlling, hysterical, masochistic, withdrawn, paranoid, or grandiose. Pure forms of these types are uncommon, and many patients will have a number of such features.

Understanding some of the conflicts and fears, and attention to management may pay great dividends for caregivers. Clinicians are often quite surprised when patients do not act as they would. The techniques and insights described should not be used to judge or stereotype individual patients, but rather should serve as guidelines to assist in the management of these patients in an empathic and successful manner. The ability of clinicians to identify these character styles will provide greater facility in aiding each patient to cope successfully during psychiatric or medical illness.

SUMMARY

Even though it appears that elderly patients are underutilizing outpatient psychiatric services for a number of reasons, much can be done to help individual patients improve their lives. It has been suggested that four common principles underlie the process of all psychotherapeutic approaches in the elderly: (1) fostering a sense of control, self-efficacy, and hope; (2) establishing a relationship with the caregiver; (3) providing or elucidating a sense of meaning; and (4) establishing constructive contingencies in the environment.

Recurrent themes in older people include: dysfunctioning of one's body, independence and dependence, concerns with time, and stereotypes of the young. Questions concerning meaningfulness of life and feelings of uselessness are also common, and therapists may help the elderly patient resolve existential crises through reminiscence and self-evaluation.

Some authors offered practical suggestions for dealing with the elderly such as having some time during each visit for social conversation and touching the patient sometimes so that the elderly patient has a sense that he or she is in a caring and meaningful relationship with the caregiver.

Since the problems of old people are likely to be social as well as intrapsychic, practical interventions are important, and the therapist should have a knowledge of community social agencies and referral sources. Programs that use the elderly as teachers, advisors, consultants, or even foster grandparents have been successful. Pets may enhance the life of an elderly patient.

When people become ill, certain aspects of their individual personalities may become accentuated and patients may behave in puzzling if not destructive ways. Illness may result in an intensification of a characteristic personality style and patients may become more dependent, controlling, hysterical, masochistic, withdrawn, paranoid, or grandiose. Pure forms of these types are uncommon, and many patients will have a number of such features. The effects of character type on coping ability and particular strategies that the clinician can use to maximize coping are reviewed as these issues arise daily in psychiatric and medical practice with elderly patients.

REFERENCES

Blume JE, Tross S: Psychodynamic treatment of the elderly: A review of issues in theory and practice, in Eisdorfer D (ed): *Annual Review of Gerontology and Geriatrics*. New York, Springer, 1980, vol 1.

Burnside IM: Principles from Yalom, in Burnside IM (ed): *Working with the Elderly: Group Process and Techniques*. North Scituate, Mass, Duxbury Press, 1978.

Busse EW, Pfeiffer E: *Behavior and Adaptation in Late Life*, ed 2. Boston, Little, Brown, 1977.

Butler R: Intensive psychotherapy for the hospitalized aged. *Geriatrics* 15:644, 1960.

Butler RN: Toward a psychiatry of the life-cycle: Implications of sociopsychologic studies of the aging process for the psychotherapeutic situation. *Psychiatr Res Rep* 23:233, 1968.

Butler RN: Psychotherapy in old age, in Arieti S (ed): *American Handbook of Psychiatry*, ed 2. New York, Basic Books, 1975, vol 5.

Butler RN: Psychiatry and the elderly: an overview. *Am J Psychiatry* 132:893, 1975a.

Geringer ES, Stern TA: Coping with medical illness: The impact of personality types. *Psychosomatics* 27:251–261, 1986.

Goff DC, Jenike MA: Treatment-resistant depression in the elderly. *J Am Geriatr Soc* 34:63–70, 1986.

Grotjahn M: Analytic psychotherapy with the elderly. *Psychoanal Rev* 42:419, 1955.

Hirschowitz RG: Foster grandparents program: Preventive intervention with the elderly poor. *Hosp Community Psychiatry* 24:418–420, 1973.

Kahana RJ, Bibring GL: Personality types in medical management, in Zinberg NE (ed): *Psychiatry and Medical Practice in a General Hospital*. New York, International Universities Press, 1965, pp 108–123.

Kahn RL: The mental health system and the future aged. *The Gerontologist* 15 (Part II):24–31, 1975.

Lago D, Connell CM, Knight B: Initial evaluation of PACT (People and Animals Coming Together): A companion animal program for community-dwelling older persons, in Smyer M, Gatz M (eds): *Mental Health and Aging: Programs and Evaluations*. Beverly Hills, Cal, Sage, 1983.

Linden ME: The promise of therapy in the emotional problems of aging. Paper presented at the Fourth Congress of the International Association of Gerontology; July 1957; Merano, Italy.

Mulligan MA, Bennett R: Assessment of mental health and social problems during multiple friendly visits: The development and evaluation of a friendly visiting program for the isolated elderly. *Int J Aging Hum Dev* 8:43–65, 1977–1978.

Saltz R: Fostergrandparenting: A unique child-care service, in Troll LE, Israel J, Israel K (eds): *Looking Ahead: A Woman's Guide to the Problems and Joys of Growing Older*. Englewood Cliffs, NJ, Prentice-Hall, 1977.

Sherman EL: *Counseling the Aging: An Integrative Approach*. New York, The Free Press, 1981.

Steuer J: Psychotherapy for depressed elders, in Blazer DG (ed): *Depression in Late Life*. St Louis, CV Mosby, 1982.

Vandenbos GR, Stapp J, Kilburg RR: Health service providers in psychology: Results of the 1978 APA Human Resources Survey. *Am Psychol* 36:1395–1418, 1981.

13

Use of Neuroimaging Techniques in the Elderly Patient

Over the past decade a number of sophisticated neuroimaging techniques that have become available allow the examination of brain structure (CT and MRI) as well as brain function (regional cerebral blood flow, single photon emission computed tomography, PET).

Techniques for examining structure permit the study of brain anatomy and possible anatomic abnormalities while methods that evaluate function allow study of the brain at work through the measurement of metabolic activity and neurotransmitter systems (Andreasen, 1988). The potential of these techniques is just being realized as clinicians are now able to map certain aspects of brain structure and function in normal subjects as well as in those with mental and physical brain disorders. These techniques will continue to expand knowledge of the pathophysiology of mental illnesses by demonstrating structural, metabolic, and neurochemical abnormalities in a wide range of disorders (Andreasen, 1988).

Currently, three types of energy sources are used in brain imaging including: x-rays, radioactive isotopes (including single photon emitters or positron emitters), and the energy response of tissues in large magnetic fields (MRI). Based on the energy source, imaging methods are grouped into two basic categories: transmission tomography and emission tomography. Transmission tomography is represented by CT and is based on the differential tissue absorption of externally administered energy in the form of x-rays. The x-rays that are transmitted through the tissue are measured and the resulting tomograms present information about the structure of the brain (Metter, 1988).

Emission tomographic techniques measure the distribution of energy sources that can be produced by natural internal energy sources as in MRI or radionuclides (ie, an isotope that emits detectable radiation) that are injected or inhaled. Radioisotopes can be attached to a variety of molecules to create radioactive compounds. Regional cerebral blood flow, single photon emission computed tomography, or PET utilize externally supplied energy sources that are injected or inhaled and then are distributed through the body based on the physiological process being measured (Metter, 1988).

COMPUTERIZED TOMOGRAPHY

One of the oldest imaging techniques, CT, developed in the early 1970s, is a proven method of measuring brain structure. Soon after development, the CT scan was used in psychiatric patients and demonstrated ventricular enlargement, and presumably decreased cortical mass, in a subgroup of patients who had schizophrenia, suggesting that this illness involves not only functional abnormalities, but also perhaps abnormalities in brain structure (Andreasen, 1988).

In addition to schizophrenia, abnormalities have been reported in patients with bipolar disorder, depression, alcoholism, anorexia nervosa, Alzheimer's disease, and multi-infarct dementia. It is invaluable in assessing mass lesions, such as meningioma or metastatic tumors, in patients with mental or neurologic symptoms.

Prior to the availability of CT scanning, the study of age- and disease-related changes of the brain was primarily accomplished by two means: pneumoencephalography and autopsy (Albert and Stafford, 1988). The majority of studies of healthy adults across the age range have reported that the size of the lateral ventricles increases with age. There are, however, conflicting reports concerning the age at which significant increases in ventricular size occur; Albert and Stafford (1988) noted that these "normal" individuals often had some findings, such as headache, or some chronic disease. When patients with chronic diseases are included in studies of "normal" subjects, age and disease are confounded. Results of studies using very strict criteria for normality found that ventricular size as measured by CT remains fairly stable throughout early adulthood and then increases exponentially at an older age beginning around the age of 60 to 70 years.

CT scan measures in patients with Alzheimer's disease have been extensively studied (see Albert and Stafford, 1988, for review). Early studies and newer sophisticated computer-assisted enhancing techniques concur in finding a significant difference between the ventricular size of patients with presenile (onset before the age of 65) and senile (onset after 65) dementia of the Alzheimer type and age-matched control subjects. Longitudinal studies have shown that the ventricles of Alzheimer patients increase as the disease progresses (Gado et al, 1983; Brinkman and Largen, 1984), supporting the idea that ventricular enlargement is a reflection of the progression of Alzheimer's disease.

Weinberger (1984) proposed indications for the use of CT scans by psychiatrists: unexplained confusion, dementia, movement disorder, psychosis, anorexia, or catatonia; late-onset affective or personality disturbances; and atypical symptoms or course of chronic psychiatric illness. Other authors suggested that abnormal results from neurologic (Larsen et al, 1981) or mental status (Beresford et al, 1986) examinations should serve as indicators for the cost-effective use of CT to identify brain disease in psychiatric patients, as CT most often yields useful information when such abnormalities are present.

MAGNETIC RESONANCE IMAGING

Mechanism of Action

MRI, a technique that does not use ionizing radiation and has minimal risk, has become widely available since the mid–1980s and has a number of advantages over the CT scan. MRI uses information derived from the decay of resonant energy signals emitted by hydrogen nuclei (has a single proton as a nucleus), which act as tiny bar magnets and align themselves (Conlon and Trimble, 1987) in a magnetic field after stimulation by pulsed radio waves (Pykett et al, 1982; Garber et al, 1988). In order to generate a measurable signal, the property of resonance is utilized. If a pulse of (radiofrequency) energy is applied perpendicular to the long axis of the nuclei (bar magnets) some deflection will occur. When the natural frequency of the nucleus is chosen for the deflecting pulse, resonance occurs, similar to the vibration of a tuning fork (Conlon and Trimble, 1987). After the pulse is turned off, the nucleus gradually returns to normal alignment, losing energy which is emitted as a measurable signal.

By manipulating the sequence of the radiofrequency pulses, three different parameters can be measured (Conlon and Trimble, 1987). First is proton density, which reflects the density of the mobile hydrogen nuclei in the area under study. Second is spin-latice relaxation, alternatively known as the time constant, T1, which is a measure of the relaxation time of the hydrogen nuclei in the longitudinal plane and depends on the interaction of these nuclei with other surrounding molecules (the "lattice"). Third is spin-spin relaxation, more commonly called the time constant, T2, which is a measure of relaxation time in the transverse plane and depends on the interaction of the nuclei with each other. Thus, proton density, T1, and T2 are the output parameters that form the image.

It is difficult to translate from these technical terms into biological or clinical language; the interacting variables are complex and a complete understanding requires knowledge of quantum physics (Conlon and Trimble, 1987). In simple terms, MRI usually measures the activity of the hydrogen nucleus. T1 measurements are influenced by the ratio of free to bound water which depends on the water content of the tissue, the binding affinity of the molecules, and chemical environment. Mobile hydrogen nuclei are found in lipids in the body. For practical purposes proton density and T1 and T2 measurements are thought to reflect the interrelationship of free water and lipids in tissues, thereby relating to local physiological activity. For example, because of the differences in lipid concentration, likely as a result of myelination, white and grey matter are well differentiated in MRI pictures and thus, in demyelinating disorders, such as multiple sclerosis, the free water to lipid ratio is altered, and the actual plaque may be visualized.

Variations in water-protein and water-lipid interactions produce signal differences that often reflect anatomic and pathologic tissue changes. Computer analysis generates clear and detailed images of the brain that can localize and characterize normal or abnormal brain structure without exposing patients to significant risks.

Advantages of MRI

Unlike CT, which is limited to imaging brain regions in a transverse plane, MRI can image in all planes, including sagittal and coronal as well as transverse (Andreasen, 1988). For visualizing frontal and limbic regions, coronal images are ideal. In addition, MRI allows excellent gray-white resolution and permits an accurate three-dimensional reconstruction of brain structures. MRI also allows visualization of areas not easily studied on CT scan, such as the corpus callosum, hippocampus, amygdala, and other temporolimbic structures.

Preliminary data suggest that MRI may allow study of not only brain structure but also some aspects of function and even possible pathologic tissue through measurement of T1 and T2 relaxation times and other parameters (Andreasen, 1988). In such functional studies, physiochemical differences in regional brain areas may be reflected in altered proton density or relaxation times which can be quantified. These studies to date are few but the potential to study subtle change, especially when gross pathological lesions are absent, has particular appeal in psychiatric research (Conlon and Trimble, 1987).

MRI can be superior to CT in demonstrating pathologic tissues associated with many neurologic disorders, including tumors and infarctions, demyelinating diseases, and seizure disorders (see Garber et al, 1988, and Conlon and Trimble, 1987, for reviews). Garber and colleagues (1988) presented a number of cases of patients for whom MRI was useful in neuropsychiatric evaluations because it detected neuropathologic tissues better than CT scans. One patient was a 49-year-old woman who had recently had visual hallucinations, generalized seizure disorder, progressive dementia, and depression with delusions and who had normal findings on physical and laboratory examinations, lumbar puncture, and a CT which demonstrated nonspecific moderate cortical atrophy and periventricular hypodensity. The rapid onset of dementia and atypical psychotic symptoms (visual hallucinations) could not be explained until MRI revealed multiple areas of abnormal signal in cortical and subcortical structures consistent with an angiopathic encephalopathy not seen with CT. The second patient, a 69-year-old hypertensive woman, had a CT scan for recent depression and memory disturbance with falling episodes and weakness in her left leg. CT showed only slight left-ventricle prominence of uncertain significance; MRI demonstrated multiple foci of increased signal in the periventricular white matter of both cerebral hemispheres, posterior temporal-occipital regions, and left central pons, again consistent with angiopathic encephalopathy. A third patient, a 56-year-old man, presented with initial onset manic syndrome and focal motor seizures and evidence of dementia. Neurologic investigations, including a lumbar puncture and EEG, were unrevealing; CT scan showed slight cortical atrophy but no focal abnormalities. After his right arm became weak and numb, a repeat CT scan showed an area of enhancement in the left parietal cortex consistent with hemorrhage. Carotid angiography revealed a left posterior mass, suggesting vascular abnormality or metastatic tumor. Although five CT scans showed gradual resolution of the edema and ventricular compression, the area of x-ray density could not be definitively diagnosed. The atypical presentation of mania and unexplained dementia prompted study with MRI, which clarified the diagnosis of a cryptic arteriovenous malformation that had previously hemorrhaged. Periventricular and subcortical areas of increased signal in the internal capsule and basal ganglia indicated an angiopathic encephalopathy not seen with CT.

Although the presence of subcortical arteriosclerotic encephalopathy in the cases just described makes vascular dementia more likely than Alzheimer's disease, both can occur in the same patient (Garber et al, 1988; Gerard and Weisberg, 1986; Erkinjuntti et al, 1987). White matter abnormalities indicative of mild subcortical arteriosclerotic encephalopathy (Binswanger's disease) and periventricular hyperintensity may not be associated with dementia; they are, however, associated with risk factors for cerebrovascular disease and their prevalence increases with age. MRI is more sensitive than CT for detecting white matter disease in dementia and other disorders (eg, multiple sclerosis).

In the cases of Garber and colleagues (1988), there were clear indications for the use of imaging techniques to define brain lesions. Signs of structural CNS disease (seizures, stroke, dementia, focal motor abnormalities) were present and prompted study with MRI after CT. They noted that such features are not present in the majority of "typical" psychiatric disorders (eg, uncomplicated schizophrenia and affective, personality, or anxiety disorders).

MRI provides a life-like picture of the brain in three dimensions with excellent resolution. Confirming earlier speculation that schizophrenic patients had abnormalities of frontal lobe function and structure and enlarged ventricles, MRI has demonstrated that schizophrenic patients have smaller frontal lobes and larger ventricles than normal control subjects (Andreasen, 1988).

Indications for Magnetic Resonance Imaging

In an attempt to clarify guidelines, Garber and associates (1988) listed the following indications for obtaining brain imaging: unexplained dementia, late-onset mania, atypical symptoms (eg, visual hallucinations), and unusual course of illness. Since these indications suggest only a need for investigation of brain structure, further criteria are needed to decide when MRI or CT scanning is most appropriate. In an attempt to tease apart the indications for MRI and CT scans, they noted that bone artifacts obscure CT images of many areas, including the anterior temporal lobes, cerebellum, subcortical structures, brainstem, and spinal cord—areas that can be visualized quite clearly by means of MRI.

MRI is particularly useful for examining midline structures, the temporal lobes, and high cerebral convexities since it can generate images in any plane as opposed to the CT scan, which is generally limited to transverse views of the brain. Clinical evidence suggesting involvement of any of these areas would be a good reason for obtaining MRI instead of CT. If the results of a CT study are abnormal but not diagnostic, MRI is indicated when it can better define the CT abnormality. MRI may also be of value after abnormal CT results are obtained, by following the progression of a known lesion. Garber and associates (1988) noted that MRI generally should not be used after a normal CT result unless there is a clear indication such as an atypical course or symptom or the suspicion of a disease likely to be better seen with MRI.

MRI provides greater contrast between gray and white matter and is more likely to detect lesions in white matter, particularly infiltrating tumors, central infarctions, and lesions resulting from demyelinating disorders, including multiple sclerosis (Garber et al, 1988). Most noncalcified vascular malformations and focal lesions provoking seizure disorders are best studied with MRI. If lesions are calcified, CT may be superior to MRI since calcium does not produce a resonance signal. Also, peripheral infarctions of the cortex and small lesions in the pituitary currently are equally or better defined with CT than MRI.

At present the cost of an MRI is two to three times that of CT. MRI requires longer time (30 to 45 minutes) than CT (15 to 20 minutes) and availability of MRI may be a problem in some communities (Garber et al, 1988). In addition, MRI involves closer confinement and potential for claustrophobic reactions; there is, however, no exposure to ionizing radiation or intravenous injection of contrast material, as with CT.

The primary contraindications to MRI involve patients who have metal fragments or aneurysm clips in the head which may move in response to a powerful magnetic field. Also, desynchronization has occurred in patients dependent on a cardiac pacemaker.

REGIONAL CEREBRAL BLOOD FLOW

Techniques using regional cerebral blood flow (RCBF) were the earliest to allow some estimate of brain function. Blood flow has most often been measured from the rate of disappearance of inhaled xenon–133 as recorded by sodium iodide photon detectors placed around the head. Sometimes other radioactive tracers are used.

The advantage of the RCBF technique is the relative inexpensiveness of the equipment and materials. The disadvantages are that counts obtained from extracerebral blood flow (eg, face and scalp) are added to the counts from the brain and that this technique primarily measures brain surface activity and gives little information about deep subcortical structures. Currently, an inhalation technique is the most popular because of its simplicity and low morbidity; injection methods are occasionally used.

With RCBF, areas of hypoperfusion and hyperperfusion can be identified by relative amounts of radioactivity detected over specific areas of the scalp. Presumably areas of higher radioactivity reflect increased blood flow and enhanced cerebral metabolic activity.

A number of investigators have demonstrated "hypofrontality" in patients with schizophrenia (see Andreasen, 1988, for review). In normal subjects this technique has been used with some success to evaluate aspects of attention and speech. Tests that require sustained attention and pattern recognition activate the frontal lobes and increase cerebral blood flow over these areas. Others have demonstrated that schizophrenic patients do not activate their frontal lobes when undergoing these tests, further suggesting frontal abnormalities. Left hemisphere abnormalities have also been noted in schizophrenics, consistent with observed language and auditory abnormalities (Andreasen, 1988).

Most studies of Alzheimer's patients, including some for whom diagnosis was confirmed at autopsy, showed a moderate decline in the global cerebral blood flow when they were compared with studies of normal subjects (see Metter, 1988, for a review). The most frequently observed regional blood flow abnormality is a decline in RCBF over the temporal lobes. In activation studies with Alzheimer's patients, in which the patient does a specific task, demented subjects showed less changes in RCBF than control subjects did.

POSITRON EMISSION TOMOGRAPHY

At the present time PET is the most elegant of the available brain imaging techniques. While RCBF and single proton emission computed tomography (SPECT) studies rely on the detection of single photons, PET localizes activity by recording the position of two photons that are emitted after a positron strikes an electron and produces an annihilation of both (Andreasen, 1988). When a positron combines with an electron and annihilates, it forms two photons, which are emitted in directions 180 degrees apart (Metter, 1988). Two detectors electronically linked in coincidence are used to detect both photons and accurately determine the line of origin.

Resolution with PET is far better than resolution with single photons. Since PET requires the generation of positron-emitting isotopes, an on-site cyclotron is needed as well as a support team consisting of physicists, radio-chemists, and experts in computer modeling. Since the isotopes have very short half-lives (from several minutes to two hours), they must be produced by a cyclotron either on the day of the scan for $_{18}F$, or constantly during scanning, for $_{15}O$. PET is therefore extremely expensive to operate; however, it surpasses all other brain imaging techniques in sensitivity and flexibility (Andreasen, 1988).

PET has two major applications—the assessment of metabolic activity and the measurement of neurotransmitter function. Various isotopes are available for PET imaging. In early studies, measurements of cerebral metabolism with deoxyglucose, which could be labeled with $_{18}F$ or $_{11}C$, were commonly used. Newer studies have used short half-life isotopes such as $_{15}O$ (inserted into either water or carbon dioxide) to serially compare perfusion and metabolism in a variety of conditions (eg, before and after cognitive challenges). Spiroperidol labeled with $_{11}C$ has been used for measuring dopamine receptors and a number of other compounds are currently under development.

The ability to visualize a structure depends on object size, shape, and the influence of neighboring structures (Metter, 1988); that is, if two or more structures or cerebrospinal fluid and tissue occupy a given measured volume, the measurement will be an averaged value of each tissue (or the tissue and fluid) and their isotope concentration. Despite recent improvements in PET, most diencephalic and midbrain structures are not well resolved, although this may improve in the future.

PET studies reflect the functional state of the brain during the scanning procedure; thus, changes in resting states can result in variability in regional glucose metabolism. Results of stimulation studies have shown selective brain activation to specific tasks (Metter, 1988). For example, varying visual input has been found to change the level of primary and associative glucose metabolism of the occipital lobe and auditory stimulations caused different patterns of metabolic activation depending on the stimulus and, in some cases, the perceptual or cognitive strategy employed in carrying out a task. Verbal stimuli produced diffuse increases in glucose metabolism in the left hemisphere, bilateral transverse, and posterior temporal areas. Nonverbal stimuli (chords) produced diffuse right temporal and bilateral inferior parietal activation (see Metter, 1988, for review of studies). Those subjects using highly analytical strategies had greater left posterior temporal activations, while those using nonanalytical strategies had right-sided activation.

In schizophrenic patients, a relative increase in metabolic activity in subcortical regions as well as an inability to activate frontal areas has been demonstrated (Andreasen, 1988).

A specific area of hyperactivity has been identified in the right parahippocampal gyrus in patients who are susceptible to lactate-induced panic attacks (see Andreasen, 1988, for review). Since this is an important region for encoding memory, this finding is particularly interesting, in that the experience of panic either may be triggered by old anxiety-producing memories or may involve the encoding of new memories that may later trigger subsequent panic attacks. In patients with obsessive-compulsive disorder, patterns of increased metabolic activity have been observed in the frontal lobes and basal ganglia.

Studies using $[_{18}F]$ fluorodeoxyglucose PET have shown a decline in glucose metabolism in Alzheimer's patients compared with aged normal subjects, often with the parietal cortex showing the greatest decline (Metter, 1988). Relative to age-matched normal subjects, Alzheimer's patients showed a 54% decrease in parietal cortex metabolism, 48% in dorsolateral occipital metabolism, 37% in superior frontal metabolism, 32% in temporal metabolism, 29% in calcarine mebtabolism, 27% in motor-sensory metabolism, and 23% in inferior frontal cortex metabolism. Smaller decreases were found in subcortical structures, such as the caudate and thalamus (see Metter, 1988, for review). Of interest, patients with early or mild dementia were found to have metabolic rates that overlapped with those of control subjects, while severe dementia was associated with a marked metabolic decline.

In correlations of blood flow alterations to clinical findings in subgroups of patients with Alzheimer's disease, those who have difficulties with language early in the course of their illness have been shown to have a greater reduction in glucose metabolism in the left than in the right hemisphere. Other patients who present with constructional apraxia have a greater reduction in glucose metabolism in the right hemisphere. Patients with just memory difficulties with fairly intact speech and constructional skills had symmetrical alterations in blood flow (see chapter 5 for more details). This variability may be clinically important since some treatment approaches may affect one subgroup of patients with Alzheimer's disease and not others.

Patients with dementing illnesses other than Alzheimer's disease have been studied. Subjects with multi-infarct dementia show scattered focal defects throughout the cortex and white matter. Many of these lesions are not found on CT scans. Patients with Pick's disease differ from those with Alzheimer's disease in the presence of prominent frontal declines in RCBF. Patients with Parkinson's disease have generally been shown to have lesser degrees of global decrements in blood flow, as measured by xenon RCBF or by glucose PET, than patients with Alzheimer's disease. Regional differences are reported in some studies but not in others (see Metter, 1988, for review). Patients with progressive supranuclear palsy have a prominent decline in local glucose metabolism as shown on PET scan and patients with Huntington's disease demonstrated caudate metabolic decline as measured by PET prior to any structural changes on x-ray CT scan. These abnormalities were found in some asymptomatic subjects.

With the present availability of ligands for the study of dopamine (D1 and D2), serotonin, benzodiazepine, opiate, and muscarinic receptors, study of neurotransmitter systems in the brain with PET is likely to be rewarding (Andreasen, 1988). The blockade of dopamine D2 receptors by neuroleptics has been demonstrated through PET, by giving patients labeled neuroleptic when their receptors were already blocked by previous neuroleptic and finding that the labeled drug would not bind to the receptors even though it did bind prior to pretreatment with neuroleptic.

The advantage of PET over earlier techniques, such as measuring metabolites in the cerebrospinal fluid, is that it allows researchers to bypass peripheral measures and study the brain directly in a number of clinical and research settings. The identification of abnormalities in specific neurotransmitter systems or of subsystems within specific brain regions may permit the development of more specific pharmacologic agents for treatment.

SINGLE PHOTON EMISSION COMPUTED TOMOGRAPHY

SPECT is another technique that allows estimations of brain function. SPECT uses radionuclides that radiate single photons. Detectors count the emitted photons and use statistical techniques to predict the plane of origin; when enough counts are made, a matrix can be constructed of the predicted origins of each photon. This is a scanning technique that uses the computerized tomographic reconstruction method originally developed for CT and MRI in combination with the detection of single photons emitted through an exogenously administered tracer.

Although its resolution is not equal to that achievable with PET, it may prove sufficient for many applications. Since commercially available tracers with long half-lives are used for SPECT, and it does not require the on-site presence of a cyclotron or a team of physicists and chemists, it is a far less expensive technique than PET. In the near future, radionuclides suitable for imaging neurotransmitter systems may be available and may make it possible to monitor the effects of treatment and mechanisms of drug action by means of SPECT.

Tracers for dopamine and acetylcholine receptors currently exist, and one report has indicated increased dopamine receptors in the basal ganglia that were observed with SPECT (Andreasen, 1988). SPECT has also demonstrated a pattern of hypoperfusion in posterior temporoparietal regions that appear to be specific to and characteristic of Alzheimer's disease (Bonte et al, 1986). In depression, flow patterns appear to be different; if such differences are confirmed, the observation of blood flow could be very useful for the differential diagnosis of dementia versus depression in the elderly who present confusing clinical pictures.

SUMMARY

The future of neuroimaging appears unlimited and the science of neuropsychiatry is being advanced at an unprecedented rate by these techniques. The long-term promise of brain imaging is substantial as it will permit the mapping of cerebral function in normal individuals so that researchers can achieve a better understanding of normal brain structure, physiology, chemistry, and functional organization. On the basis of this knowledge, the abnormalities underlying major mental illnesses may also be mapped.

REFERENCES

Albert MS, Stafford JL: Computed tomography studies, in Albert MS, Moss MB (eds): *Geriatric Neuropsychology*. New York, Guildford Press, 1988, pp 211–227.

Andreasen NC: Brain imaging: Applications in psychiatry. *Science* 236:1381–1388, 1988.

Beresford TP, Blow FC, Hall RCW, et al: CT scanning in psychiatric inpatients: clinical yield. *Psychosomatics* 27:105–112, 1986.

Bonte FJ, Ross HH, Chehabi MD, et al: *J Comput Assist Tomogr* 10:648, 1986.

Brinkman SD, Largen JW: Changes in brain ventricular size with repeated CAT scans in suspected Alzheimer's disease. *Am J Psychiatry* 141:81–83, 1984.

Conlon P, Trimble MR: Magnetic resonance imaging in psychiatry. *Can J Psychiatry* 32:702–712, 1987.

Erkinjuntti T, Ketonen L, Sulkava R, et al: Do white matter changes on MRI and CT differentiate vascular dementia from Alzheimer's disease? *J Neurol Neurosurg Psychiatry* 50:37–42, 1987.

Gado M, Hughes CP, Danziger W, et al: Aging, dementia, and brain atrophy: A longitudinal computed tomographic study. *Am J Neuroradiol* 4:699–702, 1983.

Garber HJ, Weilburg JB, Buonanno FS, et al: Use of magnetic resonance imaging in psychiatry. *Am J Psychiatry* 145:164–171, 1988.

Gerard G, Weisberg LA: MRI periventricular lesions in adults. *Neurology* 36:998–1001, 1986.

Larson EB, Mack LA, Watts B, et al: Computed tomography in patients with psychiatric illness: advantage of a "rule-in" approach. *Ann Intern Med* 95:360–364, 1981.

Metter EJ: Positron emission tomography and cerebral blood flow studies, in Albert MS, Moss MB (eds): *Geriatric Neuropsychology*. New York, Guildford Press, 1988, pp 228–261.

Pykett IL, Newhouse JH, Buonanno FS, et al: Principles of nuclear magnetic resonance imaging. *Radiology* 133:157–168, 1982.

Weinberger DR: Brain disease and psychiatric illness: when should a psychiatrist order a CAT scan? *Am J Psychiatry* 141:1521–1527, 1984.

Cycloplegic, 297-298

Dalmane. *See* Flurazepam
Dantrolene, 222
Day-care for demented patients, 188
Deafness, 99
Death. *See also* Suicide
  of spouse, 110-111
  terminally ill patient and, 39-40
Deficiency state, 42
Degeneration, neuronal, 228
Degenerative dementia, 128
  Alzheimer's disease as. *See*
    Alzheimer's disease
  carbamazepine and, 236
Degenerative neurologic illness, 161
Delirium, 289-309
  alcohol withdrawal and, 315, 316
  causes of, 294-303
  clinical features and, 291-293
  diagnostic criteria and, 290-291
  mechanisms of, 293-294
  treatment of, 303-305
  withdrawal and, 318, 320
Delirium tremens, 325-326
Delusion
  paranoid, 209-210
  schizophrenia and, 204
Delusional depression, 97-99
Dementia. *See also* Alzheimer's
  disease
  agitation in, 235-236
  alcoholism and, 317, 318
  anxiety and, 266
  buspirone and, 239
  depression and, 53
  dexamethasone suppression test
    and, 50-51, 157-158
  frontal lobe and, 131-135, 136
  imaging techniques and, 379
  Mini-Mental State Exam and, 9
  Parkinson's disease and, 108, 177
  psychotic symptoms and, 241
  serotonergic agents and, 238-240
Demographics, 2-3
Dependence, 311, 312
Depression
  Alzheimer's disease and, 179-181
  antidepressants and, 57-68, 80-81
  cognitive changes and, 52-55
  delirium and, 295-296
  dexamethasone suppression test
    and, 46-52, 157-158

diagnosis of, 40-43
duration of treatment for, 90-92
electroconvulsive therapy and, 92-97
grief and, 111
lithium and, 81-86, 89-90
mania and, 83
mnemonic for, 13
monoamine oxidase inhibitors and,
  68-81
neurochemical changes and, 55
obsessive-compulsive disorder and,
  352
psychostimulants and, 86-89
psychotherapy and, 55-57
psychotic, 97-99
recognition of, 34-40
suicide risk assessment and, 43-46
thyroid hormone and, 89-90
Desipramine
  anticholinergic potency of, 102
  antimuscarinic potency of, 302
  blood levels for, 63
  characteristics of, 58
  delirium and, 298
  Parkinson's disease and, 109
Desyrel. *See* Trazodone
Dexamethasone suppression test,
  46-52
  depression and, 157-158
Dextroamphetamine, 88-89
Diabetes mellitus, 95-96
Diazepam
  antidepressants overdose and, 66
  anxiety and, 260
  distribution of, 26-27
  sleep disorders and, 285
Diazoxide, 73-74
Dietary factors
  anxiety and, 256
  monoamine oxidase inhibitor and,
  74, 76-77
Digitalis, 300
Digoxin
  renal excretion and, 29
  trazodone and, 61-62
Diphenhydramine
  abuse of, 332
  anxiety and, 264
  delirium and, 298
  drug-induced dystonia and, 223
  insomnia and, 282
  parkinsonism and, 223
  sleep disorder and, 284

Disinhibition syndrome, 71-72
Disopyramine phosphate, 68
Distribution of drug, 26-27
Diuretics, 300
Donation of blood, 155-156
Dopamine
   anxiety and, 256-257
   monoamine oxidase inhibitor and,
      70, 71
   pathologic laughing and crying and,
      240-241
   PET studies and, 379-380
Dopamine antagonist, 229
Down's syndrome, 160
Doxepin
   anticholinergic potency of, 102
   antimuscarinic potency of, 302
   blood levels for, 63
   characteristics of, 58
   depression and, 59
   frontal lobe atrophy and, 87
   overdose and, 64
Dream anxiety disorder, 276
Drug abuse, 330-335
Drug interactions, 267
Drug-induced depression, 42
Drug-related anxiety, 256
DST. See Dexamethasone suppression
   test
Durable power of attorney, 182-183
Dyskinesia, tardive, 225-230
Dyssomnia, 273-275

ECT. See Electroconvulsive therapy
EDTA. See Ethylenediaminetetraacetic
   acid
Elavil. See Amitriptyline
Electrocardiographic changes, 64
Electroconvulsive therapy, 92-97
   dexamethasone suppression test,
      158
   obsessive-compulsive disorder and,
      347-348, 356
Electroencephalogram, 234
Encephalopathy
   subcortical, 151
   Wernicke's, 327
Endocrine disorder
   anxiety and, 256
   delirium and, 294
   depression and, 42
   dexamethasone suppression test
      and, 48-49

Environmental modifications
   delirium and, 303
   dementia and, 165-166
Enzyme, hepatic microsomal, 28
Epilepsy, 83
Epileptiform discharges, periodic,
   302-303
Erection, 60
Ergoloid mesylates, 170
Eskalith. See Lithium carbonate
Ethchlorvynol, 257
Ethylenediaminetetraacetic acid, 172
Euthanasia, 173-174
Exposure therapy, 349
Extrapyramidal disorder, 152-153
Extrapyramidal effects, 216, 218,
   223-230
Eye
   lithium and, 85
   neuroleptics and, 219

Family
   delirious patient and, 304-305
   demented patient and, 181-188
   obsessive-compulsive disorder and,
      351-352
Fluid, cerebrospinal, 151-152
Fluorodeoxyglucose PET, 379
Fluoxetine, 62, 75
   depression and, 59
   monoamine oxidase inhibitor and,
      81-82
   obsessive thoughts and, 353-354
   obsessive-compulsive disorder and,
      355
Fluphenazine
   antimuscarinic potency of, 302
   delirium and, 299
   equivalent doses of, 217
   side effects of, 216
Flurazepam
   anxiety and, 260
   distribution of, 27
   insomnia and, 282
   sleep disorders and, 285
Fluvoxamine, 354
Folate deficiency, 301
Folie à deux, 211
Frontal lobe atrophy, 87
Frontal lobe dementia, 131-135,
   136
FTA-ABS test, 149
Furosemide, 73-74

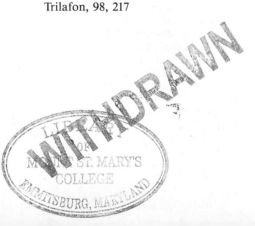